Social and Behavioural Sciences for Nurses

Mame and Pape, not forgotten; Sophie Béphage and Eppie Béphage, my daughters, with love from Papa

For Churchill Livingstone:

Commissioning Editors: Ellen Green; Jacqueline Curthoys
Project Manager: Gail Murray
Project Development Manager: Valerie Dearing
Illustrator: Ethan Danielson

Social and Behavioural Sciences for Nurses

An Integrated Approach

Gaëtan Béphage BA(Hons) CertEd DipN(Lon) Cert Social Studies RGN RMN
Lecturer in Social Sciences and Nursing Studies, School of Health, University of Hull, Hull, UK

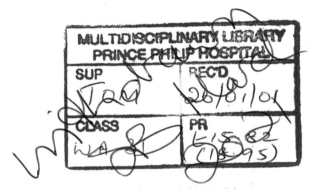

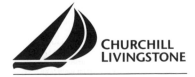

CHURCHILL
LIVINGSTONE

EDINBURGH LONDON NEW YORK PHILADELPHIA ST LOUIS SYDNEY TORONTO 2000

CHURCHILL LIVINGSTONE
An imprint of Harcourt Publishers Limited

First published 2000

ISBN 0 4430 5719 2

British Library of Cataloguing in Publication Data
A catalogue record for this book is available from the British
Library

Library of Congress Cataloging in Publication Data
A catalog record for this book is available from the Library
of Congress

Note
Medical knowledge is constantly changing. As new
information becomes available, changes in treatment,
procedures, equipment and the use of drugs become
necessary. The author and the publishers have, as far as it is
possible, taken care to ensure that the
information given in this text is accurate and up to date.
However, readers are strongly advised to confirm that the
information complies with latest legislation and standards
of practice.

Printed in China

Contents

Preface

As we proceed into the new millennium, it is certain that care professionals will increasingly be expected to apply an eclectic approach in their interventions. This is becoming imperative as users of care develop high expectations from their care providers. Not surprisingly, the health care profession is constantly undergoing major changes to meet such demands. Parallel to these developments, curriculum design has to keep pace and reflect adaptation to changing needs and problems in society. Social change impacts on both clients and care organizations, which has implications for practice.

The rationale for this book lies in the recognition that social phenomena affect the individual in many ways, and that multiple agencies have responsibilities to intervene collaboratively to achieve the best outcomes for their clients.

While the social sciences literature has contributed much to raising our understanding of social factors and their effects on a healthy lifestyle, the content has somehow lacked emphasis on circumstances and their effects on psychological well-being. I have attempted to redress the balance by incorporating a psychology section. Moreover, throughout the book I have indicated, where appropriate, the interactions between the social and the psychological. Further, the section on social policy aims to establish the fact that as individuals we function within a wider framework – a socio-political one – and that our actions are more or less guided by policies designed at a higher level of society.

During writing, I have been acutely aware of issues related to the theory–practice gap, which receives regular attention from clinicians. I have therefore integrated, where relevant, case studies, suggested activities, and questions to aid reflective practice.

While the translation of theory into practice is not always an easy task, my purpose has been to provide the reader with a tapestry of contemporary issues that health care professionals encounter not only in the literature, but in their daily interactions with clients and their significant others.

The evolutionary nature of health care in the UK and worldwide demands that the care provided be sensitive to population needs. Consequently, I have endeavoured to highlight perennial problems, and suggested ways to confront them. Most importantly, my aim is to stimulate debate among professionals engaged in providing sensitive care in a variety of settings.

Although this textbook is primarily designed to meet the needs of health care professionals in clinical practice, and students following the higher education diploma in nursing courses, I hope that students of social work will be able to tap in to the many social issues I have brought to the fore in this volume.

And finally, writing a book always seems like an endless journey with many hours of aloneness. I am indebted to the following people who made that journey easier: Ellen Green, who showed the way; Valerie Dearing, who was always at the end of the phone to answer my queries; Gail Murray, who managed the production stages of the project; the health care library staff in Butterwick

House, Scunthorpe; Linda Bell, Judith Proudley, Deirdre Welch and Muriel White; and Mary Ullfors and her staff at the East Riding campus, Willerby. With thanks to Debra Barrie, too.

Scunthorpe 1999   Gaëtan Béphage

1

Society, health and illness

This section places into context issues of health and illness as they affect specific groups in society. An eclectic approach in discussing health and illness issues demonstrates the interplay of sociological factors with psychological issues concerning the well-being of individuals in society.

Introduction to sociology

To gain an awareness of sociology as a concept, some of its main attributes are considered in this chapter. It is therefore essential that some classical theories are examined and their relevance to nursing and health care explained. The focus is on the individual's relationship with the social structures that impinge on human behaviour. Emphasis is also made of the fact that a dynamic, two-way relationship exists between groups and social structures. While social structures can be transformed by human action, humans are also subject to change and adaptation.

SOCIETY AND HEALTH CARE

SOCIETIES AS SYSTEMS OF SOCIAL ORGANIZATION

All human societies comprise social groups. When groups are formed, there is usually a purpose behind such formation. Individuals have needs that must be met: survival needs, for example, motivate people to organize their social lives, so that optimal benefits can be derived by the utilization of one's resourcefulness to cope with living conditions.

Our ancestors, as hunters and gatherers, worked in groups as they searched for food. Subsequently, once food was obtained, decisions had to be made with regard to its distribution to group members and their families. Hence a system of social organization developed over time.

Viewing a society as a set of systems implies that such systems possess some determined characteristics, such as:

- group cohesion aimed at achieving specific goals
- human groups operate within definite structures
- the systems possess distinct functions
- there is a state of interdependency between social structures.

Once social systems have been designed and are fully operational (e.g. community care systems, economic and political systems, kinship systems etc.), the behaviour of the group is seen to be regulated by unambiguous patterned social regularities. For example, social life is governed by the need to earn one's living: this is achieved by gaining employment. Social life is also governed by rituals and cultural practices which provide a definable framework of social behaviour in particular circumstances: birth, marriage and death, for instance. One may therefore argue that the structures of society exhibit recurrent arrangements of social functioning, which Lawson and Garrod (1996) describe as the constancy of social features. The same authors argue that social structures, which are permanent, differentiate themselves from the characteristics of people who are members of their social structures. They explain that a common facet of any society is the death of individuals, while social structures outlive human groups. One may refer to family systems, education systems and community systems, all of which are social structures and which remain permanent.

Structuralism

In studying and analysing society the concept of structuralism is often affiliated with its nature and is one of the sociological theories frequently considered. Some theorists may therefore argue that human behaviour is influenced by social structures, denying that human social action or activity has no influence over these structures (Haralambos et al 1995). Linked with the concept of structure is the idea of permanence, which

means change is not anticipated. This notion is, however, considered to be unrealistic since social groups, which are aspects of the social structure, form the core elements of dynamic social processes. When one considers, for example, family systems and their structures, ample evidence exists showing that they are constantly undergoing changes. For example, it is nowadays becoming increasingly common to have same-sex (non-heterosexual) partners as heads of families.

Marriage structures are also experiencing changes: this is evident in homosexuals fighting for their rights to be married and to look after children. An increase in cohabitation is another example of this change in structure. The Central Statistical Office (1993) stated that 23% of non-married women aged 18–49 were cohabiting in 1991 compared with 11% in 1979. Divorced women are more likely to cohabit, but statistics reveal that single women are also showing trends of increase in cohabitation.

Structuralism is a theoretical viewpoint emphasizing the patterned regularities of human social behaviour. It is a perspective that found its origins in structural linguistics (New Encyclopaedia Britannica 1992). Thoughts are expressed through language, which has a structure. This principle is adapted to explain social and cultural life as it operates under specific norms, values and beliefs and from which emanate clear-cut expressions of social activities.

Some communities, for instance, have set rituals when disposing of the dead, organizing religious activities or their socio-economic and political systems. The key features of structuralism as a sociological concept are considered to be the ethos of permanence or continuity, a degree of interdependence (social structures are all interconnected) and functional regularity (social structures, like the internal mechanisms of a clock, have set patterns of movement).

Another viewpoint was provided by Parsons (1961) whèn he argued that social structures do possess features that show 'constancy', while on the other hand, the 'functional' characteristic of the social system is related to its 'dynamic' processes.

These processes evolved from the social organization of human groups, and the 'personalities' of its individual members. Social change (caused by members who become agents of social change, for example pressure/interest groups) may impinge on social structures, establishing what Parsons called 'equilibrium' of the social system. As society faces an increased crime rate, the need may arise to re-evaluate the credibility of law enforcement institutions and to implement changes as required (Box 1.1).

Social systems, therefore, are systems of structures that embrace the human aspects of social organization by influencing its group members. Parsons made reference to the personality

Box 1.1 Institutional racism

British law enforcement agencies are facing criticisms from communities, politicians and the media, since the murder of a black youth several years ago. They are being accused of institutional racism because of failures in the systems. A new report issued provides detailed guidelines of structural changes needed to improve the system.

'structure' of the individual, which is shaped by the cultural values, norms and beliefs of social systems (Fig. 1.1).

In this context one cannot demarcate individuals from the structures influencing their

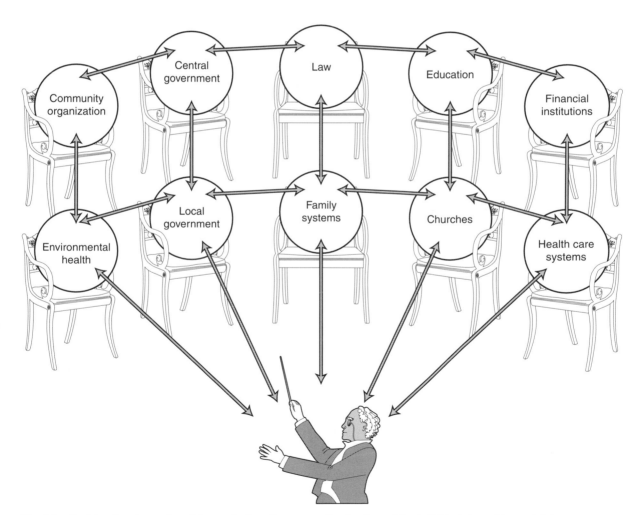

Fig. 1.1 Society of systems of social organization: the personality structure of the individual shaped by societal norms, values, beliefs etc.

behaviour and vice versa. Utilizing structuralism as a social theory to explain macro-structures of society may convey impressions that the human factor is insignificant in the framework (Outhwaite & Bottomore 1994). Giddens (1979, 1994) argued that social structures do not function in isolation regardless of social groups, but are dependent upon such groups, which as social actors have capacities to mould the structures they live within.

Social groups have knowledge about their societies and how these are organized. This 'knowledgeability', Giddens postulated, gives them the skill to produce and reproduce (by using specific 'formulae' and under identified 'rules') social circumstances that will cause some effects on their social structures. The assertion he made fully explained that, without the collectivities (communities as a whole), structures will cease to exist. Conversely, some characteristics of social structures can also exert specific effects on individuals.

Johnson (1995) argued that some features of the economic systems create social inequality and underachievement among some groups. Other changes (caused by advancement in technology and science) interfere with the labour markets, altering job structures and causing some occupations to become outmoded. Johnson used the term 'new structuralism' concerning these social changes. Such changes, however, are not new developments that encroach on human lives. The growth of industrialization has altered social structures and living conditions since the late seventeenth century, creating wealth for many nations, while simultaneously increasing the cost in relation to human suffering (Guinness Encyclopaedia 1990).

Hence, social structures may cause 'incompatibilities' and 'contradictions', and stimulate social action and change by social actors who strive to alter the existing state of affairs (Mouzelis 1997).

What are the functions of society?

As early as the seventeenth century, sociologists were asking whether society has any purpose

Activity 1.1

1. During your neighbourhood trail project identify the structures/social organizations that have influence over the behaviour of local people.
2. Talk to neighbours and friends during informal interactions about their perceptions of their social environment.

??? Question 1.1

1. What is your personal view of the relationship between social structures and social groups?
2. Do you agree that social organizations have influence over people in society?

and goals, whether what was happening around them had any functions. Social structures, as discussed in the previous pages, serve the purpose of maintaining continuity in relation to social life.

Social life, as interpreted at the time of social thought development during the parallel evolution of the natural sciences, could be explained in an analogical way with the latter. Thus, if the structure of the human body (the skeletal system) is commensurable with its biological systems, which are in a state of homeostatic interdependence, one should therefore be able to transfer this principle to society as a whole. Society can be said to possess similar features:

a. it has structures and systems (kinship, family, communities, religion, law, education etc.
b. structures and systems are interconnected and interdependent
c. human groups, which are part of the structures, are the collectivities with roles to perform in order to maintain social homeostasis: to keep the social system in a state of equilibrium.

This school of thought is known as the theory of 'functionalism'.

Functionalism, as a social theory developed by Talcott Parsons in the 1940s, has stimulated a series of debates in sociological fields. It is pointed out that the origin of functionalism can be found in the work of anthropologists such as Radcliffe-Brown on social structure, and Bronislaw Malinowski on culture, values, norms and social relations (Scott 1995). While the term 'functions' is of customary usage in daily conversations, its meaning is not so loosely applied to explain the meaning of functionalism among sociologists.

Scott (1995) explained that, from a sociological stance, functionalism refers to the interconnected parts of society and to the nature of the state of interdependency between the parts. These parts in combination form the whole, which when analysed individually can be identified as systems.

Since systems consist of human groups, it is their action on the social structure that *functions* to create a consequence and vice versa (Fig. 1.2). Law enforcement agencies (statutory structures of society), for example, have a duty to respond to a general public outcry on the increase in paedophilic activities and child abuse. A response in this context is sociologically interpreted to mean a 'structural–functional' tendency to restore order, control, adaptation and adjustment (to use some Parsonsian terminologies).

Parsons' theory of the social system from a functionalist perspective has been criticized for its reliance on 'normative regulation' (an action that conforms to people's expectations of behaviour and, in the process, serves to control by

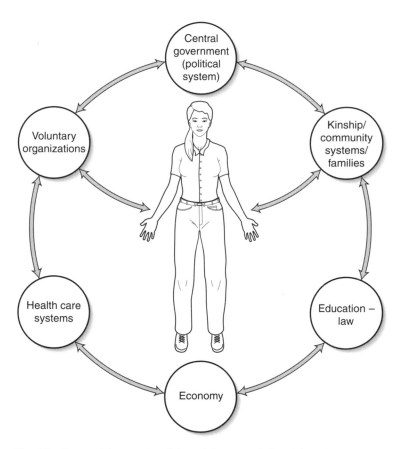

Fig. 1.2 Parsons' theory of society as interconnected social systems.

rules, leading to adaptation to the environment). This approach, which stipulates a degree of consensus of the collectivities, fails to acknowledge evidence of social conflict, disequilibrium and the collision of systems within the social structures, as in the strife between various religious factions throughout the world.

The representation of society and its functioning parts to maintain group solidarity and cohesion neglects the existence of dissent. Craib (1997) points out that functionalists are inclined toward seeing society as a stabilized whole, leaving issues of social conflict out of the equation. Contradictions and incompatibilities, as Mouzelis (1997) puts it, are perennial social realities that function by causing systemic alterations, but not without prior dissent and instability.

Social groups are not solely passive, harmonious social actors working hard at integration and adaptation, but are also agents of social changes, aiming at altering the 'contradictory status quo' (Mouzelis 1997). An understanding of the issues outlined above should help to explain the meaning attached to the concept of sociology (Box 1.2).

Moore (1987, 1988) explained that as our insight increases about the nature of our social world, through sociological knowledge, we become more aware of the order and meaning provided by cultural norms, values and beliefs. This knowledge improves our understanding of the world (Cox 1983).

Social knowledge, however, as pointed out by Sharp (1995) is 'multi-paradigmatic' in comparison with the natural sciences, since the social world is left open to a multitude of interpreta-

Box 1.2 What is sociology?

Some authors (e.g. Cuff et al 1990) argue that an attempt to define the term sociology will only lead to the formulation of more concepts, which subsequently will require further clarification and definitions, and may not necessarily increase understanding of the subject matter. Definitions of concepts are important. They provide a basic framework that can be explored at the reader's will.

To argue that sociology is a branch of the social sciences, concerned with group processes and relationships with social structures (Groenman et al 1992), provides the reader with the first step on a long journey of discovery concerning the many attributes of this relevant social science. Sociology may be defined as the study of the social framework developed by groups of individuals over time (Béphage 1997).

To study sociology is to increase one's awareness of an individual as a social person who has been socialized by the norms, values and beliefs of society. It also helps us make sense of the social world (Joseph 1990). Sociology can refine our sensitivity to the social behaviour, problems and daily activities engaging humans daily, with repercussions on their social lives. For example, when the Minister for Education says that a sum of £1000 will have to be paid by students who want to go into higher education, many parents and students feel that such a decision would reduce incentive and motivation to progress to higher educational awards. Society, as already pointed out in the previous pages, is made up of structures that, in combination, form the social system. Hence, studying sociology will develop our awareness of the nature of society.

The word 'society', however, can be interpreted to mean the following:

a. complex systems of human organization
b. diverse human relations
c. social structures that are in a state of dynamism.

Abercrombie et al (1994) indicate the interdependent nature of all parts of the system with each other, showing the organismic nature of society. Society can also be interpreted as structures of social conflict (Box 1.3).

Activity 1.2

1. Collect some local and national newspapers. What comments do politicians, pressure groups, educationalists and ethnic minority groups make on aspects of society (e.g. the poor, the economy, the education system)?
2. In small seminar groups, have a debate on the application of social system theories to the realities of social life.

??? Question 1.2

1. Do you agree that conflict is a common social feature?
2. How do people and organizations function in society?

Box 1.3 Society as structures of social conflict

This model of societal representation commonly referred to as 'conflict theory' or dissent in society – to be distinguished from the integrative and adaptive model of the functionalists – found its origin in the philosophical and sociological thinking of its proponent, Karl Marx (1818–1883).

Marx's revolutionary approach to an understanding of society was founded on his observations of dramatic social changes taking place in the late eighteenth and nineteenth centuries. Craib (1997) traced the roots of these important landmarks in social development from early communist societies, whose main feature was the fair distribution of surplus goods to maintain their societies (Alaszewski & Manthorpe 1995a), to a social condition characterized by relationships of owners of production (ruling classes) and 'sale of labor power' (the working classes) (Wright 1996).

Some key concepts emerge from this theory:

a. Owners of production (the landed aristocracy as owners of machinery, land and factory).
b. The means of production (the production process: machines and tools used by labourers/workers).
c. The relations of production (relationships between the workers and the owners, usually defined as a state of subservience, dependency, oppression and exploitation) (Fig. 1.3).
d. The division of labour (loss of craftsmanship due to the separation of individual tasks, accomplished by several workers, instead of one person).
e. False consciousness (this is a state of unawareness which prevails among the working classes, concerning their oppression by the owners of production).
f. Conflict and contradictions (a conflicting relationship between employers and employees, due to inequalities fostered by class position differences).
g. Anticipated revolution of the working classes to fight capitalism (the struggles of the poor, from which will emerge the eradication of capitalism, the rise of communism/socialism and classlessness).

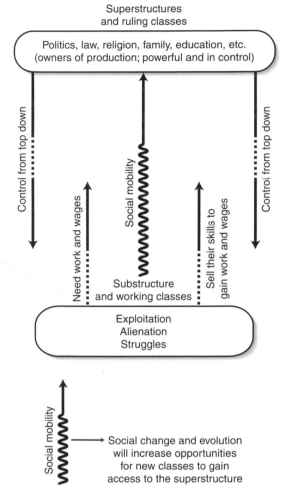

Fig. 1.3   Superstructures and ruling classes.

tions. This is evident in the numerous social theories and perspectives on society, generated by sociologists throughout the world.

It must be pointed out that, at the time of Marx's writing, drastic social changes were taking place, impinging on the livelihood of the rural agricultural workers. Industrialization and increased machinery production stifled traditional methods of agriculture, prompting the migration of workers to towns and cities to seek employment.

Marx's vision of the collapse of capitalism and a classless society has not materialized. The collapse of communist regimes, Turner (1996) argued, is sometimes associated with the death of Marxism. Turner, in addition, made the following assertions:

1. Socialism becomes a reality only when capitalism has exhausted its 'capacity' to maintain a monopoly over the means of production.
2. Marxism and its development continues to be a popular social science theory.
3. A re-evaluation of Marxist theory is needed parallel with social change, with some 'reconstruction'.

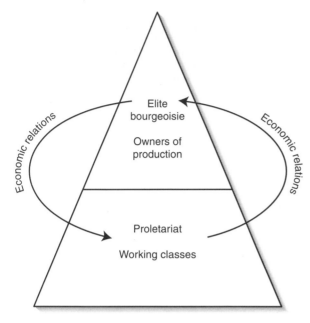

Fig. 1.4 Marx's theory of society, i.e. relationships between owners and workers.

Marx's theory of class struggles and contradictions in relationships is based on economic principles (Fig. 1.4). But the concept of class, as Turner (1996) found out, becomes irrelevant when other social issues (e.g. class and the sexual division of labour) are examined. For example, in the USA and Sweden, Turner observed that among many families, Yuppie husbands and their working class counterparts do equally little work within the home.

Social order

The essence of social order (societal structures and their organization) in the Weberian tradition is interpreted to differ from Marxist views in the following ways:

1. Societal group divisions are identified in the ways they are *politically* divided or stratified.

2. Social *honour* and *prestige* are equally important aspects, dividing groups in respect to their *grades*.

3. Although class analysis is important in discussing stratification, the concepts of political division and social honour can be considered on their own merit, as social processes that show divisions and classifications of human groups.

4. To Weber, a person's *economic* position in society (e.g. a chief executive of a petroleum company) represents his economic class (Fig. 1.5). Similarly, a channel tunnel engineer's economic position reflects his economic class.

5. Weber identified *status* position to be a social class – a type of social classification to be distinguished from Marx's definition, which relates to relationships between the elite (owners of production) and the workers.

6. Economic class and social class (status position) may not be neatly intertwined, but examples may be found in society to illustrate the linkage and non-linkage. For example, sex workers are usually perceived to be of working class, but their economic position could be high.

Activity 1.3

Make an appointment with trade union officials in your organization. What are their views on employers' and employees' relationships? Do they identify any conflictual relationship in the workplace?

??? Question 1.3

What do you consider to be the major differences between functionalism and conflict theory?

Economic position = Economic class

(businessmen and women; merchants, traders; bankers, shareholders)

Social status = Prestige, honour or a lack of these

(the poor, homeless, undesirables (e.g. caste systems), aristocrats, etc.)

Fig. 1.5 Weber's theory of society, i.e. class and status.

7. Status groups develop exclusive communities that impart differentiated forms of lifestyles in comparison with other status groups, based on their economic position and prestige etc. (e.g. material possessions: swimming pool, Rolls Royce, shopping at exclusive and expensive shops).

8. One's social status – the 'market situation' – can be classified as a class position. If one owns properties, has goods and services to provide to others, this implies that a person's market situation allows for some specific social action to take place, leading to earning financial rewards. When an individual or group shows these characteristics, it demonstrates their market situation. There are variations in market situations. In society one finds, for example, large and small shareholders, self-employed businessmen managing small companies and others managing huge corporations. Craftsmen using traditional methods in their work constitute another group.

9. Weber considered *social action* to be an important sociological concept; by social action he meant the meaning people give to their daily social interactions (Fig. 1.6).

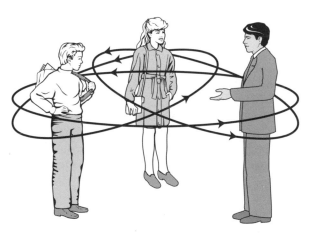

Group processes: interactions between people demand understanding of meanings attached to such interactions (e.g. a police constable conversing with two teenagers; a head teacher talking to two pupils; a father talking to his two children, etc.)

Fig. 1.6   Weber's theory of social action and meaning.

How do people view their working conditions? What meanings do they attach to the way society is evolving around them? This particular approach is often used in the field of social anthropology. The term used is 'emic' which applies to the person's subjective experience. 'Etic' on the other hand refers to the observer's interpretation of others' behaviour.

Social facts and social solidarity

The way society is organized is given a different interpretation by the French sociologist Emile Durkheim (1858–1917). His interest in analysing society led him to conclude that human beings share common values and beliefs, which cement group relationships. Group cohesion is engendered during social interactions. Shared values promote integration and social solidarity.

On *social facts*, which many writers allude to, Durkheim affirms his perception of society by arguing that an individual is subjected to constraints in many ways, within social structures. These structures are social facts, while what happens to the individual is also a social fact.

To Durkheim, social facts are the many embracing features of social life. Every human activity reflects a social perspective, unless of course, one is observing the individual either from a biological or psychological perspective, or both.

When people behave in a particular way, Durkheim argued that they are responding to an objective external social reality: laws, customs, beliefs and practices of a society. For example, no matter how much we want to throw a brick at a shop window, we don't do it, because we will surely be arrested and fined. Therefore, the law has a constraining effect on our behaviour. It is this coercive power which imposes itself on its citizens. Individuals have a need to conform to society's rules to avoid sanctions and disapproval from agents of social control.

The nature of social facts (Fig. 1.7), according to Durkheim, rests on the 'imposition' of cultural values – as an external reality – from the processes of socialization. Children are socialized to behave according to societal expectations. Any

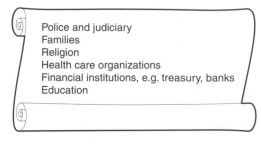

Police and judiciary
Families
Religion
Health care organizations
Financial institutions, e.g. treasury, banks
Education

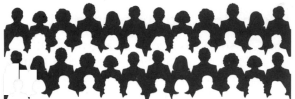

Fig. 1.7 Durkheim's theory of society.

tendencies toward deviation will be reprimanded. Durkheim expressed the view that a social fact has many characteristics:

1. Individuals have a need to conform due to society's power and coercive inclination.

2. Power is exercised when sanctions occur and rules are enforced.

3. When people violate the rules of society, those in power (e.g. criminal justice system, law enforcers) will oppose deviant behaviour.

4. A social fact has an external feature (Craib 1997) – an objective reality and a controlling influence.

5. Social facts are to be regarded as *objects*. Craib (1997) explained that, by regarding social facts as objects, we are identifying their quality as objects (objectivity) and not relating to 'an attitude of mind' (subjectivity).

6. Constraints as social facts may sometimes appear as *social currents*. Durkheim explained this by using suicide as an example (Box 1.4). He argued that, when major and accelerated social changes occur, some people are driven to suicide. Social change causes social currents, which impose constraints and drive behaviour.

7. Collective consciousness is another social fact. This term applies to the integrative functions of groups bound by common shared values, which maintain and constrain the group to cohere.

Box 1.4 Durkheim's classification of suicide

- **Altruistic suicide:** this type of suicide is precipitated by a condition of unselfishness; a state of concern for others. Self-inflicted starvation is one example; a hunger strike to force a change in people's attitudes, for the benefit of others.
- **Anomic suicide:** anomic is a word of Greek origin (anomia, anomos), which means lawless; the French version is anomie. Durkheim was referring to conditions (e.g. urbanization and the consequences of industrialization – see Case example 1.1) whereby usual social and ethical standards among groups were lacking. When a society is undergoing extreme social change, as in industrial and political developments, some people are prone to commit suicide.
- **Egoistic suicide:** groups sharing similar values (e.g. soldiers who are prepared to die for their battalion).
- **Fatalistic suicide:** when rules or norms of a particular society constrain behaviour to the extreme, there are expectations of complete disregard for oneself. For example, in some Hindu cultures, the practice of a widow immolating herself on her husband's funeral pyre.
- **Assisted suicide:** in addition to the above, in some societies (e.g. Holland and the USA) – (see Case example 1.2), assisted suicide is becoming an issue of importance for moral and legal reasons.

As a functionalist, Durkheim (1950) saw society as an organism, with many interdependent features, functioning to maintain group solidarity. Collective consciousness is an external reality which pulls people together for a common goal.

Activity 1.4

Ask community workers (community psychiatric nurses, district nurses, health visitors, community midwives etc.) their views on the extent of suicide rates in their catchment area. Is there any difference in the rate of suicide between ethnic groups and non-ethnic groups?

??? Question 1.4

1. How do you perceive the differences in the way Parsons, Marx, Weber and Durkheim understand society?
2. The media informs us about socio-political changes. To what extent do these changes affect our daily activities? Can you give some examples?

Case example 1.1 The effects of social change on the individual

Fraser (1984), in his study of the urbanization and industrialization process of the eighteenth and nineteenth centuries, observed how British society had to adopt new social policy measures, which impinged on the individual, his work and working environment.

Social change, Fraser pointed out, due to urbanization and new manufactures, drove members of society to re-examine their relationships with others, and with new representations of social authority.

The change process, he argued, led migrants from rural areas to the manufacturing cities, with feelings of employment insecurity. The change and the new systems of working in an 'evolving' urban setting precipitated alienation and anomie within British society.

Case example 1.2 Assisted suicide

Increasing attention is being given to assisted suicide in some countries, such as Holland and the USA, according to Scanlon and Rushton (1996). Evidence is found in these countries, from their legislation, initiatives, research and court decisions. Assisted suicide, however, places health professionals in a maze of moral and professional issues, which challenge their roles in critical care settings.

SOCIOLOGY AND NURSING

There is ample literature on the subject of sociology and its relevance to nursing. The major debates reside in arguments highlighting sociology as a social theory that will facilitate student nurses' learning with regard to the context in which health care takes place (Theodore 1989, Alaszewski & Manthorpe 1995b), or whether the application of sociology in nursing curriculum is a help or hindrance (Sharp 1995). Alternatively, some argue that sociological truth (Lambert 1993), which enlightens one's awareness of social phenomena, will guide health care workers in establishing links between the causation of disease and ill-health as social constructs.

Nursing as a practice-based profession evolves within a social framework. Family nursing (care delivered by family members when someone is sick at home), community nursing (statutory care from health care professionals: district nurses, midwives, health visitors, community psychiatric nurses etc.), hospital- and nursing homes-based nursing represent the social realities (social facts). Nursing is occurring not only in a health care context but a social one too, since the care organized and delivered comes from specialized groups in society. It is also a fact that individuals are constantly exposed to their social structures, which are in a state of continuing change 'for reasons of efficacy or political determination' (Lambert 1993).

Social change, which runs parallel with social conflict, can affect physical, mental and social well-being. An awareness of sociological issues, and their implications for nursing practice, Theodore (1989) argued, will develop better understanding of clients' problems and needs. The process of assimilating sociological knowledge, however, with the aim of transfer to the clinical setting, has been criticized with too much emphasis on micro-sociological interactions (client–nurse interactions for example) at the expense of the macro perspectives (Cooke 1993a).

It is argued that a failure to consider wider social and organizational structures affecting professionals in their work will narrow their outlook, causing neglect of socio-political issues pertinent to their practice. By increasing the focus on symbolic interactions between clients and nurses, Cooke (1993b) argued that the boundaries between public (macro-sociology) and private (micro-sociology) can only become blurred.

The recognition of wider social influences, which many will argue can cause inequality, social conflict and occupational discontent, is important. Nevertheless, since nursing is practice-oriented, health care professionals' concentrated efforts on daily basic interpersonal reactions and interactions with their clients can be understood. This does not imply, however, that they are not concerned with how socio-political decisions and policy-making machinery are continually impinging on their practice. Porter (1996) rightly argued that there is growing evidence in the literature of professionals analysing their position in society in a critical way.

Although instrumental (clinical skills) knowledge is essential for nurses, Porter (1996) argued, sociological knowledge becomes one of the main ingredients of holism to guide and develop reflective practice.

A knowledge of sociology may not be needed to set up an intravenous infusion or to give an injection. It is nevertheless imperative to use sociological knowledge to anticipate a client's social and psychological reactions to a blood transfusion (e.g. a Jehovah's Witness). Alternatively, some patients may refuse to have an injection if they believe that their medications have *hot* or *cold* properties.

With regard to the relationships between individuals and wider social issues, Porter and Ryan (1996) asserted their position, explaining that nursing research can still retain its integrity by analysing social structures while not losing sight of its individual members. It is acknowledged, for instance, that the relationship between an individual and the social framework is a two-way process.

While social structures influence individuals, they are at the same time being shaped and re-designed by the actions of members (Porter & Ryan 1996). This is evidence that society is dynamic and in a state of evolution. Porter and Ryan additionally alluded to the theory–practice gap issues, supplying some arguments founded on a small research they did. They pointed out – after their observations on one ward area – that lack of resources (underfunding) and human capital constrain nurses' clinical effectiveness in applying theoretical knowledge fully into their practice (Case example 1.3).

NURSING AND SOCIETY

Today's nursing has to progress in line with developments in society as a whole. New technologies, advanced scientific space explorations, proliferated industrialization – with accompanying environmental pollution – and demographic changes, demand that the implementation of

Case example 1.3 Resources constraints and their effects on practice

National newspapers and professional literature constantly report bed closures and the ineffectiveness of some National Health Service Trusts in managing their budgets. Some Trusts have been known to overspend. The consequences are reported to be:

a. restrictions on staff recruitment
b. pressure to exercise personal accountability on budgeting issues at differing departmental levels, and pressure to reduce spending. Marginalizing the purchasing of equipment (e.g. specialist beds for the prevention and treatment of pressure sores) therefore occurs
c. low staff morale
d. increased sickness rates
e. increased stress levels.

Activity 1.5

Formulate some objectives you want to achieve on clinical placements based on the following:

1. an understanding of care organization
2. how nursing staff apply theory to practice
3. mentors' and assessors' views on organizational constraints
4. staff awareness and knowledge of wider social and political issues.

??? Question 1.5

How important is it to recognize the effects of social issues on clinical practice?

nursing care is driven by professionals who have a deeper and broader knowledge base. To acquire this 'fullness of knowledge', as Lafferty (1997) suggests, professionals in nursing have to refine their understanding of humanistic nursing: the integration of culture and interpersonal relationships at the point of care delivery becomes a desirable goal. To achieve this objective, Lafferty argues that the features of nursing as an empirical reality (science of nursing) and the art of nursing (aesthetic nursing) must be recognized.

Other dimensions, such as evidence-based nursing, become essential requirements in nursing practice, to ascertain that care 'does the patient no harm'. In this context, the ethical (moral) and personal dimensions (self-knowledge) enhance the whole process of nursing. The representation of self-knowledge as a personal dimension can only be consolidated through evidence-based approaches to care, with sensitivity to ethical issues.

In the public domain of the social system it is an expectation that clients will be cared for by highly skilled, competent practitioners. It is for this reason that some writers (e.g. Fralic et al 1997) emphasize that practitioners must be prepared to meet the nursing needs of society. The authors posit, however, that such needs can only be met by nurses in society who become 'critical thinkers', managing a diversity of care prerequisites.

While traditional training has fostered 'risk avoidance', they argue that professionals' risk-taking role should be developed to help them manage in unstable environments caused by social changes. To attain this goal, however, knowledge must be advanced through scientific research enquiry.

Researching one's profession in a modern context – to promote knowledge – is concerned with an exploration of societal influences. Cultural diversity is one aspect, while acknowledging the presence of other factors – technological developments for instance (Lister 1997) – and medical advances that impinge on practice.

It has already been acknowledged (Sharp 1995, Porter 1996) that instrumental knowledge (hands-on-nursing) is necessary. Nursing theory, however, according to Cash (1997), when critically examined shows that:

1. there is a tendency to believe that professionalization of nursing will emerge secondary to formal knowledge
2. society legitimizes the competent practitioner to practise
3. technical knowledge (nursing theories) demarcates itself from public domain knowledge (lay or informal knowledge).

Nursing boundaries are hence created with the establishment of a power structure
4. nursing continues to be significantly associated with women's work. Cash pointed out that its social identity can be traced from traditional patriarchal sexual division of labour.

As nursing evolution is sociologically situated, it is argued that its key underpinnings should be explored by critically evaluating social theory (Wilson-Thomas 1995). By using sociological theories (Box 1.5) the practitioners will be better equipped to question assumptions made about their practices.

The application of social knowledge in a care setting is, in addition, one of the tools that can enhance reflective practice.

FAMILIES IN SOCIETY

Modern society is witnessing rapid changes in the structure, composition and functions of families. Most noticeable is the changing definitions of what constitutes a 'family'. Even more remarkable in the sociology of the family is the varying nature of 'families', to the extent that using the singular (a family) is now considered inappropriate.

Most stereotypic images of family structures conjure up the concept of men and women (husbands and wives) with children, thus making the former mothers and fathers. Parenthood in this context – a popular image – becomes a social expectation. The role of mothers is seen as nurturing, while fathers are viewed as exerting control over the young. However, in reality both parents exert control over their children. Brannen et al (1994) argued, however, that since mothers spend more time with their children, they exercise more control over them than fathers. One explanation for this could be due to the fact that men are more likely than women to be in full-time employment. This employment situation, Kiernan (1992) explained, will hence impinge on the degree of contact between fathers and their children. Moreover, fathers' control over their

Box 1.5 Parsons, Marx, Weber and Durkheim: a nursing and health care perspective

Parsons

It will be remembered from the previous account that Parsons' view of society consists of systems, which maintain social stability/equilibrium; health care systems are such organizations. Their aim is to rehabilitate the sick so that they can regain their full potential to resume their normal socio-economic activities.

The 'sick role' assumes a person's new status while under care. The patient is relieved of social and economic responsibilities. At the micro-sociological level, care specialists (nursing, medical, paramedical personnel etc.) aim to alleviate the suffering of the sick. They are the care agents, trained according to a statutory code of conduct laid down by society's health care organizations.

Marx

Contradictions and conflict exist in health care. We are all familiar with the hierarchical system of the National Health Service. The Department of Health has control and responsibilities over care organizations. Marxists will argue that this governmental superstructure is the owner of health care production. The infrastructure consists of all the bedside health care personnel in direct contact with their clients. The prestigious position of medical personnel is in sharp contrast with the subservience of the nursing organization. Nursing care is initiated following medical diagnoses. Medical training is seen to be more technical, concerned with complex pathological processes, whereas nurse training is focused on basic activities of daily living.

Weber

To use a Weberian perspective, within the health care organization, varied economic positions (economic classes) and social statuses can be identified. A consultant's economic position and social status are in contrast with a ward manager's economic stature. Similarly, a ward housekeeper is in a different economic and status position.

What is more important in the nursing context is the *social action* of individuals. Understanding the meanings patients give to their situations is an essential responsibility for care personnel. How do patients view their health status? What interpretations do they give to the nursing and medical interventions? How satisfied are they in relation to their holistic needs being met? What rationale do they give when they refuse to take medications?

Durkheim

Since one of Durkheim's social theories rests on social facts and their constraining effects on individuals, health care organizations, according to this view, are social facts.

Constraints are exerted over health care personnel. Their practice has to adhere to strict guidelines from a professional code of conduct, designed by their professional bodies (e.g. United Kingdom Central Council (UKCC), British Medical Association (BMA) etc.). On the other hand, social facts can also be identified to comprise collective sentiments and customs of health care organizations. Customs and health beliefs in combination have integrative functions for groups. For example, when a multidisciplinary team is mobilized (Case example 1.4), it reflects the shared values, beliefs and vision of the group to attain a specific goal: to promote the health of their clients. Moreover, the group may consider, in addition to other issues, how best to work collaboratively.

Case example 1.4 Collaborative work

The Chief Executive of a National Health Service Trust organizes a meeting with nursing and medical personnel to discuss a strategy, with the aim to reduce conflict in the workplace, and to enhance communication between nursing and medical staff.

A workshop is organized. The themes for discussion include holistic approach to patient care, and multidisciplinary team intervention; analysis of social and economic constraints; and assessment of patient's level of satisfaction with the care delivered.

Activity 1.6

Organize a mini-seminar with your peers to debate the importance and relevance of applying classical social theories in clinical settings.

??? Question 1.6

1. In what way would you improve therapeutic relationships in practice by applying social action theory?
2. What do you consider to be the main rationale for professions to work together?

children is further reduced in divorce situations when children live apart.

The nuclear family as described above is a common family composition. In the winter of 1994–1995, 27% of families in Great Britain com-prised couples with dependent children (Central Statistical Office 1996). According to this source, families will also comprise a cohabiting couple with or without children, or a lone parent with children. Single people living on their own are not considered to be families.

COHABITATION

It is affirmed that unmarried couples living under the same roof are cohabiting. Cohabitation is not a new social phenomenon. People have been cohabiting for many years. It is a situation on the increase due to developing changes in beliefs systems, concerned with personal life experiences regarding living arrangements.

Statistics for people aged between 16 and 59 years show that, between 1991 and 1993, 9% of all people in this age group in Greater London were cohabiting, while in North England 6.3% and in East Anglia 8.5% of all people aged 16–59 were cohabiting during this 3-year period. If one looks separately at each country comprising Great Britain, one finds that England had the highest rate (7.8%) of cohabitation between 1991 and 1993; 7.2% in Wales; 5% in Scotland; and 1.9% of people in Northern Ireland aged between 16 and 59 were cohabiting from 1991 to 1993 (Central Statistics Office 1995).

Increase in cohabitation is, to some people, a reflection on the erosion of 'normal' family values (Muncie & Sapsford 1995) and structure. Other social factors, such as lone parent families and increased divorced rates, add to these beliefs. Many possible factors can be associated with reasons given for cohabiting (Box 1.6)

Latest figures (Central Statistical Office 1997) show that the proportion of all non-married women aged 18–49 who were cohabiting in Great Britain has doubled since 1981, to 25% in 1995–1996.

Attitudes towards cohabitation vary. Marked differences are found among groups born before 1930, and those born between 1960 and 1978. In the former, according to (Central Statistical Office 1997) based on a British Household Panel Survey (BHPS) data analysis, 40% of men thought cohabitation was wrong; in the latter group, only 7% thought it was wrong.

LONE PARENT FAMILIES

Lone parent families are on the increase. This trend is particularly noticeable over the past 25

Box 1.6 Reasons for cohabitation

- **Tension and conflict** in the family of origin, e.g. teenagers leaving the parental home to live with partners.
- **Physical and psychological abuse** of children/young adults, precipitating their migration to big cities where they may cohabit with individuals with similar experiences.
- **A belief model** based on cultural practice: identifying with one's parents' social practice (i.e. cohabiting parents).
- **An experimental** living arrangement prior to marriage.
- **Enforced cohabitation**: a situation whereby a person who is socio-economically deprived relies on a partner (who does not want to get married) for survival, and has to live with that person.
- **Failed marriages**: many divorced couples live together prior to marriage. Divorced men tend to cohabit more than divorced women (Central Statistical Office 1997).
- **Illicit cohabitation** (pseudo-cohabitation): couples who are already married living away from their official husbands or wives. Their extramarital family arrangements may reflect personal problems within their marriage.
- **Extramarital birth** (e.g. teenage pregnancies): although some cases lead to marriage, this is known to be linked to cohabitation.
- **Fear of divorce**: cohabiting is perceived as safer than getting married – a view based on ideological grounds and a belief that the institution of marriage is 'oppressive' (Roberts 1995).
- **Financial constraints**: getting married is expensive.
- **Lesbianism and homosexuality**: parental and wider kin hostility impel non-heterosexual couples to leave family homes and live together.

years, according to the National Statistics Office (Central Statistical Office 1997).

In 1994, 23% of all families in Great Britain were headed by lone parents with dependent children, an increase since 1971. Lone mothers form the majority of lone parent households. In 1995–1996, two-fifths of lone mothers were single, while a smaller percentage were divorced. Unmarried mothers with dependent children are perceived in a negative light, according to a British Social Attitudes Survey (BSAS) (Central Statistical Office 1997). Thirty-two per cent of respondents felt that unmarried mothers who find it hard to cope should blame themselves; on the other hand, 26% felt that unmarried mothers should be better understood by others in society.

Many single mothers fail to gain employment. Pyke (1997) pointed out the socio-economic differences between lone mothers and double-earner families, arguing that the former are getting poorer, while the latter are more successful in the job market. As high income families increase in numbers, their stature overshadows the plight of the work-poor families, along with unemployed mothers who are dependent on state benefits. Slipman (1994), from the National Council for One Parent Families in London, argued that there are at least 1.3 million one parent families in the UK. He asserted that their needs are exerting a strain on Government's welfare benefits systems.

In spite of the Government's philosophy of retaining old traditional family values, lone parents' plight remains a reality. Leach (1997) claims that a new approach using family-friendly employment policies would encourage lone parents to participate in the labour market. Moreover, tax and benefits allowances introduced in the 1999 Government Budget should support parents in the cost of care. In the field of housing, child care and education, for example, strategies aimed at the roots of social inequalities could be implemented.

Activity 1.7

Assess the impact of unemployment on lone parents in your area. Seek the help of community health workers to achieve this objective.

??? Question 1.7

According to National Statistics (Central Statistical Office 1997), there are more lone mothers with children than lone fathers with children. What explanations can you give for this trend?

ASPECTS OF FAMILY LIFE IN OTHER CULTURES

Wife-sharing

Wife-sharing is a familiar phenomenon in 34% of 101 cultures (Broude 1994). Although in Britain, and some other Westernized countries, 'wife swapping' – as it is colloquially known – takes place, it is nevertheless a covert practice, which occasionally is exposed in some tabloid newspapers.

Wife-sharing, however, is a social norm in other cultures. It is, for example, usual for the Banen of Cameroon not to prevent their wives from having sexual relations with other men. West African Mende husbands may share their wives or *lend* them to some male relatives from time to time (Broude 1994). A son may be allowed to sleep with one of his father's wives, but not his own mother. In old age, a Nigerian Tiv man may allow his sons sexual access to his wife. Exchange of wives may take place between two married Alaskan Kaska men.

Wife-sharing in these cultures helps to strengthen kinship bonds, the cementing of relationships and to prevent or diffuse hostilities, as amongst the Aranda of Australia.

Work activities

In British culture, a stereotypic image is of the housewife attending to the daily household management: washing and cleaning, child-rearing etc., while the husband goes to work. During the weekend, if he has the skills, he engages in do-it-yourself jobs around the house: repairs, lawn cutting etc.

If his wife is ill a man will most probably take over the tasks she normally does. In Mexico, however, a Tepotzlan husband will avoid doing housework or looking after children (Broude 1994). It is considered odd for men to do women's jobs. In cases of sickness he will ask a female relative to undertake his wife's tasks.

A Kiwai wife in New Guinea is expected to carry heavy loads of goods without help from her husband, unless she has an unusually long way to go.

Ifaluk wives in Micronesia will work with no help from their husbands, who spend their time around 'canoe houses doing nothing'. In Indonesia, Alor women are expected to undertake hard physical labour.

Intimate marriage and aloof marriage

An intimate marriage relates to the degree of physical and social closeness in the relationships between a married couple and other members of the family. The Rajput of Khalapur, India are examples of aloof marriages. Women's role is to be segregated from their husbands and others. The Hindu ethic places great emphasis on the husband's (son's) attachment to his mother. Wives in these living conditions only have sexual and reproductive functions (Broude 1994). The degree of companionship is almost non-existent until the husband's mother dies.

The Kapauka of New Guinea lead aloof lives. Husbands and wives sleep in separate rooms. Children sleep in the same room as their mother. Leisure activities are also undertaken separately.

Activity 1.8

Inform your neighbours and friends you have to write a project on family life. Seek their cooperation in identifying their views on the evolution of family relationships over the years. Compare their ideas with sociological theories.

??? Question 1.8

1. What do you consider to be the major differences between Western and non-Western cultures' understanding of the role of the family?
2. In what ways would you improve the social situation of lone parent families?

THE FUNCTIONS OF THE FAMILY

Families have set functions in society; the maintenance of health through caring (Box 1.7) is one. Families also have socio-economic and reproductive functions. Functionalists argue that families maintain a society's economy by their productivity in the work environment. Reproduction ensures the continuation of the species. The rearing of children prepares them for the world of work. To many, the family is a sanctuary

---

Box 1.7 Family health

The functional family aims at integrating their individual activities to meet the demands and pressures of modern life. Although the division of labour in the home has been criticized by feminist writers, the activities performed by a family are directed at ensuring the safety of its members. A caring behaviour is hence the expected norm of any family.

The survival of a family relies on its socio-economic functions. When a family member is sick, health-oriented behaviour is demonstrated and there is the mobilization of human and financial resources. Health maintenance, therefore, rests on the act of caring.

Caring and nurturing are two attributes very often linked to the feminine role (MacDougall 1997). Men, however, are just as capable of showing a caring attitude.

Participating in leisure activities (riding, swimming, walking etc.) are aspects of family life practised by many individuals to maintain personal health integrity. Further, how individuals perceive their own health and their families' health is important. Thus being able to work, and to continue with their hobbies, whilst achieving independence and health for their families, are values expressed by some Finnish people (Häggman-Laitila 1997).

When, however, independence is disrupted through ill-health, requiring hospitalization, the emotional, physical and socio-psychological attachments of the adaptive family are fragmented. Family nursing should therefore be implemented – with the whole family in mind – to prevent neglect of family members. The latter have an important role to play in strengthening the potential of the sick person to get better (Asted-Kurki et al 1997).

A family-focused nursing care (Collier & Schirm 1992) should circumscribe to the many faceted perspectives of caring. Whilst effective communication and emotional support are essential in care delivery, it is pointed out (Callery 1997) that the nature of maternal knowledge can help professionals to understand the 'norm' about a child who is sick.

Similarly, this principle can be applied in a variety of settings where adult nursing is taking place. The seeking of information (from significant others) will help identify behavioural norms of the individual client. Care plans should hence reflect these strategies.

---

where tension and the pressures of life can be attenuated.

Marxist sociologists view the family as a unit that produces a future workforce to maintain the elite classes in a dominant position. On the other hand, feminists will argue that the family is an expression of women's oppression in a patriarchal society, and that it functions by allowing men (husbands/partners) to hold a dominant role.

THE DYSFUNCTIONAL FAMILY
The dark side of the family

If the aim of families is to function by ensuring that healthy behavioural patterns are maintained by its members, families whose practices consist of violence, abuse and neglect (physical, psychological and emotional) of its members (Case example 1.5) are described as dysfunctional.

Case example 1.5 The isolated family

The villagers often talked about the 'odd' couple living at the end of the village, and their two little children, Mary (5) and Danny (6). They always looked unkempt and uncared for as they played in the front garden. They were not allowed to play with other children and, in addition, they did not attend the local school. There were doubts that they ever went to school. The health visitor had tried on many occasions to meet their parents, but without success. She was concerned for their safety.

When she finally gained access to the house, the health visitor was appalled at their living conditions. The parents would leave the children to sleep on a mattress on the floor; their diet was poor; there were no books for them to read; they lacked communication skills; and they looked distressed and apprehensive in the presence of their parents. The latter ignored their children's emotional needs. They, in fact, were aloof toward their children.

The dark side of the family is often exposed by the media. Violence against women in the home is a recurring theme. The scope of the problem is pervasive in its nature, embracing diverse socio-economic and ethnic groups (Campbell & Landenburger 1995).

The ultimate violence against women is rape, followed by murder. Wife-battering, husband-battering, rape, sexual harassment and psychological abuse are common occurrences in the homes of many families. These practices are not frequently reported since there is a fear of reprisals. Additionally, there is stigma attached to abuse in the family.

Violence against husbands in the family, although a social reality, does not attract similar attention and does not seem to generate intense emotive reactions. The stereotypic image of men as physically strong clouds the notion that they may be abused by their wives and children. Alcohol and drug dependence are possible factors that may predispose to this social condition. Moreover, husbands who are abused may feel embarrassed to officially report their situation. Exposing their plight may be perceived by others as being of a weak personality.

Child abuse makes the headlines regularly. There are many unreported cases, however. It has been known for children and teenagers to be sexually assaulted by their parents, murdered and then buried underneath the floorboards of their bedrooms. Babies may be left asphyxiated in drawers and cupboards.

When parents interfere with their child's health in subtle ways (i.e. the fabrications of symptoms (Repper 1995) and causing the simulation of illness (Facey 1989), it is termed *Munchausen syndrome by proxy*.

Abuse also takes place between siblings. Sibling abuse, Johnstone and Marcinak (1997) argue, is another component of domestic violence.

Activity 1.9

1. Do a literature search on Munchausen syndrome. Discuss your findings with peers.
2. Talk to your local newspaper publisher/editor. How many cases of domestic violence have been reported recently?
3. Ask community health professionals for their views on family nursing. Can they pinpoint some of the pertinent issues they encounter?

??? Question 1.9

1. Do you agree with the suggestion that families have a 'stabilizing' role in society?
2. What possible arguments can you give to explain the presence of the dysfunctional family?

SUMMARY

In this chapter some broad sociological concepts in relation to the organization of society, and the ways it can be understood and interpreted have been considered. It has been concluded that society is made up of social structures that have influences over groups, while being simultaneously prone to changes themselves as a consequence of human action.

An awareness of sociological theories helps in understanding the workings of society. The application of sociological theories in health care settings contributes to developing insight into the taken-for-grantedness activities of social practice, which is situated within a wider context. The analysis of clients' needs and problems must be implemented within a robust social science framework.

GLOSSARY

Communism   the idea that control and ownership of resources are within the grasp of all the people, sharing the benefits

Constructs   conceptual framework; a set of ideas

Empirical reality   practical experience

Holism   a whole. A contemporary term used in health care that considers the whole person

Macro-sociology   a sociological approach that considers the major structures in society and their functions. The opposite of individual action

Macro structures of society   major organizations in society (e.g. Department of Health, Law Corporations, Central Government etc.)

Market situation   personal buying and selling capacity: ownership, economic power etc.

Micro-sociological   sociological study that focuses on group processes, their interactions etc.

Multi-paradigmatic   a contemporary social science terminology, which means a set of concepts with many features

Organismic nature   acting as an organism with systems of homeostasis

Patriarchal   male oriented; male dominated

Social actors   a term used in sociology referring to society's members who act on their social systems

Stratified   a sociological term borrowed from geology, that refers to the hierarchical layers in society (e.g. class systems)

Structural–functional   an overlapping of structuralism with functionalism theories. Structures with specific functions

Symbolic interactions   the social meanings and interpretations that people give to their social interactions, which to some people may symbolize something

Weberian tradition   the theory that society is best studied by looking at individual actions and meanings attached to it; and people's status according to their economic/market situation

REFERENCES

Abercrombie N, Warde A, Soothill K et al 1994 Contemporary British society. A new introduction to sociology, 2nd edn. Polity Press, Cambridge

Alaszewski A, Manthorpe J 1995a Social Marxism, class conflict and health care. Nursing Times 91(20): 36–37

Alaszewski A, Manthorpe J 1995b Weber, authority and the organisation of health care. Nursing Times 91(29): 32–33

Asted-Kurki P, Paunonen M, Lehti K 1997 Family members' experiences of their role in a hospital: a pilot study. Journal of Advanced Nursing 25(5): 908–914

Béphage G 1997 Social science and health care: nursing applications in clinical practice. Mosby, London

Brannen J, Dodd K, Oakley A, Storey P 1994 Young people, health and family life. Open University Press, Buckingham

Broude G 1994 Marriage, family and relationships. A cross-cultural encyclopaedia. ABC Clio, Santa Barbara, CA

Callery P 1997 Maternal knowledge and professional knowledge: cooperation and conflict in the care of sick children. International Journal of Nursing Studies 34(1): 27–34

Campbell J, Landenburger K 1995 Violence against women. In: Fogel C, Woods N (eds) Women's healthcare: a comprehensive handbook. Sage, Thousand Oaks

Cash K 1997 Social epistemology, gender and nursing theory. International Journal of Nursing Studies 34(2): 137–143

Central Statistical Office 1993 Britain 1994: An Official Handbook. HMSO, London

Central Statistical Office 1995 Regional Trends 30. HMSO, London, p 52

Central Statistical Office 1996 Social Trends 26. HMSO, London, p 53

Central Statistical Office 1997 Social Trends 27. HMSO, London, p 45

Collier J, Schirm V 1992 Family-focused nursing care of hospitalised elderly. International Journal of Nursing Studies 29(1): 49–57

Cooke H 1993a Why teach sociology? Nurse Education Today 13: 210–216

Cooke H 1993b Boundary work in the nursing curriculum: the case of sociology. Journal of Advanced Nursing 18(7): 1990–1998

Cox C 1983 Sociology: an introduction for nurses, midwives and health visitors. Butterworth, London

Craib I 1997 Classical social theory: an introduction to the thought of Marx, Weber, Durkheim and Simmel. Oxford University Press, Oxford

Cuff E C, Sharrock W W, Francis D W 1990 Perspectives in sociology, 3rd edn. Unwin Hyman, London

Durkheim E 1950 'What is a social fact?' In: Worsley P (ed) 1991 The new modern sociology readings. Penguin, London, p 29–33

Facey S 1989 Munchausen syndrome by proxy. Nursing Times 89(4): 54–56

Fralic M, Brothers D, Keeling E, Torkelson D 1997 Critique of Schlotfeldt on knowledge, leaders and progress. Image: Journal of Nursing Scholarship 29(2): 126–127

Fraser D 1984 The evolution of the British welfare state, 2nd edn. MacMillan, Basingstoke

Giddens A 1979 Central problems in social theory, action, structure and contradiction in social analysis. MacMillan, Basingstoke

Giddens A 1994 Elements of the theory of structuration. In: Giddens A, Held D, Hubert D et al (eds) The polity reader in social theory. Polity Press, Cambridge, p 80–88

Groenman N H, Slevin O, Buckenham M A 1992 Social and behavioural sciences for nurses. Campion, Edinburgh

Guinness Encyclopaedia 1990 Guinness Publishing, Enfield

Häggman-Laitila A 1997 Health as an individual's way of existence. Journal of Advanced Nursing 25(1): 45–53

Haralambos M, Holborn M, Heald R 1995 Sociology themes and perspectives, 4th edn. Collins Educational, London

Johnson A 1995 The Blackwell dictionary of sociology: a user's guide to sociological language. Blackwell, Oxford

Johnstone H, Marcinak J 1997 Sibling abuse: another component of domestic violence. Journal of Pediatric Nursing: Nursing Care of Children and Families 12(1): 51–54

Joseph M 1990 Sociology for everyone, 2nd edn. Polity Press, Cambridge

Kiernan K 1992 Men and women at work and at home. In: Jowell R, Brook L, Prior G, Taylor B (eds) British social attitudes: the 9th report. Dartmouth, Aldershot

Lafferty P 1997 Balancing the curriculum: promoting aesthetic knowledge in nursing. Nurse Education Today 17(4): 281–286

Lambert C 1993 Plato, sociology and nursing. Nurse Education Today 13: 445–450

Lawson T, Garrod J 1996 The complete A–Z sociology handbook. Hodder & Stoughton, London

Leach P 1997 What price home visiting and family support? Health Visitor 70(2): 72–74

Lister P 1997 The art of nursing in a 'postmodern' context. Journal of Advanced Nursing 25(1): 38–44

MacDougall G 1997 Caring: a masculine perspective. Journal of Advanced Nursing 25(4): 809–813

Moore S 1987 Sociology alive! Stanley Thornes, Cheltenham

Moore S 1988 Sociology GCSE passbook. Charles Lett, London

Mouzelis N 1997 Social and system integration. Sociology 31(1): 111–119

Muncie J, Sapsford R 1995 Issues in the study of the 'family'. In: Muncie J, Wetherell M, Dallos R, Cochrane A (eds) Understanding the family. Sage, London

New Encyclopaedia Britannica, Vol 27 1992 University of Chicago, Chicago

Outhwaite W, Bottomore T 1994 The Blackwell dictionary of 20th century social thought. Blackwell, Oxford

Parsons T 1961 The four functional imperatives of the social system. In: Worsley P (ed) 1991 The new modern sociology readings. Penguin, Harmondsworth, p 532–536

Porter S 1996 Why teach sociology? A contribution to the debate. Nurse Education Today 16: 170–174

Porter S, Ryan S 1996 Breaking the boundaries between nursing and sociology: a critical realist ethnography of the theory–practice gap. Journal of Advanced Nursing 24(2): 413–420

Pyke N 1997 'Single mothers fail to get the jobs'. Times Educational Supplement 13th June, 22, col 1

Repper J 1995 Munchausen syndrome by proxy in health care workers. Journal of Advanced Nursing 21(2): 299–304

Roberts C 1995 Whatever happened to marriage? In: Clulow C (ed) Women, men and marriage: talks from the Tavistock Marital Studies Institute. Sheldon Press, London, p 13–28

Scanlon C, Rushton C 1996 Assisted suicide: clinical realities and ethical challenges. American Journal of Critical Care 5(6): 397–405

Scott J 1995 Sociological theory: contemporary debates. Edward Elgar, Aldershot

Sharp K 1995 Sociology in nurse education: help or hindrance? Nursing Times 91(20): 34–35

Slipman S 1994 One-parent families: some contemporary issues. Professional Care of Mother and Child 4(6): 163–164

Theodore J 1989 Sociology by any other name. Nursing Times 85(19): 74–75

Turner S 1996 Social theory and sociology: the classics and beyond. Blackwell, Cambridge, MA

Wilson-Thomas L 1995 Applying critical social theory in nursing education to bridge the gap between theory, research and practice. Journal of Advanced Nursing 21(3): 568–575

Wright E 1996 Marxism after communism. In: Turner S (ed) Social theory and sociology: the classics and beyond. Blackwell, Cambridge, MA, 120–145

FURTHER READING

Doyal L 1983 Cancer in Britain: the politics of prevention. Pluto Press, London

Giddens A 1971 Capitalism and modern social theory: an analysis of the writings of Marx, Durkheim, Weber. Cambridge University Press, Cambridge

Marx K, Engels F 1964 The German ideology. Lawrence & Wishart, London

May T 1996 Situating social theory. Open University Press, Buckingham

Navarro V 1982 Imperialism, health and medicine. Pluto Press, London

Parsons T 1943 The structure of social action: a study in social theory with a special reference to a group of recent European writers, 2nd edn. Glencoe Press, New York

Parsons T 1951 The social system. Routledge & Kegan Paul, London

Parsons T 1967 Sociological theory and modern society. Glencoe Press, New York

Porter S 1995 Sociology and the nursing curriculum: a defence. Journal of Advanced Nursing 21(6): 1130–1135

Sharp K 1994 Sociology and the nursing curriculum: a note of caution. Journal of Advanced Nursing 20(2): 391–395

Sharp K 1995 Why indeed should we teach sociology? A response to Hannah Cooke. Nurse Education Today 15(1): 52–55

2

Families and health care

It is becoming widely recognized and accepted by health care professionals in a variety of health settings that holism in clinical practice is incomplete without a meaningful and purposeful focus on the clients and their social networks. The aim of this chapter is to highlight the multidimensional nature of the concept of 'families'. Emphasis is placed on the phenomena of families in clinical setting. Their specific needs and care are discussed within the broader social context, concurrently with their special needs as they relate to specific clinical situations in which they find themselves.

FAMILIES IN HOSPITAL

Caring for families in the familiar surroundings of their own homes is a worthwhile philosophy. It is, however, a goal that cannot always be attained entirely, as when family members who are ill have reached a stage in their illness requiring not only statutory community nursing services but the intervention of hospital-based nursing and medical personnel. Many families do their best to maintain responsibility for the care of their relatives at home, avoiding as long as possible admission to hospital with all its unfamiliar environment. Hospital avoidance may be a reflection of the fears and anxieties the hospital generates because of clinical procedures. In addition, the beliefs among some people that institutional care means the old workhouse care cause some to avoid hospital. Moore (1994) argued that care in the 1990s is still deeply embedded in institutional care. While some families for varying reasons will rely on their own resources to care for their members, others will request admissions for their relatives, despite fears of hospital.

Several reasons may be identified leading to the admission of a person into hospital, thus causing a fragmentation of the family kinship connection:

- mental ill-health – thought disorders, perceptual alterations, violent behaviour due to sociopathic traits, brain failure, severe mood disturbances
- physical pathology – renal failure, metabolic disorders, brain pathology, myocardial disorders.

FAMILY PHENOMENOLOGY

Families' involvement in care intervention within the hospital setting is a new phenomenon. In the past the family of the sick person had marginalized contact with their relative in hospital. Restricted visiting times discouraged many family members from maintaining regular contact with their next of kin. Their presence is now being felt due to open visiting. This new development entails that relatives are more likely to witness the full impact of the disease process on their loved ones. Additionally, they are in many instances the witnesses of the vast array of routine nursing and medical interventions. Although their participation is encouraged in some health care settings, it is nevertheless restricted to basic aspects of care (hand washing, changing clothes, bedbathing, nail cutting, assisting to eat etc.). Such activities, nevertheless, are meaningful to the recipient of care, and conversely to the caregiver, whose kinship bond is being expressed and maintained. This availability of kinship networks – at the scene of clinical practice – means that families whose main objective is to support the sick person will likewise experience trauma in observing progressive deterioration of their kin. Although physical or psychological deterioration may not be apparent,

hospitalization due to pathology generates a multitude of emotions and fears amongst families and patients.

It is argued (Theobald 1997) that health care professionals lack insight into some wider issues related to the feelings of families in clinical situations where their loved ones are being cared for. Theobald pointed out that in intensive care settings, for example, where patients with cardiac conditions are admitted the psychosocial needs of families should be considered. While hospitalization and acute illness have an impact on both patients and their relatives, the emotional turmoil affecting the latter can have a devastating effect on their future lifestyle. Fear about the future, concerns regarding the ability to cope and to resume a normal way of life and being able to make adaptation to one's routine to meet with new pressures, are some aspects of the social and emotional experiences of families. Theobald argued that families are in need of support and that they very often rely on other family members and friends or in their religious beliefs. Health care professionals can consolidate this support by ensuring that:

- families in clinical settings receive unambiguous information avoiding technical terminology
- information given is continuous and related to the patient's progress
- some relatives may be satisfied to receive information secondhand from other relatives; others, however, may prefer to 'obtain this information directly from their partner'.

SOCIAL NETWORK AND SOCIAL SUPPORT

If family-focused care is to be implemented effectively, a strategic care planning should be designed to include the participation of informal lay support groups. Support group presence in family care (clients' social network: family, friends, neighbours, working colleagues) could be utilized alongside professional support. This approach, it is argued (Hildingh et al 1995), will facilitate the empowering of patients. Recognizing the important roles of clients' social networks and seeking their participation in providing emotional support is a nursing strategy that can be developed with the aim to enhance care implementation. Hildingh et al believe that by making use of lay mutual support groups, their presence will exert a buffering effect on the traumatic experiences of patients in care, thus establishing a social condition likely to increase the individuals' well-being. It becomes imperative therefore for care professionals to identify the existence of any social networks, and to assess their integrity as well as the group's willingness to provide support as needed (Case example 2.1).

Inviting familiar, mutual self-help groups in clinical practice does not discount the professional and technical expertise of the professional. It adds a new dimension to not only patient-focused care but also to family-focused care. While a human support group is an important facet in the implementation of family nursing strategies, some individual patients' social networks comprise animals: pet cats and dogs, for example. Where appropriate, after discussions with nursing personnel, a patient's animal companion may be brought in at visiting times.

Additionally, during visiting times, close but discreet observations of the number and frequency of visitors at the clients' bedside should be noted. The rationale behind this approach is:

- to identify new social network formation
- to identify clients who may not be receiving family social support
- to assist personnel in their decisions to update their care plans
- to direct their technical (professional) support to specific client groups who may need such support
- to enhance health care professionals' systematic assessment.

Careful assessment of clients' interactions with significant others is essential. Besides, nursing and medical staff need to assess their own interactions with the client while engaging themselves in daily conversation with them. The aim of such interactions is twofold:

1. purposeful interactions provide a direct or indirect variety of meaningful support to the client
2. daily conversation familiarizes the practitioner with the clients' thinking, needs and their relationships with visiting relatives (Case example 2.1).

Case example 2.1

John Tampleton is a 70-year-old retired farmer. He lost his wife in an accident 10 years ago. He has a son and a daughter who live five miles away in the next village. He lives with his housekeeper in an old farmhouse. Although retired, he still helps out on the farm, tending to the sheep with the help of a young shepherd. In the game season he goes pheasant and woodpigeon shooting, taking his two labradors. In the evening he meets with the local farmers in the village pub; sometimes his housekeeper will accompany him. He whiles away the evening talking to his fellow farmers and the landlord about the good old days. Occasionally his son and daughter will visit him at home, bringing in home-made pies and cider, which he likes.

It is important for hospital staff to encourage visits from Mr Tampleton's family, housekeeper and fellow farmers while he is in hospital, in order to continue the links with his social network.

Activity 2.1

During visiting times, observe the number of patients without visitors. Inform your mentor. Formulate a plan of action with your mentor and peers which will aim at ensuring that lone patients in your area will have someone to talk to.

??? Question 2.1

1. What is the importance of lay support for patients who are in hospital?
2. What is your role as a member of the ward team in ascertaining that accurate assessment of clients' interactions with their families is made?

The integration of lay support in care provision should be seen as a collaborative partnership between professional and informal groups.

Hildingh et al (1995) assert that these groups represent phenomena 'that should be brought up for discussion in nursing as well as other health professions today'.

Family nursing

Traditional hospital-based nursing practice has, in most cases, focused on the client from a medical-oriented care approach, at the expense of the social context of care and the psychological needs of patients. Family nursing is concerned with the individual (the sick person) as well as the importance of families in nursing practice (St John & Rolls 1996). It is acknowledged that families have positive effects on the health outcomes of the sick person (St John & Rolls 1996), that their importance must not be underestimated and better understanding of their roles is needed through development of family nursing knowledge (Rennick 1995). A knowledge of the dynamic processes of the family as a unit of care will increase sensitivity to a wider dimension of patient care. A model of care encompassing both patients and their kinship systems is a prerequisite. The focus is hence on the family: the patient and significant others.

Interactive social and psychological processes in a family model of care requires meticulous analysis (Fig. 2.1). The challenge to health care professionals is how to judge the level of support required by a family during a relative's hospitalization (Carr 1997). In many instances, the family of the sick person, who may be a child, an adolescent, an older member of the family, feels it is their duty to be at the bedside as constantly as possible. Carr (1997) refers to this attitude as 'family vigilance'. It is a natural response complementary with the severing of kinship bonds caused by the emotional traumas of hospitalization. For this reason, in many clinical settings provision is made for families to remain overnight in a room specially prepared for their needs in the ward area.

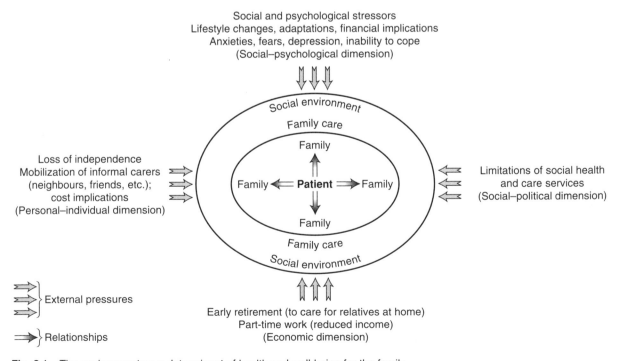

Fig. 2.1 The environment as a determinant of health and well-being for the family.

The constancy of family contact under this arrangement allows the professionals to assess the level of support needed. The support needed may possess multiparadigmatic features:

1. A family may feel psychologically and physically weakened by the onslaught of their lived experience: distressing events in clinical practice; increased stress in the home environment. They require the support of health care professionals to enable them to undertake their functions as resource mobilizers, which will strengthen positive links not only with their hospitalized kin but with the multidisciplinary team.

2. Recognition that caring for one's relative in hospital is an expression of family values and responsibility, a cross-cultural basic phenomenon rooted in the family as a powerful social force.

3. Where the patient is showing signs of cognitive dysfunctions, family members may need help in the task of functioning as advocates. As Carr (1997) emphasized, a multitude of issues will concern the family such as:
   a. monetary matters
   b. living arrangements
   c. the preparation of a will
   d. contact with legal advisers
   e. home adaptations if discharge is being planned.

4. In stressful situations, families may experience difficulties in identifying their own needs with regard to the amount and frequency of information required. Careful and sensitive assessments of their responses during interactions must be carried out so that information giving is correspondent with their needs. Factual information will facilitate their decision-making concerning personal issues.

5. The health status of relatives can suffer due to the stressors of caring. Some individuals' health belief may consist of showing 'independent coping' (Häggman-Laitila 1997). Such inclination, however, may mask underlying psychological and physical problems (i.e. depressive states, sleep disturbances) due to situations that present a threat to one's coping abilities.

LIFE-THREATENING ILLNESS AND FAMILIES

To many families, being confronted with an illness may seem life-threatening, in spite of reassurances from health care professionals to the contrary. There are many instances, nevertheless, in clinical practice which evoke fear of death: a myocardial infarction, a life-threatening ruptured aortic aneurysm, a brain tumour, a fulminating systemic infection, or a cancerous disease. A cancer diagnosis can exert far-reaching effects on families (Crosby 1994). Family interpersonal relationships may become strained. Marital breakdown – separation and divorce – very often are prominent social features.

Hence, families in this situation become fragmented, and their socio-psychological and physical make-up weakened. A feeling of hopelessness can prevail. The experience of losing hope is linked to events beyond one's control. Disease, ill-health and admission to hospital annihilate one's structured, orderly living arrangements. People spend their lives living in hope. In clinical settings this hope loses its intensity. Families are often seen weeping at the bedside. Others manage to exhibit a brave demeanour, controlling their emotions. On the other hand, their dying relative may still harbour feelings of hope and the belief that they still have a contribution to make before dying: discussing or talking about future plans of the family; talking about past memories; making arrangements concerning children's needs; and reassuring relatives.

Although hope can be destroyed by a diagnosis of a life-threatening illness (Wilkinson 1996), evidence in clinical practice shows that many individuals diagnosed as terminally ill have survived beyond medical and nursing expectations. Wilkinson argued that hope, in this instance, has become a powerful motivator to survive against adversity. Some families, when confronted with adversity, adopt varying strategic defences: withholding information concerning a diagnosis and denying the realism of the life-threatening illness. Such an attitude has a negative impact on the concept of hope as a powerful motivator.

Honest communication (Wilkinson 1996) will enhance the sick or dying person's 'expectation that life can be lived as fully as possible in whatever time is left'.

To achieve such an objective the recipient of care requires 'social support', which Chiverton (1997) defines as the inclusion of non-verbal approaches to care such as 'listening', expressing 'concern', and 'intimacy' in interpersonal behaviour, with the aim to sustain the individual's 'emotional' stability.

While the benefits of social support have been emphasized, it is sometimes assumed by families and care professionals that relatives must be seen at the patient's bedside regularly to undertake their responsibilities as agents of support. It is a practice that may affect some patients' well-being. Frequent visitations can be detrimental to health. The person who is confronted with pathology and attempting to cope with the exhaustion caused by the disease may develop what Lazure (1997) calls a 'sense of helplessness'. This feeling can be triggered by a 'lack of control over the entry and timing of visitors' (Lazure 1997). Lazure argued that her research (a two-group experimental study in a Coronary Care Unit, California), showed a two-dimensional perspective on the effects of family visiting on patients:

1. some undesirable side-effects have been noted: increased patients' heart rate and blood pressure, as well as cardiac arrhythmias
2. visits can benefit the patients by stabilizing the cardiovascular system, reducing anxiety and inducing calmness.

A balanced and critical assessment of the needs for family support during visiting times is necessary. A patient-led approach, under close guidance of health care professionals, with emphasis upon the individualization of visiting policies, will help clients and their relatives to tailor a visiting programme to match their needs. Their involvement in care planning will promote empowerment (Box 2.1).

A model of care in practice should contain the following features:

1. the patients' preferences (where to die; frequency of family visits etc.)

Box 2.1

In a care triangulation (Fig. 2.2) professional care-givers act as facilitator, observer, counsellor and care-giver as required, dependent on patients' and family needs. They are a supportive presence characterized by silent companionship; the verbal expression of humane understanding concurrent with genuine non-verbal communication. The combination of technical and lay knowledge (social networks) becomes imperative. This approach should be congruent with the needs of the recipient of care (Riegel 1989).

In a care triangulation, the professional acts as a facilitator, an observer, a counsellor and a care-giver, as required, dependent on the patient's and family's needs

A supportive presence, characterized by silent companionship, the verbal expression of humane understanding, concurrent with genuine non-verbal communication

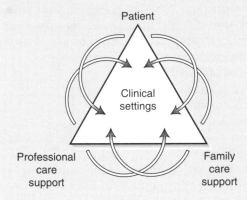

Fig. 2.2   Care triangulation.

---

2. the relatives' preferences (organization of care; types of care based on their informal knowledge of the patients' needs etc.)
3. the patients' and relatives' narration of their experiences in clinical setting: their relationships with staff members (conflict, fears, misunderstandings, expression of rational or irrational behaviour, communication needs and constraints)
4. special needs: privacy, dignity, cultural practices (needs to pray, to express sexuality and spirituality)

5. safety needs: socio-psychological and biological aspects of needs (Case example 2.2).

Case example 2.2

Mr John Talbott, aged 60, was admitted to a surgical ward at 02:00 h after he collapsed at home. He was accompanied by his wife. On arrival to the ward his blood pressure was 70/50, pulse rate 110/min, temperature 35.5°C, respiration 25–30 min. His skin was cold and clammy. His extremities were deeply cyanotic. Oxygen was administered at 2–4 l/min. His facial expression showed severe anxiety.

His wife, who stayed at the bedside while the nurse made him comfortable, was very distressed and needed reassurance. A staff nurse was assigned with the role of attending to Mrs Talbott's psychological needs, while her husband was prepared for emergency surgery. The doctor on call who examined Mr Talbott had made a diagnosis of leaking aortic aneurysm. It was explained to the patient during his preoperative preparations that he would have to be transferred to the intensive care unit from the operating theatre. Mrs Talbott was kept informed of the procedures throughout. She agreed for her husband to have the operation and signed the consent form.

Activity 2.2

1. Prepare a plan of care which highlights an assessment of the patient's social needs.
2. Explain to the relatives their roles and functions with regard to their support as social networks.

??? Question 2.2

1. What are the concepts of social support and social networks?
2. What is the role of the health care professional in care implementation during a life-threatening illness?
3. What is the importance of applying a family nursing perspective in clinical practice?

THE CRITICALLY ILL IN THE ICU

Patients' needs and the family

The high technological environment of an intensive care unit (ICU) triggers fears and anxieties among patients and their relatives. The media frequently portray the clinical and specialized activities of professionals as they attend to the needs of the critically ill. Additionally, the ICU is often associated with patients who are/have been on assisted pulmonary ventilation from a few weeks to many years. Thereafter, decisions have to be made in connection with whether ventilators need to be switched off (if recovery is not expected) or not, thus allowing the patient to die peacefully. These factors in conjunction with the social and psychological vulnerability of the patients and their families have a tendency to compound the effects of admission to an ICU.

Patients and families have complex needs. Consequently, a patient and family driven provision of care should be tailored to address these multiple needs. Wesson (1997) argued for a 'developed specialist role in intensive care nursing'.

The importance of recognizing the needs of families and patients in ICU is well documented (Halme 1990, Hickey 1990, Marsden 1992, Scullion 1994, Hammond 1995, Quinn et al 1996, Wesson 1997). As patients' families' needs are increasingly gaining attentive acknowledgement, the issues related to services which may be provided to meet their complex needs are highlighted (Box 2.2). Since their needs are as important as the sick person's in connection with the informational, social, psychological and emotional dimensions, Wesson (1997) asserted that by reflecting upon one's 'knowledge and experience', would promote the development of specialized support strategies 'for each patient and family' in the ICU, to include transfer and discharge planning in the process. Some positive measures can be taken to reduce increased stress and vulnerability levels among families in ICU setting:

1. Their needs for information can be met by active listening, to identify key issues from *their* perspectives, causing them anxiety. For example, hope for recovery, length of stay, the patient's progress or deterioration, the functions of equipment, visiting rights, overnight stay to maintain continuity of presence and close proximity.
2. The assignment of a health care professional

Box 2.2 Issues to be considered when involving families in care

- Seek the patient's consent (this is dependent on the nature of the critical illness (i.e. an unconscious patient on assisted ventilatory functions will be unable to give consent). However, the patient should be informed that family members are helping in the care as needed.
- Some relatives may adopt a non-participatory role, feeling that lay contribution may impede professional care.
- Careful assessment of family responses to critical illness: some individuals' stress levels may be deepened by direct participation.
- Some relatives may express embarrassment in connection with intimate aspects of care: bedbathing, changing soiled clothing and bedlinen etc.
- Active participation, in many cases, has the positive consequence of 'decreasing powerlessness' (Hammond 1995). Prior to participation, however, discussion with relatives pertaining to the types of care activities they wish to be involved in should be identified. In addition, the duration and intensity of the involvement should be discussed, compatible with the skills and needs of the informal carers.
- Information concerning a variety of issues, i.e. technical equipment, medical reports, radiological and haematological results etc., should be imparted concisely, avoiding the use of jargon.

to be the 'family link'. The link nurse will then undertake the responsibility to develop and maintain therapeutic interpersonal relationships with relatives. A therapeutic relationship comprises attending to the family's needs for counselling. The provision of an environment – away from the immediate clinical atmosphere of the ICU – conducive to the expressions of emotions, apprehension and frustrations is essential.

3. Regular updates with reference to altered physiology, treatment changes and investigative procedures.

4. Full explanations concerning the rationale for specific specialized interventions; for example, parenteral nutrition, cardiac catheterization, central venous pressure monitoring and haemodialysis.

5. A non-hurried, confident and calm, professional approach to instil confidence and to demonstrate that time spent with relatives is invaluable and meaningful.

6. Facilitate the family's understanding and acceptance, as well as their coming to terms with their relative's critical illness as follows:

a. explaining empathetically the effects of pathology on body systems

b. communicate in an objective way that the aim of therapy and care is to ensure the physical and psychological comfort of their relative

c. explain that effective pain control is being achieved by the administration of regular analgesia and/or supplemented with complementary therapy (e.g. acupuncture, massage, chiropractics)

d. utilize the ICU specialist (health care professional with counselling expertise) to enhance the family's coping skills and to 'facilitate the long-term development of adjustment and acceptance' (Wesson 1997)

e. obtain their views regarding individual ways of expressing acceptance of the critical illness (e.g. wish for family participation in giving physical and emotional care)

f. the encouragement of lay participatory care (under professional guidance as necessary) will 'strengthen and confirm relationships' between the ill person and relatives (Hammond 1995).

THE ILL CHILD IN CRITICAL CARE SETTING

Impact on the family

When the ill child is admitted to an ICU, this becomes a major event to the families concerned, with implications for social functioning. A process of change is set in motion. Modifications are made – to adapt to the situation – in the re-establishment of new routines so that 'time and attention could be devoted to the child' (Rennick 1995). Thus, attempts to maintain links with their children in hospital show the interdependence of family members. The responsibility of maintaining continuity and proximity with their child, however, becomes a major stressor for the family, often resulting in 'parental role conflict' (Rennick 1995).

Role erosion, caused by care control exercised by health professionals, becomes one of the factors impacting on the family process. Other factors could include the intimidating, technological environment that has taken over responsibility of maintaining vital functions.

The overall, intensive specialized care becomes a stress factor to parents. Stressors, hence, have an impact on family members. Curran et al (1997) make reference to the multi-faceted aspects of stressors. In a neonatal ICU they point out, for example, that maternal health is affected by a combination of factors. The degree of social support will impinge on not only the mother, but other family members too. Factors such as negative life events, conflict and discord in the family, separation and divorce, inability to express one's needs in relation to socio-cultural beliefs concerning child's health and needs add to the level of family stress.

Curran et al's survey of a sample of parents and infants who had been inpatients in their neonatal ICU at Rush Green Hospital, Essex, UK, reveals some interesting findings. Although the investigators were interested in the level of psycho-emotional care of parents of children, their results also gave an insight into not only the degree of psychological responses to environmental stressors, but indicate the family dynamics as well: social relationships, social needs, interactions and communication needs.

The survey revealed that seven (11%) of the 60 parents interviewed felt fear on discharge, while 14 (24%) of the 60 parents said they felt stressed. The authors concluded that care of parents on discharge should be seen as a continuing process, to ascertain their ability to cope in community settings. The implications for practice can be summarized as follows:

1. Stress and fear will undermine parents' ability in regaining previous relationships' stability.
2. Healthy family dynamics could suffer: lack of knowledge regarding their children's physiological and mental health status and how to cope

Table 2.1		
Relative	Positive effect % (*n*)	Negative effect % (*n*)
Partner	64 (39)	18 (12)
Grandparents	50 (30)	12 (8)
Other children	18 (12)	16 (10)
Other family	28 (17)	18 (12)

with unexpected changes could add strain to marital relationships, with repercussions on siblings and the convalescing child's safety.
3. A baby in a neonatal ICU showed that 'a significant proportion of parents revealed their relationships to be negatively affected by stress experiences' (Curran et al 1997) (Table 2.1).

While intervention by an experienced counsellor is beneficial at an early stage of hospitalization to reduce the stress factor, an identification of specific areas of concern for parents must be considered as a prerequisite. For example, the parent–child relationship can be improved by the 'emotional support of parents and facilitation of continuation of the parenting role where possible' (Craft 1995). Acknowledging the important contribution of parents in the care triangulation not only 'helps parents to feel a valued part of the child's care team', Craft (1995) postulated, but this approach will simultaneously alleviate anxieties experienced by both parents and child. Parental involvement in child care therefore becomes a highly positive therapeutic tool, well recognized in the literature (Sheldon 1997).

Communication becomes integral within families. Curran et al discovered that 83% (50 of 60) of parents expressed their feelings to their partners; 63% (38 of 60) utilized the family networks. The researchers emphasized, however, that only seven of 60 (11%) of parents could relate to the medical staff. Thirty-six per cent (24 of 60) of parents felt they could relate to nursing staff.

These findings have implications for nursing and medical practice. Communication enhancement is required between parents and the multidisciplinary team to ensure sufficient information is imparted, since the survey showed that 15% of parents complained about the lack of information. On the other hand, meaningful use of parents' reliance on their social networks could be encouraged. This can be achieved by:

1. Increasing parental awareness that healthy communicative systems strengthen their kinship bonds, which concurrently exerts a buffering effect against stress.

2. Explaining that some family members may possess characteristics that have potential in maintaining family cohesion:

- social skills – ability to relay information obtained from professionals in clinical settings reliably and efficiently to significant others
- practical skills – participating in informal caring as needed and managing household tasks while parents are visiting the ill child.

PROACTIVE PATIENT AND FAMILY EDUCATION

The aim of patient and family education is to increase the individual's empowerment. In a clinical setting the environment becomes a major stressor to patients and their family networks. Education in the context of health care practice potentiates the patient's and family's scope to better appreciate 'the disease process' and to develop strategies to manage the disease (Trocino et al 1997). The authors asserted that the provision of meaningful and appropriate information giving becomes a 'critical professional activity'. However, the implementation of patient and family education requires careful planning with insight into multiple factors that can impede such practice: time factor; inadequate preparation of personnel concerning their role as patient and family educators; lack of incentive; paucity of available literature to facilitate the education process.

In a survey undertaken to assess nurses' attitudes toward patient and family education, in a large health care system in central Florida (Trocino et al 1997), findings revealed differences in attitudes linked to:

- **gender** – males were more confident in their roles as family and patient educators
- **age** – older nurses (in their 50s) argued that teaching about patients' diagnosis was the physicians' responsibility; nurses in their 20s showed higher commitment in the education of patients and their families
- **years of experience** – nurses with more than 20 years' experience did not feel it their responsibility to 'explain specific aspects of patients' disease if the physician does not'. Additionally, nurses with more than 20 years' experience expressed the view that they lacked confidence in communicating with families about patients' illnesses.

Evidence from the above research clearly highlights a need for a clear distinction of one's role and attitudes in professional practice. The provision of a standard acceptable policy aimed at empowering patients and their families is required. The maximization of family potential to cope with a health crisis and to ensure patient satisfaction can be met by proactive measures:

1. Statutory educational programmes to firmly establish a foundation on which professionals can confidently develop a positive role in the education of families about disease process and self-care skills.

2. Identification of areas (e.g. teaching pain control, sexuality, sexual dysfunction), in which

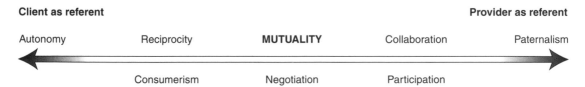

Fig. 2.3 Client–provider mutuality. Redrawn with permission of the publisher from Henson RH 1997 Image: Journal of Nursing Scholarship 29(1): 77–81.

some personnel are least confident, to develop knowledge for practice accordingly.

3. Development of communication skills to keep pace with consumer demands for information.

4. A system of mentorship/preceptorship so that practitioners with the least experience can work alongside an experienced specialist.

5. Applying the concept of *mutuality*, negotiation, collaboration and participation. Henson (1997), in his analysis of *mutuality*, defines the concept by locating its position in the centre of a continuum between paternalism and autonomy (Fig. 2.3).

Mutuality becomes the contact point between not only caregivers and care recipients (the patient) but should also encompass significant others (informal carers) (Fig. 2.4).

Family involvement is therefore necessary to complete the framework of the theory (Case example 2.3). Mutuality consists of a state of

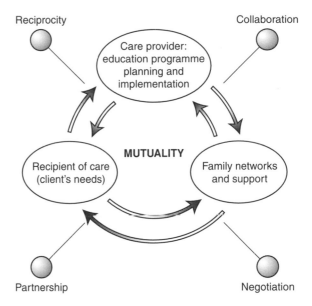

Fig. 2.4 Dynamic, flexible process of joint exchange among individuals. (After Henson 1997, with permission.)

Case example 2.3

When Amy, aged 5, was admitted to the paediatric intensive care unit (PICU) following a road traffic accident, her parents were devastated. She had sustained severe abdominal injuries: a ruptured spleen and laceration of the kidneys. Additionally, a fracture of the tibia and fibula was diagnosed. Following emergency surgery she was transferred to the unit and was placed on ventilatory support.

Her father and mother visited every day and required constant reassurance from the staff. Her mother, Emily, was asthmatic. It was therefore important for the multidisciplinary team to bear this aspect in mind in their family care process. It is known that emotional state influences asthma (Lane 1996); stress and anxiety can act as triggering factors (Barnes & Newhouse 1994, Williams et al 1996). An informal meeting was arranged with Emily and her husband John, to take place in a non-clinical environment: a specially designed comfortable parents' room away from the main unit areas. The room was tastefully decorated: there were plants, pastel-coloured wallpaper, comfortable armchairs, oil paintings on the wall, wall lights with dimmer switches and so on. The window overlooked a wide expanse of green fields.

The professional allocated to be the link person and family helper was a specialist paediatric intensive care nurse.

Research has shown that there are differences in the ways parents perceive their child's illness (Hall 1996). According to Hall it has been assumed that 'fathers react similarly to mothers at the crucial time of diagnosis' and in other social situations. Hall argued that this is not the case.

With this finding in mind, the paediatric nurse in her interactions with the parents ensured that she obtained a full assessment of each individual parent's perception of their child's condition. By actively listening, the professional gradually identified the father's and mother's experience.

By encouraging them to talk openly about their feelings she was able to differentiate the intensity of their feeling and reactions to diagnosis. Hall (1996) explained that fathers have a tendency to repress their emotions, to avoid increasing the mother's distress. Furthermore, she postulated that fathers have tendencies to experience negative feelings towards professionals.

It was therefore essential for the nurse, after having listened to the parents, to highlight her role as family support, and to reassure the parents that they are important members of the caring team. The rationale for this approach, additionally, is to nurture the parents' confidence and to encourage independence.

An important aspect of the interview for the link nurse was to explore the parents' coping strategies and their support networks, to answer queries as accurately as possible and to refer the parents to key specialists of the team (e.g. medical/surgical consultants, physiotherapists etc.) dependent on the nature of the queries.

collaborative partnership in care; its essence, however, is made up of shared understanding, a shared purpose and goal, a dynamic process facilitated by the professionals' sensitivity and 'a synchronous pattern of give and take' (Henson 1997) operating within a flexible framework for the attainment of goals identified and agreed upon by all parties.

Activity 2.3

1. Identify from literature searches the impact of the critically ill child on the family.
2. Write your findings, separating the social effects from the psychological effects. Discuss with your placement mentor a list of objectives you want to achieve in connection with your search (for example, working as a member of the team to meet the social and psychological needs of patients and their families etc.).

??? Question 2.3

1. What is the importance of applying the concept of mutuality in health care setting?
2. What are the factors that may cause parental conflict during a child's hospitalization?
3. What measures may be implemented to ensure that families of the critically ill child cope with the stressors of the intensive care unit?

FAMILY GRIEF AND BEREAVEMENT

There are times in clinical settings when families experience intense sorrow and grief, for instance when one of their loved ones (a child, a spouse or a friend) dies in hospital. A grieving family experiences a deep sense of loss. Sometimes the factors that have caused the death of their relatives are so traumatic that images and visions as well as mental rehearsals of events compound the psychological effects of the experiences.

Although grieving is a personal event, every member of the family is affected by the loss (Lendrum & Syme 1992). Grief is not only a psychological process, it has a social dimension too. Family networks are affected. For example,

parents of dying children find their daily social arrangements and relationships with others disturbed. The intensity of feelings generated by their dying or dead children impinge on their coping abilities (Adams 1990).

While parents are attempting to come to terms with their loss or impending loss, siblings too are struggling with their intense feelings of loss and dramatic social events affecting their lives. The social implications of not being able to cope psychologically are wide-ranging. Some adolescents project their vulnerability by engaging in activities such as 'risk taking in fights, driving or drug taking' (Raphael 1984), and confrontation with agents of social control, the police, magistrates and teachers for example. Raphael (1984) also made reference to evidence of truancy, stealing, shoplifting and examination failures. On the other hand, Kohner (1995) argued that some children identify with their parents' grief, and consequently are frightened by it and the death itself.

DEATH AND DYING IN HEALTH CARE SETTINGS

The terminally ill

Dying is an aspect of a living process; death terminates the process. Whether the processes occur in a clinical environment (hospital ward, neonatal or paediatric intensive care unit), hospice or home environment, the social and psychological sequelae on living members are as devastating. The grieving process, which may have begun well before a terminally ill diagnosis has been made, will affect significant relationships within the patient's family milieu (Kindlen 1994). The unique experience of grieving should be borne in mind during therapeutic interactions with grieving relatives and the terminally ill. The latter, too, is experiencing the grief process. Sometimes, however, their conditions impede their ability to verbally express their needs. Discreet observations of their non-verbal behaviour during interactions, with the help of relatives, will help in facilitating the assessment and identification of their needs.

Emotional comfort is as important as the physical dimension of care. Giedosh (1997) emphasized its importance and relevance in a life-threatening illness. Her experience in practice showed that a dying person's thought turns toward the family: a husband, a wife and any other relevant kin of significance in the person's life. In this context of uncertainty for the dying person and their family, health care professionals can enhance the integration of the patient's personal meaning of the illness and its effects on others in the family (Altschuler 1997).

Brain death: families and their needs

In clinical practice an individual may remain on life support for a number of years in a vegetative state. A recent report from a working party convened by the Royal College of Physicians of London (Black et al 1997) emphasized the essentiality of including relatives' and carers' descriptions and accounts in their examination of patients prior to making a permanent vegetative state (PVS) diagnosis. In many cases a diagnosis of 'brain death' will have been made. This clinical state is defined as evidence of a 'non-functioning brain' and replaced the 'traditional criteria of stopped heartbeat and respiration' (Giacomini 1997). It is therefore argued that, while the brain cells have relinquished all neurological functionings, other systems of the body (cardiovascular, renal and respiratory systems, for example), which are homeostatically maintained by artificial means, do not form part of the criterion of a living person.

Relatives of a brain dead person are most distressed at the news that their loved one is now medically and technically considered dead. In such a context, family burden is much increased as it arouses intense emotions and great stress (Evans 1995).

The role of health care professionals is to demonstrate empathetic communication skills in their explanations of the concept of brain death to grieving relatives. Evans argued that this situation will impact relatives, making them realize the impossibility of recovery. The discontinuation of artificial support after lengthy discussions with grieving families triggers intense release of emotional expressions. As grieving is a unique and personal experience, professionals must be receptive to families' possible cathartic reactions. Field (1993) emphasized that the socio-cultural and spiritual make-up of individuals will determine the type of responses exhibited under this circumstance.

Some relatives may express the need to communicate their feelings of despair and hopelessness to the nursing and medical personnel present. Others, on the other hand, may respond to the event by suppressing their emotions or by seeking more information on the diagnosis of brain stem death. Hence, it is important to respond to the uniqueness of each person's expressions of needs, and to implement care accordingly.

For the families concerned it is a time of crisis (Evans 1995), and according to Field (1993), families of brain stem dead patients have multiple needs:

- **cognitive needs** – information seeking, advice
- **emotional needs** – expression of feelings, to be close to the dead patient, some control and participation in care, spiritual care and needs
- **personal needs** in relation to looking after one's physical needs: comfort, rest, food
- **intimacy security**
- **partnership security**
- **reciprocity security**.

Cognitive needs

It is imperative that families have a realistic understanding of the situation. Communicating frankly, consistently and with sensitivity will help alleviate anxieties and any misunderstanding.

Emotional needs

Relatives should be encouraged to enunciate their feelings and to express their needs pertaining to wishes to be in proximity of their loved one. Participating in care could also mean working with nursing and medical staff concerning decisions to withdraw treatment from either a critically ill adult or child. As Purcell (1997) explained concerning the latter, parents can be empowered to actively participate in the decision process. The spirituality of care needs should be assessed from the relatives' interpretation of spirituality.

Personal needs

When families are confronted with emotional turmoil they often neglect their own physical needs for rest, sleep and food. Arrangements should therefore be made to ensure that facilities are provided to meet their specific needs.

Intimacy security

To feel intimately secure in a technological environment, relatives should feel comfortable to informally communicate with the staff and to feel accepted as members of the ward team. Field (1993) postulated it is a two-way process of communication. Interactions with relatives, however, should be based on trust and understanding. The giving of false hope should be avoided (Evans 1995); but hope, according to Gamlin and Kinghorn (1995), can be fostered, is part of the process of caring and should be dependent upon individual families' needs. Grieving families often experience a trajectory of hopelessness: helping them to refocus on positive aspects of life will help them to regain understanding and control over their capacity to survive the uniqueness and loneliness of their grief.

Partnership security

It is imperative for relatives to feel secure in an alien environment. To achieve this goal the fostering of intercollaborative partnerships is required. A nurse's caring behaviour has enhancing effects on the 'spirit of the family group' (Warren 1994). Caring behaviour, Warren argued, has many facets. To communicate openly and honestly promotes trust and confidence. When professionals utilize their communication skills, in particular their non-verbal behaviour: eye contact and 'varied facial expressions' (Warren

1994), relatives feel reassured. Respecting families as individuals with unique needs and experiences, lays the foundation for the development of partnerships in care. Warren asserted that 'family members' personhood' should be recognized. Partnership behaviours therefore rely heavily on verbal and non-verbal expressions of needs from not only family members but also from care professionals.

Information-giving and attention (Geary et al 1997) are two of the many dimensions to be taken into account. As Field (1993) posited, developing intimacy between relatives and the nurse, so that feelings can be expressed with 'security and openness', requires the integration of meaningful professional collaboration with the family's informal and unique personal experiences. Consistent dialoguing followed by encouragement are some of the professional objectives to be attained, with the aim to create an atmosphere of trust, enabling families to regain their full potential for coping.

Reciprocity security

Field (1993) defines 'reciprocity security' as the mutuality of the relationship between the nurse and family, as health-enhancing behaviours. Meaningful interactions act as buffering agents in times of stress. To consolidate reciprocity security, professionals must attempt to gain insight into relatives' constructions of death and dying. Similarly, professionals' self-awareness in regard to their perception of death and dying must be identified.

Research findings on the impact of death and dying on nurses (Copp 1997) show that nursing staff experience uncertainty, apprehension and feelings of guilt. Inadequacy tendencies generated by unresolved personal beliefs and feelings impair their ability to act objectively. Empathy, which is an aspect of professional care, is not easily demonstrated (Simpson 1997).

Attempting to deal with their own grief, Simpson argued, impedes the nurses' capacity to demonstrate the 'support and understanding' the families need. The implications for practice are evident. There is a requirement to recognize that families have complex emotional and social needs (Ovenden 1997), which must be met empathetically and efficiently. Furthermore, nurses' development of their own self-awareness (Field 1993) of their feelings and perceptions regarding issues about death and the nature of dying (Taylor et al 1997), as well as 'ambiguous decision-making' carried out by medical staff (Simpson 1997), impinging on their own self-beliefs will ensure objectivity in their rapport with families. As Simpson argued, families are often 'confused' by events, and his observations show that some nurses experience difficulties in relating to families when attempting to explain situations they are unable to comprehend themselves.

The difficulties encountered by some professionals in relaying information to grieving relatives may be compounded by cultural issues too. Individuals' behaviours are influenced by their socio-cultural beliefs, which have an effect on the way they view their social world (Nyatanga 1997). In their interactions with families, health care professionals' knowledge of multicultural and ethnic issues should be put into practice, so that 'the original (purist) value and belief system of each individual patient's culture' is respected. Is is hence necessary to examine one's preconceived beliefs to ensure that perceptions of families' and patients' behaviours are not misunderstood, thus increasing sensitivity to their cultural and emotional needs (Nyatanga 1997).

ORGAN DONATION AND FAMILY NEEDS

Critical care staff have a role to play in obtaining the family's consent for organ donation (Siminoff 1997). Additionally, assumptions must not be made that families will respond positively to organ donation. Time should therefore be spent with families, to identify their views, with staff being 'positive about the donation option' (Siminoff 1997).

Research findings based on exploratory retrospective designs indicate that families have multiple needs triggered by their confrontation with clinical events (Pelletier 1992). Their perception of stressful situations during the organ donation experience creates implications for clinical practice.

An awareness of situational factors causing family stress is essential. Pelletier's study of seven families from New Brunswick, Canada, revealed that the families identified the life-threatening illness affecting their loved ones, and interactions with health professionals, as stressful. Some factors related to the inconsistency, insufficiency and, in some cases, excessive information-giving by the staff as anxiety provoking. Most family members reported on the 'insensitivity' of the staff, evident in the 'hurried, busy, abrupt and matter-of-fact behaviour of some health professionals'.

Other issues centred on being confronted with a diagnosis of brain death, with a lack of sufficient information about both the meaning of brain death and the issues surrounding organ/tissue donation, and the waiting time associated with the latter being retrieved (Case example 2.4). Pelletier also identified a series of inconsistencies in relation to the processes of organ donation:

Case example 2.4 Diagnosing brain death

Penn Grafoe, aged 50, was admitted to the intensive care unit following a physical assault by a gang of four youths. He sustained severe blows to the head, caused by a blunt instrument, probably a hammer, according to the pathologist. There was evidence of superficial skin lacerations. On admission he was reported unconscious and was immediately connected to a ventilator by the anaesthetist.

Mr Grafoe's head injury had resulted in severe damage to the brain, causing severe hypoxaemia. Prolonged hypoxaemia can cause irreversible damage to the brain (Goldstone & Moxham 1994). Two independent, experienced medical observers were called to make an assessment of brain stem injury. Mr Grafoe showed all the features of irreversible brain damage, namely, deep coma with no response to peripheral and central stimuli, absence of corneal, gag and tracheal reflexes, no eye movement in response to ice-cold water irrigation to the external ear, and no respiratory efforts when the ventilator was switched off, in spite of hypercapnia. A repeated investigation 24 hours later showed similar results. Brain death was subsequently confirmed.

1. Failure to thoroughly involve the families in discussing 'which organ/tissue could be donated' and to whom.

2. Failure to identify the brain dead person as a potential donor in good time for families to make decisions.

3. Lack of enthusiasm and motivation from health care professionals when three family members asserted their wishes to donate their loved one's organ/tissue.

4. Failure of health care professionals to voluntarily approach families regarding the possibility of 'donating their loved one's organs/tissue'.

5. Long waiting time concerning tests and final retrieval of organ/tissue. This unexpected aspect disturbed family members.

It can be argued from the above findings that the phenomena of organ donation has multi-dimensional repercussions which health care professionals must contemplate to secure competent family care (Box 2.3).

Box 2.3 Family-centred care: the role of health care professionals in organ donation

1. Explain the meaning of brain death, using non-technical language.
2. Ensure that the process of information-giving takes place in a relaxed atmosphere away from the immediate clinical environment.
3. Show a genuine concern and a supportive approach consistent with professional conduct.
4. Active involvement with families is necessary to capture their phenomenology, and meaningful intercollaborative partnership with medical personnel to identify donors.
5. Identify the family's views pertinent to their needs concerning the types of organs/tissues they can donate, and who the recipients are likely to be, if known at the time.
6. Select a member of the staff prepared to serve as a patient–family advocate, who will also act as a resource person to families, ensuring communication is concurrent with their expressed needs.
7. Formulate realistic objectives with the personalities of individual family groups in mind, so that they receive what Butterworth (1996) calls the 'support of well qualified and clinically expert professionals … mindful of the wider system of circumstances which surround them'.

Activity 2.4

1. Liaise with the ward manager and the theatre staff while you are on placement, concerning your wish to observe procedures in theatre during organ/tissue retrieval.
2. Write notes on the observations you make.
3. Identify the methods used to store the retrieved organ or tissues.
4. Collect data concerning the management of the patient throughout surgery and postoperatively.

??? Question 2.4

1. What features are associated with the multiple needs of families in organ donation?
2. What is the importance of sensitive care management of patients and their families in organ donation?

INTRA-UTERINE DEATH
Parents' needs and care

Perinatal death is a tragedy that affects both parents and their wider kin networks. The traumatic effects, on parents, following a diagnosis of fetal death can be identified as follows: bewilderment, a deep sense of loss, grief, uncertainty, a depressive state that may be followed by emotional cathartic behavioural expressions, confusion, distrust in the ability of medical and obstetrics staff, self-blame, feelings of unworthiness and decreased self-esteem. Perinatal death (Fox et al 1997) is of frequent occurrence, and has been identified as a precipitating factor in the causation of psychological morbidity. Death in the perinatal period affects the caring team too (Bryan 1995).

Professionals may feel unable to cope with the grief reactions of parents. Staff may, therefore, use denial as a defence mechanism, attempting 'to ignore or even forget' (Bryan 1995) the realism of the situation. Denying, either inherently or outwardly (non-verbal expressions of disbelief) the evidence of intra-uterine death, will interfere with their capacity to exercise objectivity in supporting parents at a time when their coping mechanisms are fragmented.

Approaches to care should follow strict, but flexible, guidelines to ascertain that parents and their family networks receive adequate support to help them cope with the loss, their grief, and to meet their mourning needs. Fox et al (1997) argued that an important aspect of care management is to offer choice to parents. The choice to decide, for example, when to be admitted to hospital for delivery; who should be present during the procedure (i.e. a known midwife who has maintained therapeutic contact throughout the pregnancy; the husband, a relative or a close partner); to discuss prior to the delivery procedure whether to hold the dead baby; the choosing of a name or not; decision whether to have a post-mortem examination (Fox et al 1997); and the collection of mementos if desired.

Bryan (1995) argued that parents should be allowed space to express their grief reactions, without restraints, avoiding at all cost, tendencies to make misguided remarks such as 'how lucky that you still have a healthy baby' (in cases of one twin baby intra-uterine death). Procedures, such as ultrasonography, and physical examination must be undertaken with sensitivity and tact, ascertaining throughout that the mother and father are kept informed. When the image on the monitor confirms that death in utero is evident, some parents' emotional responses may be overwhelming to the staff. Allowing the free expression of grief is essential. Liossi and Mystakidou (1997) recommend the therapeutic and beneficial effects of cathartic reactions by stating that release of pent-up emotions helps individuals to achieve 'mental rearrangements'. They point out too, that when professionals are confronted with distressed parents and their relatives, they may feel the urge to 'overdistance' themselves 'from their feelings', suppressing their own emotions, and in the process convey the attitude that violent expressions of emotional distress are to be controlled.

Avoidance reactions from professionals will undermine the positive effect of spontaneous emotional expression. Crying, which is a basic biological and instinctual behaviour, should not be discouraged. Verbal support, i.e. talking as appropriate and reflecting the parents' moods and feelings, is important. Physical support is also necessary; close proximity, but respecting individuals' private space, by holding hands or touching the shoulder may be necessary, while being sensitive to the person's socio-cultural practices in relation to physical contact.

The supportive presence of the midwife and obstetrician, characterized by skilful management of parental anger, is necessary so that distress is freely ventilated. Other measures could include the privacy of a sideroom for the mother and father to have time for 'intimacy and quiet reflection' (Fox et al 1997).

Families' need for reassurance could be expressed in ways that may go unnoticed by care professionals. For example, repetitive questioning in connection with the diagnosis as well as the delivery of the baby and its features, or on one's ability to sustain healthy conception in the future. Additionally, questions can be focused on the delivery procedures: the duration, post-delivery pain experiences, discharge planning and the fear of not being able to cope on leaving the baby behind.

In order to ensure that parents' needs for reassurance are met, the role and responsibility of professionals are to ascertain that intervention is consistent with clinical guidelines and tailored according to individual needs:

1. Maternal safety: physical and psychological safety become priorities. Decision-making processes should be reliant on accurate investigative findings demonstrating no evidence of a life-threatening condition, thus allowing the mother to spend some time at home with her partner prior to delivery, to discuss social rearrangements; this will allow opportunity for reflection and for the family to give unqualified care to each other, thus reinforcing psychological security. Secondly, parents have the opportunity to unite significant others in their wider kin networks who would be prepared to support them in the management of the household, caring for the children, for example. A degree of social safety is hence guaranteed.

2. As Fox et al (1997) stated, the management of intra-uterine death is complex, and the

involvement of a multidisciplinary team is expected. For this reason, collaborative care planning is a prerequisite. The principles underpinning collaborative care ensure a systematic approach to patient and family care, but are dependent on professionals working as a team (Scott & Cowen 1997).

3. Parents' wishes must be recorded in detail, the information being relayed thereafter clearly – in writing – to team members. Wishes may encompass provision for a private room with amenities: a telephone, bathroom facilities and a cot for the baby if so desired. Some parents may wish to keep little mementos of the child, for example, 'photographs, ink prints of the palm and sole' (Fox et al 1997). Some parents may ask for a post-mortem examination. Information should be made available to help them reach a final decision.

4. In cases of twin death, with one survivor, the parents' mourning process may be helped by encouraging them to talk about their feelings for the dead baby. Bryan (1995) posited that attempting to redirect the mother's thought on the 'healthy child to the exclusion of the dead baby' has psychological and social implications for the surviving baby. The mother may begin 'idealizing' the dead baby and reject the survivor by distancing herself.

Complex issues in connection with family care are linked to the concept of intra-uterine death. Once discharged from the labour ward or gynaecology department, the mother and her family will require careful follow-up. Mobilization of community midwifery resources is necessary so that professional support is maintained according to needs.

TRANSFERS AND DISCHARGE PLANNING

INVOLVING FAMILIES

Planning for transfers and discharges should be seen as an important procedure, not only for the patients but also for their families. It is distressing for relatives to discover on routine ward visiting that their partners, spouses or children have been transferred to another department without them being informed. Sometimes constraints in clinical settings – bed shortages, emergency admissions and incoming day cases – signify the transferring of patients urgently and at short notice to create bed vacancies. In the urgency of the situations, relatives are sometimes neglected, by failures to update them of changes likely to affect them.

If attempts to contact relatives fail, a nurse should be delegated to inform the relatives immediately on arrival to the ward, before the absence of their kin is noticed. Explanations should be given for the reason of transfers – to reduce any apprehension – concerning their sick relatives' condition. When transfers are planned in advance, patients and their relatives should be fully involved in the process. Such an approach will help to alleviate any undue stress and anxiety.

Effective liaison procedures between wards, departments and other organizations is essential to ascertain smooth transfers and optimal staff awareness and knowledge of bed occupancy changes.

Similar approaches should be adopted when planning discharges. The implications of early discharge (Gillan 1995) on patients and their families are numerous. Discharging patients, Gillan (1995) argued, is a complex and diverse process. A failure to implement strategic and effective administrative discharge planning policies, incongruent with needs (Ahulu 1995) will have implications for families too. Early discharge means expecting families to cope, when they have not been fully briefed and educated in relation to care management while their loved ones are 'still in need of extensive rehabilitation' (Ahulu 1995).

There is evidence that assumptions are made concerning families' willingness and ability to care for the discharged patient once they get home (King & McMillan 1994); in reality, many relatives lack physical strength (due to being old and frail themselves) to give care. Social circumstances should be thoroughly assessed, involving carers during 'admission assessment and discharge process planning' (King & McMillan 1994). This implementation would help to increase control and the coping skills of individuals concerned (Wiffin 1995). Their involvement in the decision-making process (Ryan 1994) is one of the key attributes of discharge planning. The aim is to make sure that transition from hospital to home is as smooth as possible. This requires clear communication and intraprofessional cooperation (Nazarko 1997), involving community services. A home profile can subsequently be developed for patients and their families.

Although the above discussions relate to discharge planning affecting the older person, evidence shows that in a paediatric orthopaedic ward discharge instructions to parents caused them unnecessary anxieties while at home (Robinson & Miller 1996). This was due to ambiguous presentation of information and the technical jargon used, making the information inaccessible. Other writers (Bull & Jervis 1997) make reference to the lack of information on diet, medications and community services, thereby preventing chronically ill older women and their care-giving daughters from making a smooth transition during post-hospital discharge. Health care professionals should be mindful of an interdisciplinary discharge process.

Interdisciplinary discharge process features in patients' and families' care

Traditionally, patients have been discharged from a variety of care settings with minimal involvement in the process, while their families have been expected to maintain care continuity by whatever strategies at their disposal. The NHS and Community Care Act (1990) stimulated and mobilized widespread multiprofessional organizations (health and social care) to function collaboratively and to coordinate care pertinent to individuals' needs and their families.

One important aspect of care demanding immediate priority concerns discharge planning to be initiated at the time of admission (Chipps et al 1997). As these authors postulate, fragmented

and inadequate communication between 'in-patient and community staff means that adequate community services and equipment are often not available when required'. Family burdens are therefore likely to increase, since the lack of coordinated support services between agencies leave them to improvise their own care. Remedial action should accordingly consist of a collective effort to unite health and social services so that families' (including their sick members) inherent potential can be optimized. The discharge planning process can become clinically effective when the features outlined in Box 2.4 are integrated in the all-inclusive framework.

LONE PARENT FAMILIES

Lone parent families are stereotypically perceived as a distinct grouping that is removed from the customary interpretation of a family unit: a wife, a husband and children. Various viewpoints have been expressed:

- these families are disenfranchised minorities with special needs (Ford-Gilboe & Campbell 1996)
- some families headed by a single mother have difficulties with reading and language (Dunscombe 1985)
- this family form, although legitimate, does not match societal norms, and is accordingly viewed as a 'deficit model' (Butcher & Gaffney 1995)
- lone parent families are 'dysfunctional' (Leach 1997)
- single mothers are prone to psychological problems (Hall et al 1991), and are subjected to negative health and socio-economic consequences (Hao & Brinton 1997)
- low status makes single mothers a victimized group within the socio-political framework (Slipman 1994)
- lone parents are penalized through budgetary control of benefits (Berenson 1997).

The negative portrayal of lone parent families augments their unequal position in society, while simultaneously failing to identify their positive social and behavioural characteristics;

Box 2.4 Essential features of the discharge process

1. Developing effective communication networks between inpatient staff and other agencies (e.g. hospice) (Chipps et al 1997).
2. Clear-cut clinical guidelines on assessing and evaluating the role of next-of-kin, and their ability to cope and to manage care on clients' discharge. An assessment of *carers' dependency* on the discharged client should also be included. Clinical guidelines should contain specific information related to the individual client's condition (McClarey & Duff 1997).
3. Initiation of discharge planning process from time of admission to include clients' perspective of needs.
4. Involving carers (family networks) so that they receive first-hand information on the extent of care needed by the convalescing client.
5. Teaching and education: for example self-administration of medicine, such as managing with inhalers.
6. Maintain a standardized liaison with health visitors, district nurses, midwives, social services etc., dependent on clients' and relatives' needs.
7. Inform relatives well in advance about possible discharge plans so that they can make necessary social arrangements.
8. Organize a family interview to gain insight into their living experience of managing the post-discharge client. A family interview will also provide information on their experiences of health and well-being (Astedt-Kurki & Hopia 1996).
9. Benchmarking: the application of knowledge gained from other organizations to the efficient management of resources to ensure best practice (Ellis & Morris 1997).
10. The implementation of prompt follow-up visits after discharge (e.g. after accident and emergency visit) (Runciman et al 1996), to prevent re-admission.
11. Respect for the socio-cultural beliefs of families, as well as care to match their expectations (Bull & Jervis 1996).
12. Monitoring care daily to identify incongruencies through collaborative care principles (Scott & Cowen 1997).

an approach that reinforces their marginalization in parallel with their unrecognized diversity (Ford-Gilboe & Campbell 1996).

Lone parent families have needs that require assessment from a broader social context. Social constraints (poverty, unemployment) can impose limitations on their coping abilities. Nevertheless, in spite of negative life influences, many families grow and develop (Ford-Gilboe & Campbell 1996), and engage in personal productive activities. At the same time, lone parents often receive support from caring parents and relatives in the form of 'kin co-residence' (Hao & Brinton 1997). The strengths of lone parent families include better problem-solving skills and a high level of adaptability (Butcher & Gaffney 1995).

However, in spite of some positive behavioural characteristics, a study of 225 mothers showed that 59% displayed high depressive symptoms (Hall et al 1991). The mothers' depressive states made them socially withdrawn from families and friends. Additionally, the researchers concluded, 'aversive child behaviours' sometimes aggravated the depression as mothers felt incompetent to cope with the situation. Lack of informal support increased the stress level, precipitating the use of 'avoidance as a strategy' (Hall et al 1991).

The unique experiences of lone parent families must be borne in mind when planning their care, demonstrating congruence with individual group needs (Box 2.5).

Box 2.5 Measures that can be implemented when caring for lone parent families

- Child–parent relationships can be improved by utilizing parent groups on positive parenting, using the STEP method (Systematic Training For Effective Parenting) (Angeli 1997).
- Health visiting initiative with integrated visiting and community development work, advocated by Brown (1997).
- The marshalling of voluntary and statutory services to assess parents and communities in need:
  - developing social networks and parenting skills
  - raising awareness of local groups (e.g. toddler groups) and how to access them
  - focusing on disadvantaged families.
- Educating parents and developing existing family health-related behaviour patterns and the utilization of networking systems.
- Fiscal management and benefits awareness.
- Early identification of family conflict and evaluation of key figures within families' support systems, using an 'eco-systemic approach' (Friedmann & Andrews 1990).

Caring for lone parents

It is a prerequisite of effective care planning and implementation to have not only an awareness of single parents' socio-economic position but a thorough understanding of their unique and diversified needs. It is therefore important to avoid stereotypical attitudes and any preconceived ideas.

The nursing assessment should comprise the more 'critical elements' (Burke 1983), namely the emotional climate: degree of stress and quality of child-rearing. Emotional deprivation can be caused by faulty child-rearing practice. A child from an emotionally deprived background is prone to *psychosocial dwarfism* (Stanhope et al 1994). A failure to grow is the manifestation of this condition, which Stanhope et al believe is caused by a lack of love from the parents. An identification of the parents' reasons for their inability to express overtly their affection for the child is necessary. Stress factors (i.e. antipathetic children's behaviours) and family conflict are possible precipitating factors. Although psychosocial dwarfism is not easy to diagnose, health care professionals should exercise professional judgement and a constant awareness of this possibility.

The aim of care is to potentiate families' existing strengths and to utilize life experiences as appropriate. Frequently, this entails adapting different approaches 'to the bad conditions' so that their skills are enhanced to manage the children's needs and to increase their confidence (Salter & Widenmann 1997).

Stress prevention and parents' adjustments become possible when the wider social context is examined (Friedemann & Andrews 1990) (Case example 2.5). For instance, rallying informal support networks to help with child-rearing will allow mothers to participate in productive employment.

Early detection of needs and problems requires a multidisciplinary approach. Families' needs may circumscribe such dimensions as housing and employment (Gaze 1997), financial support, mental well-being, education, informal support (friends, relatives, neighbours), safety (social, psychological, environmental) and the need to discuss openly psychosocial concerns (Glascoe 1996). Families' dependence on state benefits (Nazarko 1997) and public support (Davies 1994) needs acknowledging. Such needs can be dis-

cussed during 'non-stigmatizing home visiting' (Leach 1997), combined with the promotion of a healthy lifestyle (Butcher & Gaffney 1995).

Case example 2.5

Jon Finely and his wife Mary moved from Barnsley with their two children to settle in London. They wanted to start a new life in a city where job opportunities are greater. They lived in a ground floor flat that was rather cramped. Jon worked as an assistant manager in a bookshop.

A year later, Jon and Mary decided to apply for a mortgage to buy a small terraced house. Prior to exchange of contract Jon told his wife that he could not cope anymore with the pressures of city life, that he was not managing well at work, and that moving house was proving highly stressful. After a fierce quarrel with his wife, Jon left the house. She had not heard from him and had been living on her own with the two children ever since.

Activity 2.5

Organize a meeting with the health visitors from the local NHS Community Trust. Identify the percentage of lone parent families in the area. Discuss the support services available. Assess the extent of psychosocial problems amongst the families identified. Debate on the families' health-related behaviour and health outcomes.

??? Question 2.5

1. What is the role of professionals in collaborative partnerships in the assessment of families' social and health needs?
2. What interventions can be implemented to ensure that lone parent families' needs are met?

SCHIZOPHRENIA AND THE FAMILY

The clinical manifestations of schizophrenia embody such terms as delusions, thought disorders, altered perception, incongruity of affect, motor abnormalities, passivity phenomena (thought disorders subjectively interpreted by the sufferer) (Brennan 1997). To families whose members exhibit the above features, the disruption of normal family life caused by the client's symptoms becomes a stressful life event. The effects are mostly felt when the sufferer's social functioning is markedly impaired so that their safety and significant others' safety is jeopardized.

Families are the primary observers of gradual mental and physical deterioration (Brennan 1997). Social withdrawal, self-neglect and malfunctioning of interpersonal skills are noticeable manifestations. Brennan argued that informal carers may mistakenly attribute these changes to laziness, disinterest or even shyness, when in reality there is a more sinister aetiology. Similarly, professionals may misdiagnose schizophrenia, due to improper understanding (Jones 1997) of the person's behaviour and to the inaccurate identification of specific schizophrenia variants (Gournay 1997). However, labelling individuals as 'schizophrenic' easily becomes a stigmatized social phenomena, disrupting family organizations and provoking anxiety.

In addition to the pharmacological aspects of care, intervention should include family networks. Particular focus is on the effects of the psychotic illness on the relatives as well as the patient. Psychosocial interventions in community settings are well known (Savage & McKeown 1997). Their therapeutic benefits are recognized (Brennan 1997) and are necessary in family mental health care. Families of people with schizophrenia have to adapt to changing situations and adopt coping styles to match their requirements. The role of care professionals is to obtain an accurate understanding of what the 'families want' (Atkinson & Coia 1995). They may, for instance, need information and practical advice: education in connection with the nature of schizophrenia, medication effects and dosage and the availability of local support groups or community health services. Involving the families by imparting accurate information will enhance their valuable input (Jones 1997). Families' mental health care needs are varied. Many issues must be considered by professionals when family-focused care is being planned (Box 2.6).

Box 2.6 Care planning issues

- Availability of support groups.
- Early psychosocial interventions to prevent family breakdown.
- Social skills training.
- Services to match individual needs (intercollaborative multidisciplinary team approach).
- The reduction of 'expressed emotion', by encouraging reflection and self-awareness. Expressed emotion relates to some families' 'critical, hostile or emotionally charged' behaviour, which precipitates a relapse of florid symptoms of schizophrenia in the affected person (Bradshaw 1997).
- Family interventions: with this approach educational programmes are tailored, family communication skills and problem-solving training implemented, with the aim of reducing stress in the family environment.
- Family meetings.
- Care Programme Approach: this consists of the implementation of community care policies, which ensure that a coordinated and integrated service is provided, to meet the needs of the clients and their families (Jones 1997).
- Assessment of social functioning with families' diversified beliefs, since behaviour can be influenced by social norms and expectations (Gamble & Midence 1995).

 Activity 2.6

During a community psychiatric home visit, record your observations of the client's interactions with relatives present. Make note of the topic of conversation. Identify the client's and relatives' communication skills.

??? Question 2.6

1. What is the value of psychosocial and family intervention approaches to care?
2. What is the importance of intercollaborative partnerships in mental health care planning for families?

SUMMARY

Caring for families is a multidimensional concept. The diversity of family structures makes the task of caring even more complex for professionals engaged in health and social care. Some key points that must be recognized when interacting with families are concerned with their unique life experiences and their phe-

nomenology, the value of the informal knowledge that they bring with them, and the intensity
of their apprehension, emotions and anxieties
when confronted with hospitalization and life-
threatening illnesses. Families' reactions and
interreactions vary and are context-related; for
example, the family of a terminally ill client will
respond differently to one whose member is
suffering from schizophrenia. All of these issues
must be kept in mind in health care situations.

GLOSSARY

Antipathetic   to have a strong opposition/aversion
Aortic aneurysm   a swelling in the wall of the aorta
causing ballooning
Cardiac arrhythmias   changes in heart beat due to
disturbed rhythms
Catharsis   the process of freeing pent-up emotions/feelings
Central stimuli   stimuli aimed at producing responses
from the core structures (e.g. brain and spinal cord) as
opposed to peripheral structures
Cognitive dysfunctions   disturbed mental processes (e.g.
thinking, memory)
Exploratory retrospective design   research designed to
explore past experience
Fulminating systemic infection   infection of sudden onset
and severe in nature
Haematological   related to the blood
Homeostatically maintained   a state of equilibrium and
balance

Hypercapnia   a high concentration of carbon dioxide in the
blood
Hypoxaemia   a low concentration of oxygen in the blood
Mental rearrangements   the reorganising of one's faculties;
a process of rethinking
Multiparadigmatic   a multifaceted conceptual framework
Myocardial disorders   any disease that interferes with the
functions of the heart muscle
Myocardial infarction   death of a segment of the heart
muscle due to reduced blood supply
Phenomenology   subjective and lived experience
Sociopathic traits   a term given to antisocial personality
characteristics
Ultrasonography   the production of sound waves at high
frequency to produce pictures of structures/organs to
help diagnosis

REFERENCES

Adams D 1990 When a child dies of cancer: care of the child
and the family. In: Morgan J (ed) The dying and the
bereaved teenager. Charles Press, Philadelphia, p 3–21
Ahulu S 1995 Discharge to the community of older patients
from hospital. Nursing Times 91(28): 29–30
Altschuler J 1997 Family relationships during serious illness.
Nursing Times 93(7): 48–49
Angeli N 1997 STEPS for positive parenting. Health Visitor
70(9): 336–338
Astedt-Kurki P, Hopia H 1996 The family interview:
exploring experiences of family health and wellbeing.
Journal of Advanced Nursing 24(3): 506–511
Atkinson J M, Coia D 1995 Families coping with schizophrenia:
a practitioner's guide to family groups. Wiley, Chichester
Barnes P J, Newhouse M T 1994 Conquering asthma: an
illustrated guide to understanding and self-care for adults
and children. Manson, London, p 48
Berenson N 1997 Penalising the lone parent. Health Visitor
70(2): 81
Black D, Bates D, Grubb A, London D 1997 Permanent
vegetative state. Addendum to a review by a working
group convened by The Royal College of Physicians and
endorsed by the Conference of Medical Royal Colleges.
Journal of the Royal College of Physicians of London
31(3): 260
Bradshaw T 1997 Does family intervention reduce relapse in
schizophrenia? Psychiatric Care 4(1): 30–33
Brennan G 1997 Clinical update: schizophrenia. Primary
Health Care 7(4): 17–24

Brown I 1997 A skill mix parent group initiative visiting: an
evaluation study. Health Visitor 70(9): 339–343
Bryan E 1995 The death of a twin. Palliative Medicine
9(3): 187–192
Bull M J, Jervis L L 1997 Strategies used by chronically ill
older women and their caregiving daughters in managing
post-hospital care. Journal of Advanced Nursing
25(3): 541–547
Burke S D 1983 One parent families: helping them cope.
Canadian Nurse 79(10): 33–37
Butcher L A, Gaffney M 1995 Building healthy families: a
program for single mothers. Clinical Nurse Specialist
9(4): 221–225
Butterworth T 1996 Individualised nursing care: a cuckoo in
the team's nest? Nursing Times Research 1(1): 34–37
Carr J 1997 The family's experience of vigilance: challenges
for nursing. Holistic Nursing Practice 11(4): 82–88
Chipps J, Grey A, Hilton G, Linford J et al 1997 The
discharge process for palliative care patients. Nursing
Standard 11(42): 41–44
Chiverton C 1997 Social support within the context of life-
threatening illness. International Journal of Palliative
Nursing 3(2): 107–110
Copp G 1997 Patients' and nurses' constructions of death
and dying in a hospice setting. Journal of Cancer Nursing
1(1): 2–13
Craft J 1995 The special needs of the critically ill. Care of the
Critically Ill 11(1): 13–15
Crosby C 1994 The patient with cancer. In: Alexander M,

Fawcett J, Runciman P (eds) Nursing practice hospital and home: the adult. Churchill Livingstone, Edinburgh, p 878–904

Curran A, Brighton J, Murphy V 1997 Psychoemotional care of parents of children in a neonatal intensive care unit. Journal of Neonatal Nursing 3(1): 25–28

Davies J 1994 Caring for single parents: no more shotguns? Modern Midwife 4(11): 36–37

Dunscombe V 1985 A group with a difference. Nursing Times 81(1): 26–28

Ellis J, Morris A 1997 Paediatric benchmarking: a review of its development. Nursing Standard 12(2): 43–46

Evans D 1995 Brain death: the family in crisis. Intensive and Critical Care Nursing 11(6): 318–321

Field D 1993 Care for relatives of brain stem dead patients going for organ donation. Care of the Critically Ill 9(2): 72–74

Ford-Gilboe M, Campbell J 1996 The mother-headed single parent family: a feminist critique of the nursing literature. Nursing Outlook 44(4): 173–183

Fox R, Pillai M, Porter H, Gill G 1997 The management of late fetal death: a guide to comprehensive care. British Journal of Obstetrics and Gynaecology 104(1): 4–10

Friedmann M, Andrews M 1990 Family support and child adjustment in single-parent families. Issues in Comprehensive Pediatric Nursing 13(4): 289–301

Gamble C, Midence K 1995 The assessment of social functioning conceptual and methodological difficulties. Psychiatric Care 2(2): 52–54

Gamlin R, Kinghorn S 1995 Using hope to cope with loss and grief. Nursing Standard 9(48): 33–35

Gaze H 1997 All in the family. Health Visitor 70(9): 332–333

Geary P, Tringali R, George E 1997 Social support in critically ill adults: a replication. Critical Care Nursing Quarterly 20(2): 34–41

Giacomini M 1997 A change of heart and a change of mind? Technology and the redefinition of death in 1968. Social Science Medicine 44(10): 1465–1482

Giedosh D 1997 Emotional support and the ED patient: one nurse's perspective. Journal of Emergency Nursing 23(2): 96–97

Gillan J 1995 Editor's notes. Nursing Times 91(28): 28

Glascoe F P 1996 The importance of discussing parents' concerns about development. Ambulatory Child Health 2(4): 349–356

Goldstone J, Moxham J 1994 Critical care medicine. In: Souhami R L, Moxham J (eds) Textbook of medicine, 2nd edn. Churchill Livingstone, Edinburgh, p 546

Gournay K 1997 Clinical effectiveness: what we need to do. Psychiatric Care 4(5): 221–224

Häggman-Laitila A 1997 Health as an individual's way of existence. Journal of Advanced Nursing 25(1): 45–53

Hall L A, Gurley D N, Sachs B, Kryscio R J 1991 Psycho-social predictors of maternal depressive symptoms: parenting attitudes and child behaviour in single-parent families. Nursing Research 40(4): 214–220

Hall S 1996 An exploration of parental perception of the nature and level of support needed to care for their child with special needs. Journal of Advanced Nursing 24(3): 512–521

Halme M A 1990 Effects of support groups on anxiety of family members during critical illness. Heart and Lung 19(1): 62–70

Hammond F 1995 Involving families in care within the intensive care environment: a descriptive survey. Intensive and Critical Care Nursing 1(5): 256–264

Hao L, Brinton M C 1997 Productive activities and support systems of single mothers. American Journal of Sociology 102(5): 1305–1344

Henson R H 1997 Analysis of the concept of mutuality. Image: Journal of Nursing Scholarship 29(1): 77–81

Hickey M 1990 What are the needs of families of critically ill patients? Heart and Lung 19(4): 401–415

Hildingh C, Fridlund B, Segesten K 1995 Cardiac nurses preparedness to use self-help groups as a support strategy. Journal of Advanced Nursing 22(5): 921–928

Jones L 1997 Schizophrenia. Professional Nurse 12(6): 434–437

Kindlen M 1994 The terminally ill patient. In: Alexander M, Fawcett J, Runciman P (eds) Nursing practice hospital and home: the adult. Churchill Livingstone, Edinburgh, p 921–942

King C, McMillan M 1994 Documentation and discharge planning for elderly patients. Nursing Times 90(20): 31–33

Kohner N 1995 Pregnancy loss and the death of a baby: guidelines for professionals. Sands, London

Lane D J 1996 Asthma, the facts, 3rd edn. Oxford University Press, Oxford, p 83

Lazure L 1997 Strategies to increase patient control visiting. Dimensions of Critical Care Nursing 16(1): 11–18

Leach P 1997 What price home visiting and family support. Health Visitor 70(2): 72–74

Lendrum S, Syme G 1992 Gift of tears: a practical approach to grief and bereavement counselling. Routledge, London, p 68

Liossi C, Mystakidou K 1997 Catharsis in palliative care. European Journal of Palliative Care 4(4): 133–136

Marsden C 1992 Family-centred critical care: an option or obligation. American Journal of Critical Care 1(3): 115–117

McClarey M, Duff L 1997 Making sense of clinical guidelines. Nursing Standard 12(1): 34–36

Moore A 1994 Back to basics? Nursing Standard 8(26): 40–41

Nazarko L 1997 Improving hospital discharge arrangements for older people. Nursing Standard 11(40): 44–47

NHS Community Care Act 1990 HMSO, London

Nyatanga B 1997 Cultural issues in palliative care. International Journal of Palliative Nursing 3(4): 203–208

Ovenden S 1997 Childhood cancer: helping the individual to cope within the family. Paediatric Nursing 9(7): 24–27

Pelletier M 1992 The organ donor family members' perception of stressful situations during the organ donation experience. Journal of Advanced Nursing 17(1): 90–97

Purcell C 1997 Withdrawing treatment from a critically ill child. Intensive and Critical Care Nursing 13(2): 103–107

Quinn S, Redmond K, Begley C 1996 The needs of relatives visiting audit critical care units as perceived by relatives and nurses, Part 1 & 2. Intensive and Critical Care Nursing 12(3): 168–172; 12(4): 239–245

Raphael B 1984 The anatomy of bereavement: a handbook for the caring professions. Unwin Hyman, London

Rennick J 1995 The changing profile of acute childhood illness: a need for the development of family nursing knowledge. Journal of Advanced Nursing 22(2): 258–266

Riegel B 1989 Social support and psychological adjustment to chronic coronary heart disease: operationalization of Johnson's behavioural model. Advanced Nursing Science 11(2): 74–84

Robinson A, Miller M 1996 Making information accessible: developing plain English discharge instructions. Journal of Advanced Nursing 24(3): 528–535

Runciman R, Currie C T, Nicol M, Green L, McKay V 1996 Discharge of elderly people from an accident and emergency department: evaluation of health visitor follow-up. Journal of Advanced Nursing 24(4): 711–718

Ryan A 1994 Improving discharge planning. Nursing Times 90(20): 33–34

Salter A, Widenmann M 1997 The Danish approach to supporting families. Health Visitor 70(8): 308–309

Savage L, McKeown M 1997 Towards a new model of practice for a high-dependency unit. Psychiatric Care 4(4): 182–186

Scott E, Cowen B 1997 Multidisciplinary collaborative care planning. Nursing Standard 12(1): 39–42

Scullion P A 1994 Personal cost, caring and communication: an analysis of communication between relatives and intensive care nurses. Intensive and Critical Care Nursing 9(1): 64–70

Sheldon L 1997 Hospitalising children: a review of the effects. Nursing Standard 12(1): 44–47

Siminoff L A 1997 Withdrawal of treatment and organ donation. Critical Care Nursing Clinics of North America 9(1): 85–95

Simpson S H 1997 Reconnecting: the experiences of nurses caring for hopelessly ill patients in intensive care. Intensive And Critical Care Nursing 13(4): 189–197

Slipman S 1994 One-parent families: some contemporary issues. Professional Care of Mother and Child 4(6): 163–164

St John W, Rolls C 1996 Teaching family nursing: strategies and experiences. Journal of Advanced Nursing 23(1): 91–96

Stanhope R, Wiltz Z, Hamill G 1994 Psychosocial aspects of growth. Failure to grow: lack of food or lack of love? Professional Care of Mother and Child 4(8): 234–237

Taylor B, Glass N, McFarlane J, Stirling C 1997 Palliative nurses' perceptions of the nature and effects of their work. International Journal of Palliative Nursing 3(5): 253–258

Theobald K 1997 The experience of spouses whose partners have suffered a myocardial infarction: a phenomenological study. Journal of Advanced Nursing 26(3): 595–601

Trocino L, Byers J F, Peach A G 1997 Nurses' attitudes toward patient and family education: implications for clinical nurse specialists. Clinical Nurse Specialist 11(2): 77–84

Warren N 1994 The phenomena of nurses' caring behaviours as perceived by the critical care family. Critical Care Nursing Quarterly 17(3): 67–72

Wesson J S 1997 Meeting the informational, psychosocial and emotional needs of each ICU patient and family. Intensive and Critical Care Nursing 13(2): 111–118

Wiffin A 1995 An assessment of procedures. Nursing Times 91(28): 31–32

Wilkinson K 1996 The concept of hope in life-threatening illness. Professional Nurse 11(10): 659–661

Williams D, Williams A, Croker L 1996 Asthma: the complete guide for sufferers and carers. Piatkus, London, p 20

FURTHER READING

Appleton J V 1996 Working with vulnerable families. Journal of Advanced Nursing 23(5): 912–918

Boyle M 1990 Schizophrenia: a scientific delusion? Routledge, London

Clark C C 1997 Post-traumatic stress disorder: how to support healing. American Journal of Nursing 97(8): 27–32

Lakhani B 1994 Dodging the poverty trap. Health Visitor 67(7): 243

Pilgrim D, Rogers A 1993 A sociology of mental health and illness. Open University Press, Buckingham

Pridham K F 1997 Mothers' help seeking as care initiated in a social context. Image Journal of Nursing Scholarship 29(1): 65–70

Robinson C A 1994 Nursing interventions with families: a demand or an invitation to change? Journal of Advanced Nursing 19(5): 897–904

Tunnicliffe R, Briggs D 1997 Introducing a bereavement support programme in ICU. Nursing Standard 11(47): 38–40

Children in need

CHAPTER CONTENTS

Children have differing needs to adults. Very often those needs are not fully recognized by parents and their carers. It is an aspect evident in many social settings, with wide-ranging implications for health and social care professionals. In this chapter, the main aims are:

- to draw the reader's attention to such needs
- to discuss factors in the social environment of children which render them more vulnerable to exploitation and abuse by adults
- to highlight approaches that can be utilized by care professionals to minimize the potential for children toward self-harm
- to discuss health education and promotion strategies according to specific needs
- to emphasize the need for collaborative professional partnership in prevention, care-giving and treatment
- to develop better awareness of community-based initiatives to support children in need in society.

SEPARATION AND DIVORCE

EFFECTS AND CONSEQUENCES FOR CHILDREN

Children are very often the innocent victims of marital conflict. When the culminating point of marital strife ends in the separation of partners, children experience a deep sense of grief and loss which can be underestimated. Divorce compounds these effects, which some children find very difficult to cope with. Their suffering – from having only a single parent (Allan 1995) – can be expressed in ways that are not only distressing to themselves, but to significant others in their environment.

Social distancing and withdrawal related to depressive moods are some of the social and negative psychological sequelae. Physiologically, some children experience loss of bladder control and suffer from insomnia. In addition, research shows that family conflict causing psychosocial stress is linked to slow growth in childhood (Montgomery et al 1997). Growth is also thwarted when children feel their emotional needs for love and affection are not met (Stanhope et al 1994). Decrease or absence of parental warmth – among depressed and hostile mothers (Emery & Coiro 1995) – towards their children is of common occurrence in a conflictual family environment. Moreover, Sheeber et al (1997) provide evidence from their research that family characteristics consisting of unsupportive and conflictual behaviours predispose to depressive symptomatology among adolescents. They point out that girls are more prone to depression than boys because of their propensity for more dependence on family interpersonal concerns. However, most children experience guilt complexes and self-blame, caused by their perception that the marriage break-up is due to their transgression (Allan 1995). Associated with the break-up are manifestations of social dysfunctioning characterized by overt expressions of aggression and non-compliance, evident among boys who suffer paternal absence (Mott et al 1997). This behaviour characteristic, the researchers point out, is the possible consequence of a strong 'father–son bonding prior to the disruption, a bonding that has been disrupted'. In relation to girls, on the other hand, their adjustment levels are quicker, but their social behaviour characteristics show evidence of dissatisfaction, conduct disorders and a tendency to internalize their feelings more than boys (Mott 1997). A girl without a father may experience difficulties in developing heterosexual relationships (Allan 1995). The internalization of feelings and experiences linked to girls'

inability to ventilate them, and to discuss their difficulties, interferes with social functioning. Childhood immaturity, non-existent reflective power (Hall 1996), apprehension and confusion become obstacles that further stifle communicative verbal behaviour.

When children are entangled within a cycle of hostility, suspicion, disruptive relationships and intense emotional outbursts from their parents, their psychoemotional needs receive scant attention. Parental strife blocks the social-emotional adjustments and development of the child (Kasen et al 1996). Children may seek help from other sources (friends, relatives, grandparents). Their help-seeking behaviour may, however, trigger strong resentment from the divorced parents; a situation that exacerbates their propensity for social withdrawal. Moreover, the existence of violence prior to the separation and divorce, and occasional outbursts post-divorce, may impact on the children causing confusion and emotional turmoil.

The short-term effects of domestic violence on children, according to the NCH Action For Children (1994), manifest themselves as fright, subdued and clinging behaviour, bed-wetting problems, disobedience and aggression to other children. It is not uncommon for children who live under such conditions to run away from home (NCH Action For Children 1994, Payne 1995). An emotional chasm is created between mothers and their children, lengthening the duration of the latter's absence from their homes. While runaway children are exposed to a life of poverty, hopelessness, sexual exploitation and social hardship in the big cities, the personal and social consequences of many children who remain at home are not very dissimilar. Many children of divorced parents are prone to negative life experiences. They have low self-esteem (Bynum & Durm 1996); they achieve low educational attainment (Hartnup 1996); their reading and calculation skills are of a low standard; they engage in early pre-marital sexual relationships and cohabitation (Utting 1995, Axinn & Thorton 1996). Research findings (Kiernan 1992) suggest that family disruption in childhood increases the propensity for early home and school leaving by age 16, as well as an increased tendency to enter into a cohabitation union and to have had an extramarital birth. The respondents attributed friction at home, economic disadvantages and poor accommodation as precipitating factors in their motivation to become independent and to start earning a living. Living away from the parent can reduce the stress factor existent in the relationships. Hartnup (1996) argued that divorce strained relationships between parents and their children. Parental detachment and inability to exercise discipline and to maintain stability in the home may cause a behavioural change such as 'high irritability' among children. Similarly, Elliott and Richards' (1991) study reported a high correlation between having divorced parents and disruptive behaviour in children. Other effects, according to Hartnup (1996), include deviant behaviour, anxiety and unhappiness caused by exposure to verbal and physical abuse between the parents, increased vulnerability caused by feelings of helplessness as children witness the discord within the family environment, and the collapse of the 'protective and nurturing' family networks (Case example 3.1).

The anxiety that children experience is commonly termed '*separation anxiety*'. It is a psychological disorder in response to the situation where attachment figures (i.e. mothers and fathers) have separated, so that the child becomes separated from either the mother or father, or both in some cases. Puri et al (1996) explain that the anxiety could occur because of 'real or imagined separation'.

In spite of the above negative outcomes currently being debated in the literature on separation, divorce, marital strife and their effects on children, some authors, namely Barber & Eccles (1992) argue for a more objective assessment of post-divorce influences and single parenting on children, and the identification of positive dynamic processes. For instance, while they recognize that many single, divorced parents and their children occupy a socio-economically disadvantaged position, children's experiences are enhanced by the new family situations. Furthermore, marriage

Case example 3.1

The District Judge was appalled on hearing the report produced by the Welfare Officer in Court. In 1992, Mary and Josh, with two young daughters, Josian 4 and Ellie 6, were entangled in a bitter marital conflict.

Josh was the Chief Executive of a prospering building company. Mary, on the other hand, worked part-time in the local shop, three days a week. She felt that the extra cash would help her to buy some small luxury items for her personal use, as her husband only seemed to lavish his attention on his two daughters. While Mary was at work, Josian and Ellie were looked after by their friendly neighbours, who had both retired. Mary's parents had died 4 years ago, while Josh's parents lived 100 miles away in Manchester.

The welfare officer explained that statements written by the primary school teacher and the nursery nurse exposed their concerns regarding the two children's health. They frequently looked lethargic and non-responsive in their interactions with other children. When they reported their observations on the phone to Mary, she had explained that the children did not sleep well at night; they were also having nightmares. The teachers, on these occasions, would insist that Mary take the children home since they were so tired. Mary would subsequently leave the shop to remain at home with them.

The reporting officer made allusion to the fact that these incidences occurred during, and appeared to be linked to, the times when their father worked abroad. During that time Josh would only see his daughters for four weekends during an 8-week period. His visits were always a major fracas, since his wife strongly resented his presence in the home. The quarrels were bitter, noisy and troublesome to the children and the neighbours.

Late one night, after her husband had left home, the neighbours heard the children screaming, while Mary was shouting and swearing. There were scuffles. The neighbours called in. The back door was ajar and the children were sobbing underneath the table. They had small skin lacerations on the arms and legs. They smelled of alcohol. Mary was laid across the kitchen floor littered with broken glasses. A bottle of gin was beside her. She was conscious but uncommunicative. An ambulance was called immediately. Mary was admitted to a medical ward. The two children became inpatients on the paediatric unit. They both died 2 days later...

dissolution very often ends or lessens exposure to parental conflict when the partners are apart. Accordingly, some children 'adapt with competence' (Barber & Eccles 1992) to the disruption, while developing new skills and coping strategies. Emery and Coiro (1995) make reference to how 'children can bounce back in the face of stress' and function competently after a divorce. Many children exhibit resilience and a mature approach when facing adversity compared to children from non-divorced homes (Emery & Coiro 1995). In addition, some mothers feel it imperative to seek employment to boost their financial status. In the long term, their improved economic position helps them to adjust to their new lifestyle, which benefits the children. The mothers' employment, however, very often means delegating household responsibilities to the children. The involvement of children in the management of the household increases their skills, develops self-sufficiency, and boosts confidence and self-reliance while increasing their personal strengths (Barber & Eccles 1992). Kasen et al (1996) postulate that when children are exposed to 'adult' experiences evident in their participation in sharing adult responsibilities, children's immature social skills are enhanced, and their self-worth and confidence simultaneously heightened. Additionally, according to

Tuttle (1992), children develop a strong sense of maturity about relationships under the circumstances. However, she argued conversely that, under these social conditions of increased responsibilities, children lose their freedom of childhood. Similarly, Emery and Coiro (1995) make reference to the adverse effects of responsibilities by arguing that they heighten the children's burdens.

PREVENTION AND THERAPEUTIC INTERVENTION

As discussed already, marital conflict has far-reaching consequences. Children and their parents are equally affected. The aims of prevention in this context can be outlined as:

1. intervention to prevent family breakdown and to ensure child protection
2. to prevent or reduce deterioration of relationships
3. prevention of abuse and promotion of health and safety
4. the reduction of family conflict
5. establishment of self-awareness and development of a healthy communicative framework conducive to recuperation of self-esteem.

Therapeutic interventions have many dimensions and can only be effective when targeted groups are cooperative and voluntarily participate in the therapeutic activities tailored to meet their needs. A therapeutic intervention may consist of an informal encounter with a trained volunteer, who is also an experienced parent and who may have experienced similar family problems in the past. On the other hand, a more formal arrangement may be made with a counsellor, psychotherapist, family therapist, clinical psychologist, social worker or community psychiatric nurse.

Professionals whose roles are to intervene therapeutically aim at creating a non-stigmatizing environment based on clients' or families' choice. Most frequently, meetings can be arranged within the families' own homes. Referrals are made by health visitors, the individuals themselves, social services or friends.

Activity 3.1

Organize small groups. Examine and discuss Case example 3.1. Consider the family environment in which the children were living in. What types of preventative measures would you use to ensure the children's safety?

??? Question 3.1

1. Imagine that the social and health care agencies have become aware of the children's living conditions as described above. What action do you think will be taken?
2. Do you think or believe that separation and divorce have negative as well as positive consequences on children?

Utting (1995) makes reference to a variety of organizations and initiatives which aim, first, to avoid care proceedings, subsequently reducing costs, and secondly, to facilitate the resolution of marital conflict. Thus, organizations such as Relate can provide training and education services, relationship counselling and psychosexual therapy. Their aim is to increase the locus of control within the family, by developing the parents' and children's knowledge, improving communication, thereafter facilitating parental decision-making and improving relationships.

Home Start UK, a voluntary family support organization, have trained volunteers who are experienced parents. They give practical help and advice to families who may lack specific knowledge on how to cope with their problems. Additionally, there are family centres with an open door policy which aim to support vulnerable families, by integrating community facilities such as parent support groups and nurseries with child health facilities. Other initiatives include Family-Nurturing Network, New Parent Infant Network and the Radford Shared Care Project. These organizations function by providing intensive family care interventions in their own homes, while simultaneously working in partnership with multi-agency networks (social and health care agencies) to enhance their goals in family integration.

It is not an easy task to integrate adversarial couples. Hence other alternatives may be needed. For example, it is argued that divorcing parents benefit from an impartial third party (Dillon & Emery 1996). Divorce mediation, according to these writers, benefits parents and children in the long term. They assert that parents become more forthcoming in discussing their children's needs when conflicts are diminished.

Another beneficial effect of mediation – achieved through the objective stance of mediators – is the level of cooperation between the partners, instead of acrimonious bargaining based on subjectivity, while neglecting the children's needs and rights. Mediators undertake to redress the imbalance by objective negotiation concerning legal matters related to custody and residence (Emery & Coiro 1995). Their intervention, how-

ever, is not connected with family therapy, which according to Emery and Coiro, is only reserved when parents experience deep emotional distress. There is, nevertheless, a school of thought based on the proposition that, if children's needs are to be effectively met, the mediation process should also include the expertise of a child therapist (Beck & Biank 1997). To enhance therapeutic intervention during divorce, they recommend that several key features must be borne in mind:

1. Mediators and therapists should have a good knowledge of child development.
2. The effects of separation trauma and anxiety should be identified and appropriate intervention implemented.
3. While financial matters receive due consideration in divorce cases, the assessment of children in regard to their developmental and emotional needs should receive more attention.
4. Parents are too preoccupied with their own internal strife and turmoil to realize that their children are experiencing transition anxieties. Parental education should include explanations of the effects of anxieties on children, and how their adjustment levels can be improved by giving them time, and by encouraging the expression of feelings and fears.
5. Child therapists can enhance the mediation process if they undertake mediation training. Following a child assessment, they can help parents to 'approach the parenting agreement' objectively and empathetically. By working collaboratively with the latter, they may facilitate the decision process.
6. Regular check-ups should be done prior to, during and after the divorce to assess children's development, their coping strategies and to prevent or treat any 'developmental derailment'.

IMPLICATIONS FOR NURSING AND HEALTH CARE

In view of the detrimental consequences of separation and divorce on children, who have sometimes been described as the 'invisible victims', the implications for nursing and health care need to be considered.

The divorce literature mainly focuses on parents and their children, while neglecting the fact that grandparents have been known to exert positive and negative influences on marital conflict. Care professionals have a responsibility to develop their understanding of family sociology and psychology to deepen their insight of how environmental influences can adversely affect child development. For instance, an assessment of grandparents' psychoemotional needs and coping abilities could be done by health visitors. Since some children of divorced parents may spend a high percentage of their time with grandparents, while the custodial parent is at work, a thorough consideration should be given to the quality of the psychosocial environment in which they are being brought up. Grandparents and others in the children's environment may experience ambivalent feelings: anger, fear and hopelessness. A knowledge of how they are coping with their inner turmoil and social adjustments becomes essential in health care.

To assist children and their families effectively, a coordinated, comprehensive multidisciplinary response (Tuttle 1992) is required. The mobilization of community resources (health visiting, community mental health workers, social workers and district nursing services) is imperative. Good parenting skills can be promoted, to improve social relationships and activities, preventing 'psychopathology in children' (Tuttle 1992). Furthermore, this parental care dimension (Neale & Smart 1997), which reflects the emotional and physical interactions between parents and children, should not only be encouraged, but should be recognized by the parents and significant others as crucial for the children.

Positive interactions, the avoidance of disparaging confrontations between parents (Tuttle 1992) and protection of children from parental animosity (Emery & Coiro 1995) will boost (the children's) self-image and self-esteem.

NEEDS FOR PROTECTION

While engaged in establishing positive therapeutic social health skills, health workers must exercise vigilance in relation to children's needs for *protection*. Protection from abuse (physical and emotional) and exploitation in the home (e.g. assuming adult roles and responsibilities in caring for the emotionally deprived parent) are prerequisites in health promotion.

Some authors, however, point out that, while community health workers aim to support children and their parents, the latter's perception of care professionals can be negative. Westlake and Pearson (1997) for instance, making reference to their research findings, explained that some families have a narrow view of the health visitor's role. They interpret the latter's role to be mainly surveillance in connection with child abuse. Consequently, the researchers argued, these families' 'fear of reprisals' discourage them from expressing their needs for help concerning child care.

As discussed at the beginning of this chapter, children of divorced parents have multiple needs. Although they are living with one parent, they still experience separation anxiety and separation trauma (Case example 3.2). The single parents'

Case example 3.2

Sara 5, and her sister Emy 7, both felt depressed when their father, after a long marital conflict, left home. In spite of their protests concerning the separation, their mother, who wanted a divorce, decided it would be in their best interests. It was obvious that the mother had fear of not being able to cope without the children; additionally, the desire for revenge and control led to an acrimonious defence of her position to obtain prime custody. Family mediation, as suggested by the solicitors, ensured that the father gained access to the children twice a week. However, despite the social arrangement, the children began to experience separation anxiety and separation trauma. Although their mother lived with them, her self-preoccupation and emotional instability triggered feelings of social and emotional deprivation in the children. The situation caused a psychological loss for them. On the other hand, while their father's absence and their mother's lack of warmth increased their feelings of personal abandonment, their father remained both a biological father and a psychological one. He understood their feelings, and supported them as much as he could during their brief meetings.

behaviour could easily compound the ill effects of separation anxiety, particularly when they are reluctant to seek professional help.

The provision of non-stigmatizing professional intervention is not easily achieved, despite a friendly and non-judgemental approach. Professionals, therefore, need peer support to undertake their responsibilities. Byrne (1995) proposed a model of supervision that will provide guidance for professionals engaged in child protection. The ultimate aim is to have knowledgeable practitioners with insight of deeper issues, which will serve the best interests of children and their families. It is being recognized more often that children have the capacity to make sense of medical and health concepts (Richards 1997). If this is the case, children are also able to interpret events in their social life. In cases of divorce, for example, Harold (1997) asserts that children can make connections between the effects of marital conflict on their well-being. Their perceptions of events will determine their levels of adjustment and the degree of support they will need. As witnesses of parental conflict, anger and animosity, their development may be impeded, and they can suffer psychologically – with anxiety states and depression, for example – well into adolescence and adulthood. Children can also suffer socially, with inability to form stable relationships and to cope with aspects of daily living, such as holding a steady employment and obtaining educational qualifications. Hence professionals must evaluate children from their (the children's) understanding of the situation before providing care tailored to individuals' needs.

Activity 3.2

1. Reflect upon the issues highlighted so far. Write down your viewpoints (based on personal experiences if appropriate). Attempt to recall narratives from friends, relatives etc.
2. Debate with colleagues the extent to which changes in beliefs and values in society have led to an increase in divorce rates.

??? Question 3.2

1. What are your views regarding helping post-divorce parents to adjust to their changing situations?
2. What do you consider to be the main aim of a family mediation service?
3. Do you think that there are differences between children of divorced parents and non-divorced parents?

CHILD ABUSE

Abuse of children is not a new social phenomenon, but is a social problem with a long-standing history. It is pervasive in all societies and is interpreted differently according to one's socio-cultural beliefs. Children have been, and still are being, exploited and abused by both female and male adults, siblings and other children. Social history provides numerous examples of child neglect, physical abuse, sexual abuse and child prostitution (Johnson 1990).

Many children in the eighteenth and nineteenth centuries worked long hours in factories and mines. They were expected to be up very early in the morning to go to work, and to come home late in the evening. Since most of their time was spent toiling away in the workplace, parental contact was minimal. Their socio-emotional needs, hence, were not adequately met. Johnson explained that, at that time, children were viewed as commodities, to be bought and sold. Their rights were not respected. Very often children were used for sexual gratification by adults, and eventually discarded. Since their rights as human beings were not recognized and respected, children's social conditions were impoverished.

Television documentaries using material from historical archives and social history textbooks portray the plight of begging children in the streets, leading vagrant lives. Their increased vulnerability meant that children were dependent on others to show mercy and to protect them. However, children's need for protection seldom received the respect it deserved. Parents and others, throughout the ages, have assaulted children, raped them, hanged them and burnt them as witches. Although in the late 1990s, children are not burned as witches, their ill treatment is not too dissimilar, and may be worse (Box 3.1). Not too many years ago, the Moors Murderers, Myra Hindley and Ian Brady, made tape recordings of the victims begging to be spared, to no avail.

Box 3.1

The severely neglected and abused child suffers a slow death. A child's liver can be ruptured by an aggressive mother, father, grandfather or a stepfather, with repeated deep prods with the fingers. Alternatively, the abdomen, hands, buttocks or legs may be burnt with a hot iron. Additionally, children may be bitten by adults on the neck, violently shaken causing eye haemorrhage, dislocated lens and detached retina, or thrown against a wall or some furniture, resulting in skull fracture.

Violence against children as one commentator (Gray 1987) pointed out is worsening and getting more prolonged. The methods used are in addition becoming more sophisticated, as described, and more bizarre. The effects on the person furthermore are devastating: physical traumas and emotional scars which remain present well into later life, while sexual battering which defaces their self-image, destroys their sexuality and self-esteem.

WHO ARE THE PERPETRATORS?

Abusers of children are commonly individuals in the intrafamilial environment known to the abused victim. Natural mothers and fathers, and male guardians, have all been identified in the literature as key figures in the history of child abuse (Brunngraber 1986, Moore 1991, Hobbs et al 1996). Additionally, research findings (Moncrieff et al 1996) indicate that grandfathers, stepfathers, uncles and cousins are also implicated in abusing children under their care. Moncrieff et al (1996) also highlight instances when non-family members have been perpetrators, namely acquaintances, strangers, priests and scout leaders. Similarly, Hobbs and Heywood (1997) made reference to carers, family members and acquaintances who abused children. In many cases, the least suspected individuals within the family have been known to be perpetrators: minors such

as siblings (Hall 1996, Cleaver & Freeman 1996) (Box 3.2) and adolescents (Thompson 1995a, Masson 1995). It has also been known for professionals in the caring professions to be accused of abuse, as in the example in Box 3.3.

Box 3.2 Confession of an abused sister

'I tried everything to prevent my brother from entering the bedroom at night. I locked the door, and the windows ... sometimes I would push the sideboard against the door, but to no avail. He still managed to get in. When I tried to scream he would attempt to suffocate me with the pillow ...'

Box 3.3 The eminent surgeon

The following is an account described by Cashman et al (1992). It is a story which will no doubt increase the reader's awareness and insight into the wider implications of child abuse in the fields of nursing, social work and health care.

'A 3-year-old girl raped by her father (an eminent surgeon) developed both short- and long-term symptoms':

'As soon as his penis left my mouth, I threw up ... I remember him banging trying to get into me, and then he ripped me open ... within seconds he was gone ... My mother ... found me lying in bed covered in blood and vomit ... the next memory I have is my father, whose office was downstairs, sewing my vagina back up, without anaesthetic. I was never taken to the hospital.'

Perpetrators: a profile

Although the literature makes reference to the majority of abusers being men, it is important to note that, in general, abusers manifest features of personality disorder (Gulland 1997). This does not necessarily imply that they are mentally ill: their incompetence to develop healthy, intimate relationships with individuals of an appropriate age (Hilton & Mezey 1996) reflects the inadequacy of their personality. Dependence on a child's affection and the need to exert control and exercise power over a vulnerable person are common features.

Nevertheless, it has been known for individuals with mental ill-health to abuse children as a consequence of altered perception and sociopathic traits. In acute maternal mental illness (Cassin 1996), for example, children are prone to neglect (physical and psychological) when changes occur in the mother's mental state. Buchanan (1996) argued that schizophrenia predisposes a person to maltreatment of a child, caused by their hallucinatory states and delusions. Buchanan also made reference to learning disabled parents who can abuse their children. An awareness of the causative factors is incomplete without an insight into the relationships between perpetrators and victims (Box 3.4). Child abuse literature indicates that the relationships represent states of domination and exploitation between the former and the latter, to maintain the maltreatment and avoid detection.

Box 3.4 Perpetrators' strategies to maintain the abuse

The abusing parents, siblings, relatives and others use threats, force and blackmailing tactics to exert control over the defenceless child. They may, for example, threaten to beat the other partner up, to abuse other children in the family and to murder the abused. Sometimes rewards are given in the form of money, favouritism, a reduction in the level of violence and the offer of protection. On other occasions the abusers may make reference to themselves as victims of the law and the possibility of imprisonment. Alternatively, they may threaten to divorce the child's mother or father and to commit suicide.

The prevention of disclosure relies heavily on the violence and threatening behaviour of the abuser subjugating the victim. Some abusers resort to strategies which may take years for clinicians to detect, as in cases of Munchausen syndrome by proxy (Box 3.5).

CAUSES OF CHILD ABUSE

Health and social workers, clinicians, clinical psychologists and others in the field of child abuse have attempted to find the reasons for it. Child abuse is a multifactorial social problem; one cannot pinpoint a single cause since many features have been identified in analysing why it occurs.

Box 3.5

Munchausen syndrome by proxy presents a different dimension to the classifications of child abuse as outlined in Box 3.6. This type of abuse started to hit the headlines in the late 1970s. Many writers since have attributed the syndrome to a form of child abuse, with the mother identified as the main perpetrator (Baldwin 1996). It manifests itself as the fabrication of illness caused by the caregiver (Mercer & Perdue 1993, Baldwin 1994) interfering with the child's physical health.

Overdosage or underdosage of medication, and adding a drop of blood to a urine sample are some examples. The syndrome is recognized and accepted as a potentially lethal form of child abuse (Volz 1995), since the abused is subjected to a battery of unnecessary clinical procedures, investigations and hospital admissions. Furthermore, the process, if undetected, continues for many years, baffling the nursing and medical practitioners, while the children suffer physiologically and psychologically (Klebes & Fay 1995). Very often, death is the ultimate consequence of Munchausen syndrome by proxy.

It is important to note, however, that sexual deviance is a concept that reflects one's socio-cultural beliefs and norms. What is considered to be a repugnant practice in one society, may well be regarded as health-oriented behaviour in another. For example, anthropological studies on the sexual behaviour of distant non-Westernized cultures show us that in some Melanesian cultures, brother–sister incest is normal as part of an initiation; the Sambian culture teaches young boys that the ingestion of semen (via oral sex) from older boys is socially acceptable. The ancient Egyptian royal families were well-known for their exclusive in-breeding practices. Malinowski, author of *The sexual life of savages*, who spent many years studying the Trobrianders, made reference to small children's sexual activities and foreplay as they were watched affirmatively by their parents (Malinowski 1987).

Some researchers argue that there is a correlation between the physical or psychological characteristics of children and abuse. Turk and Brown (1993), for example, explained that being deaf and having cerebral palsy increased an individual's vulnerability to being abused. On the other hand, they argued that while certain traits can predispose to abuse, the abused person can

Box 3.6 Classifications of child abuse

Physical abuse: abuse that refers to the variety of injuries that can be inflicted on the child's body. Knight (1991), a forensic pathologist, describes it as 'child or baby battering' or 'non-accidental injury'. Numerous *bruises* can be found: on the abdomen, around the genitalia, the upper arms, wrists, ankles and knees. *Fractures* are also common, but may be identified from radiological examination which will reveal callus formation from a previously healed fracture. *Eye bruises* are also evident in the majority of cases. Injuries can be caused by 'harsh fingertip pressure', slapping, knuckle punches and instruments such as canes and hair brushes. Biting, pinching, burning and scalding are other methods (McLay 1990).

Emotional abuse: abuse that is not easily defined and has not always been recognized until recently. Repeated physical abuse causes ghettoization of the child's emotions; a state characterized by the child's emotions and feelings being trapped, and unable to be expressed. Lack of parental warmth, support and affection causes emotional damage. Sometimes this feature can be observed in mask-like facial expressions, a lack of alertness and evidence of fear in the presence of adults. These features have been aptly described as 'frozen watchfulness' (Spencer 1987, Polnay & Hull 1993). A failure to respond to child's signals of distress and need for attention and stimulation, and an absence of healthy parental engagement in activities are classified as emotional abuse.

Sexual abuse: abuse that has been recognized since the early 1980s to be an accompaniment of physical abuse. Examples of sexual abuse are: ano-sexual contact, digital penetration, or the insertion of objects into the child vaginal or anal orifices, masturbation, fondling, oral sex

(Box 3.7) or attempted or achieved penetration of the mouth (Box 3.3), causing injuries to the genital areas (scalding, bruising and burning with a lit cigarette).

Ritual/Satanic abuse: repeated abuse, whether physical or sexual, is known as **ritual abuse**. Some perpetrators, in order to entice children, would dress up in robes, use altars and other paraphernalia, to convince them that they have special powers. LaFontaine (1996) argued that 'ritual' abuse has been confounded with 'satanic' abuse.

Satanic abuse: refers to cases where perpetrators organize ceremonies based on devil worship, involving children in their practices who are used for sexual purposes. Blumenthal (1994) remarked that its prevalence may be minimal; it is nevertheless a serious social problem. Close partnership between health agencies and the criminal justice system is essential for early detection (Neate & Sone 1991). Survivors of ritual abuse experience deep psychological trauma, which has implications for their social well-being (Valente 1992).

Neglect: neglect is an aspect of child abuse. The following account (Hobbs & Wynne 1996) will illustrate the concept. A male child aged 18 months was found dead in the house. An ambulance was called and he was taken to hospital. Although the examining doctor found his physical features to be compatible with 'normal nutrition', he was very cold, wet and dirty. His nappy had not been changed for several days.

Neglect gives evidence of how children are at the mercy of their parents or guardians, and can be described as the deliberate or unintentional lack of food provision. Failure to provide physical and psychological safety for the child is also regarded as neglect.

Box 3.7 Incidents of sexual abuse

Moore (1991) made reference to a health care worker who accidentally witnessed a mother having oral sex with her son. Similarly, in a different context, Hobbs and Wynne (1990) described a 4-year-old boy's behaviour and responses in a nursery. The staff were alerted when the boy exhibited precocious sexual behaviour by attempting to have intercourse with the little girls around him, and kissing them in the vulva area. When questioned about his behaviour, the boy responded that *his mother* behaved in that way normally.

Activity 3.3

Using reflective practice theories learned on the course, reflect upon issues related to socio-cultural practices, norms and beliefs of a society concerning abuse cases. Compile a list of examples related to cases of child abuse and highlight the ways the media have exposed this social problem.

??? Question 3.3

1. To what extent do you believe that society is responsible for an increase in child abuse?
2. Can you suggest some measures that can be taken to help the abused child cope with family violence?
3. Do you agree that there are many factors linked to child abuse?

develop learning disabilities as a consequence of the trauma. Children with learning disabilities present challenges to carers. If the carer's patience and coping thresholds are low, the risk of abuse increases. Some authors (Brown et al 1995) have commented how *adults* with learning disabilities can be sexually abused. It follows, therefore, that children with learning disabilities, as members of a vulnerable group, are likely to be abused by their carers, family members and others.

Children, whether disabled or not, have a propensity for seeking love, comfort, security and attention from adults. Their desire to please and to comply makes them vulnerable targets of adults whose mentality predisposes them toward abuse. Additionally, children who exhibit non-conforming and non-compliant behaviours, and who are perceived by their parents as being purposefully awkward, rude, boisterous and destructive, can suffer abuse (Iwaniec 1997).

While the personal characteristics of the abused have been identified as possible triggering factors, the family environment and socio-economic factors have also been implicated. Poverty, for example, in association with other factors can predispose to abuse (Hobbs & Heywood 1997). Overcrowding, lack of privacy, overt and deliberate exposure of children to parental sexual activities, social disorder and lack of security (Hall 1996) are all contributing factors. In particular, the degree or lack of supervision and fragmented disruptive lifestyles (Moncrieff et al 1996) are common attributes. The abused are frequently caught up in a pernicious cycle of physical and sexual abuse (Fig. 3.1), with many

becoming abusers in later life. The abused child grows up, being primarily socialized through social learning and identification with parental behaviour, believing that social malpractice (sexual deviance, partner's abuse, parental violence and child abuse) is the socio-cultural norm. Ross (1996), for example, argued that there is a correlation between adversarial couples' violence towards each other and inclination to physically abuse their children. Children hence learn at an early age that violence in the family and general neglect, in combination with a chaotic lifestyle, is the norm.

When parental skills are poor, and when there is a gap in knowledge concerning cause and effects, namely that social disruption affects the psychosocial needs of children, a situation is created whereby ignorance perpetuates the unhealthy effects of abuse on the victims. Furthermore, the absence of nurturing (Hall 1996, Iwaniec 1997) as a constant feature in the home of abused children augments the lack of subjectivity in relation to feelings and emotions of the abuser toward the abused. Therefore, behaviour becomes more callous and impartial (similar to a stranger rapist's assault), and is likely to be repeated. This form of parental violence, where couples express sexually deviant behaviour and/or physical assault, is characterized as a primary causative factor in child abuse (Taitz & King 1988).

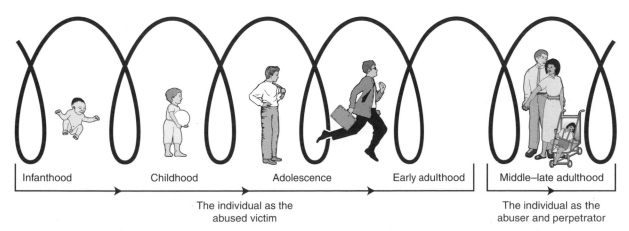

| Infanthood | Childhood | Adolescence | Early adulthood | Middle–late adulthood |

The individual as the abused victim

The individual as the abuser and perpetrator

Fig. 3.1 Pernicious cycle of abuse (from being an abused individual to becoming an abusing person).

Contrastingly, the consequences of abuse (which will be considered later) represent the secondary or aftereffects of abuse as evidence that 'actual harm' (Taitz & King 1988) has occurred.

While the personal characteristics of the abused and their family home environment are relevant features to consider in the causation of child abuse, it is as equally important to focus the discussions on the characteristics or profile of perpetrators.

VICTIMS AND SURVIVORS OF ABUSE: EFFECTS AND CONSEQUENCES

When one considers the life trajectory of abused children in society, it seems appropriate to use the terms 'victims' and 'survivors'; their chaotic lives make them the victims, their resilience against all odds makes them the survivors. They survive to tell the tale. Although many choose not to do so – because of the painful memories that are relived – those that do, present a catalogue of negative traumatic events with tragic consequences. The children are left with deep psychoemotional scars.

Many survivors find themselves caught up in the pernicious cycle of abuse. Nevertheless, despite their negative past, many survivors manage to retrieve aspects that help them to develop a more positive outlook about themselves and in their perceptions of others.

The consequences of child abuse are multifactorial. The effects that can traumatize the person are holistic in nature. The essential dimensions in assessment and care interventions are outlined below.

Physical dimension

Physical pain is experienced as the body is assaulted, and the signs and effects are manifold. Bruises and skin lacerations can become infected; head injuries, which are common, may lead to brain haemorrhage, fractures, disturbed vision, as well as detached retinas; insomnia can be a symptom of pain. Physiological battering (interference with body functions), with over- or underdosage of medication for example, can lead to fatal side-effects (e.g. coma, hypothermia, haemorrhage). Loss of bladder control can occur as a result of direct trauma or as a fear reaction. Neglect can lead to starvation and weight loss. Other physical effects include urethritis, vaginitis, anal fissure and dilatation, venereal infection of the mouth and vagina, and the possibility of HIV/AIDS.

Psychoemotional dimension

Psychosomatic effects, such as anorexia and back pain, have been reported (Cashman et al 1992). Emotional pain can be described as heartache, a nagging, hurtful feeling that cannot be described; this can be caused by feelings of being betrayed and abandoned by affectionless parents and significant people in the victim's environment: those who should have given help and support, but did not. Sometimes the abused may express feelings of heaviness and sadness. Hall (1996) made reference to 'psychic victimization': an assault on the victim's psychoemotional integrity, creating an 'emotional wasteland' and making them 'emotionally exiled'. Other psychological effects include anxiety disorder, depression and low self-esteem. When removed from the environment of abuse, individuals very often experience post-traumatic stress disorder: personality changes, nightmares, profound anxiety, fear, anger and depression (Lee 1991). Clark (1997) reported behaviour of increased vigilance, and experiences of distressing images, altered thoughts and perception, agitation, extreme sadness, panic, fury and despair. Feelings of persecution may also be present (Moore 1991).

Sexuality dimension

Many individuals experience difficulties in expressing their sexuality and in forming stable relations with peers. In some cases a deep sense of grievance directs the person into acts of sexual abuse on others. Other effects include fear of sexuality, confusion over sexual identification (Brunngraber 1986) and promiscuity.

Social dimension

One possible social consequence has already been pointed out: the cultural transmission of abuse within the family, described as 'the pernicious cycle of abuse'. This is evidenced in a replication of the offender's own experience of abuse (Hilton & Mezey 1996). Additionally, where the relationships are based on exploitation, there has been involvement in pornography and prostitution (Moncrieff et al 1996). Abuse can also result in children running away from home (Payne 1995, Hall 1996). Abused children look for an alternative, freedom from a chaotic family situation, by searching for environmental conditions that will guarantee them security and safety from abusive parents and others. Social scarring, the result of negative life experiences, leaves many children with feelings of doubt concerning their own social skills in developing healthy parental attitudes in the future. In addition, mistrust can occur in relationships; survivors experience difficulties in believing the true motives of individuals wanting to establish genuine relationships. Drug addiction and glue sniffing are known consequences of abuse (Channel 4, Innocents Lost 1997). In Guatemala, many homeless children rely on drugs to escape the painful memories of the past (Box 3.8), and on prostitution to earn a living.

Box 3.8 Life on the street

A 16-year-old boy told the reporter that he had been taking drugs for a number of years. He was homeless. He roamed the streets with other runaways, and relied on glue sniffing to escape the harsh reality that faced him (Channel 4, Innocents Lost 1997).

Positive consequences

For some, abuse in the family leads to positive consequences, dependent on the child's personality. Past experiences may increase their resilience and understanding of people's behaviour. Some survivors feel confidence in their self-image, attractiveness and sexuality, while others feel powerful and have the ability to reflect maturely upon their experiences (Brunngraber 1986), adversity helping to develop positive inner strength. Others, when they are removed from the abusive parents or relatives, may find closeness toward members of the family.

It can be deduced from the above discussions that child abuse has pervasive detrimental consequences, and that few survivors report positive effects. Professionals from all spheres of social and health care need to work together to protect the vulnerable child.

WORKING TOGETHER IN CHILD PROTECTION

Child abuse cases present professionals, and society in general, with challenges that can only be met when interagency and multidisciplinary approaches go beyond the boundaries of standard collaborative efforts. This entails seeking professional expertise from other disciplines when doubts are being expressed, to confirm the diagnosis. For example, a forensic dentist may be needed to confirm bite marks. This approach requires the combined efforts of the paediatricians and the forensic dentist (Whittaker et al 1997); their assessments and evaluations will help distinguish animal bites from human bites. Their reports, moreover, with feedback from other professionals (e.g. police surgeons, social workers) will complement previous research findings, thus empowering their position. It is known that the complementary skills of forensic medical officers are useful in assisting paediatricians and other professionals in their work (Lawrence 1997); for instance, lawyers looking for strong evidence to convict the perpetrators.

While professionals attempt to work collaboratively, it is recognized that ambiguities and disagreements concerning diagnoses among professionals in relation to physical signs of sexual abuse (Lynch 1992) can impede the process of detection. Confusion can occur, as Reardon et al (1992) pointed out, when anatomical changes due to pathology – as in cases of anal abnormalities – can lead professionals to suspect sexual abuse. This factor reinforces the notion that accuracy of clinical knowledge is required to prevent unnecessary distress to both the child and carers. Reliance on collaborative partnerships based on effective communication of research findings cannot be overemphasized.

Case conferences

Case conferences provide the arena for the team to meet and to make decisions, with the ultimate aim to ensure safety and protection for the child. Its importance is well accepted but has been criticized in cases where discussions have been 'unfocused', and when key professionals have been absent (Speight 1987), or have been unable to make decisive decisions. In a case conference, contributions from a variety of professionals are invited, e.g. community doctors, health visitors, general practitioners, social workers, police and paediatricians. Their observations and reports are vital elements in the overall framework, which may establish the missing links, thus identifying the perpetrators and securing the child's safety. Health professionals at case conferences may have to discuss strategic care assessment and planning, as in cases when a child is under an assessment order prescribed by the court. Their expertise in responding efficiently to court policies concerning the commencement of the assessment and who should be responsible (Miles 1991) is a prerequisite.

Integrated interventions

Since the children's safeguard is a dynamic discipline as well as a challenging social problem (Siddall 1997a), it is essential that other agencies, in addition to the ones mentioned above, become involved in the process. Local and central government agencies, religious groups, the media, community groups and academics all become useful allies. Bond (1997) argued for a public awareness raising campaign to highlight that families, not necessarily strangers, are abusers of children too.

PREVENTION AND CARE

Prevention only becomes effective when profes-

sionals act upon knowledge based on accurate and painstaking research findings undertaken by other professionals. In the field of domestic violence primary health care teams have a responsibility to detect the manifestations of family violence as early as possible so that appropriate measures can be taken. The stigma attached to family violence is well known (Stark et al 1997) and discourages many victims from expressing their needs for support. General practitioners and their community teams must apply sensitive, non-stigmatizing strategies in their interactions with vulnerable families. The aim of prevention is to buffer the negative effects by mobilizing available professional and informal support, and to promote parental education and training (Dubowitz & King 1995).

The above objective can be achieved by a knowledge of the aetiology of family violence, which covers such dimensions as community factors (social isolation, and poor neighbourhood); family set-up, where spousal abuse is common; and individual factors (child–parent interactions) (Case example 3.3).

Case example 3.3 Violence in the family

Tourists from the surrounding districts avoid the small town of Colville. Its 15 000 residents call it 'Colditzville': isolated, dilapidated areas where juvenile delinquents meet to sniff glue and smoke marijuana; a place where young and old alike run the risk of being mugged. Mr and Mrs X live in that town with their twin sons aged 15. Mr X is a coalminer, and an alcoholic. His wife is prone to depression, and relies on alcohol as a coping strategy. Spousal abuse is common. Violence is the norm in the household. The children suffer too. They get beaten very often. The parents' tolerance threshold is low; their parental skills are poor and the children's boisterous behaviour worsens the situation. The community team reports a history of physical abuse within the parents' own families.

While vigilance in community settings is recommended, health and social care professionals should also be vigilant in institutional settings (hospitals and children's homes), where parents have been caught abusing their children

(Gulland 1997, Sadler 1997). Dickson (1997) reports cases where children have been allowed to visit rapists and paedophiles in maximum security units. Furthermore, health care workers have been known to be perpetrators themselves (e.g. Beverly Allitt in 1983, Lincolnshire; Genene Jones in Texas) (Stark et al 1997). Evidence from real life situations and from literature reports should be utilized to guide clinical practice. An open-minded approach to prevention is necessary. House (1997) argued that patients' safety can be ascertained by preventing dangerous practices. Unsafe practices, however, will occur if inadequate health screening of personnel takes place. One cannot, nevertheless, rely solely on staff screening in prevention. A combination of screening measures and clinical supervision, as well as practice surveillance, is essential.

CARE INTERVENTIONS

Physical and psychological traumas take time to heal. Abused children need the supportive and understanding presence of people who genuinely care. Specialized help is needed. However, professionals must avoid the stereotypical argument that children are resilient, thus able to manage their own healing process (Lee 1991). An assessment of their strengths and weaknesses is necessary. Mobilizing their inner resources to improve their coping capacity, in an understanding and reassuring way, is an objective to consider.

Professional awareness and knowledge

Professionals must be aware of the features of post-traumatic stress disorder (Clark 1997). Insomnia, fears, loss of concentration, sexualized and flirtatious behaviour in children, irritability and hypervigilance are some of the features to consider in care assessment and delivery. Failure to recognize such features could minimize effective and meaningful care. Some activities may trigger images of past traumatic events in the victims, which could disturb their psychological well-being. Clark argued that care should be tailored according to individual needs. Some clients may find support among friends, relatives or professional caregivers. An identification of such needs ensures that appropriate steps are taken. The cooperation of non-abusing carers in the therapeutic approach will enhance the quality of emotional and physical support of the child (Wigglesworth et al 1996). Furthermore, the person may be helped to manage their symptoms by using some basic activities: relaxation techniques, deep breathing, writing, reading or drawing. Lee (1991) explained that the use of projective media (drawing, writing, painting) becomes a powerful tool in the expression of thoughts and emotions. Similarly, Pridmore and Lansdown (1997) pointed out that the technique of draw-and-write can facilitate the therapeutic process of releasing inner feelings, thus giving insightful knowledge of children's perceptions of their health.

Holism

A holistic approach to care focuses on the children's needs, while simultaneously considering key persons in their social environment. A child-centred approach to care consists of preventing and minimizing further traumatization. The systems of enquiries conducted by many professionals and in different settings have been criticized for adding to the emotional trauma (Siddall 1997b) of children. Advocacy centres, it is postulated, will minimize their trauma. Trained volunteers act as children's advocates, giving continuing support. Therapeutic services for the child and non-offending family members can also be provided. Continuity of lay and professional support will reduce the impact of uncertainty during and after investigations, assessment and court appearances. However, close liaison is needed among social workers, the Crown Prosecution Service, the police, medical and community health workers (Siddall 1997b). As well as the above measures, an important role of children's nurses is recognized for their proactive participation in prevention, care and education (Powell 1997).

Additionally, some older children may benefit

from innovative approaches to care such as the Opportunity Youth Programme Model, advocated by McClure (1997), consisting of peer education, with professional support. Social skills are enhanced and youngsters are given guidance in developing both coping methods to deal with their problems (e.g. abuse, homelessness, family problems etc.) and disclosure, in a safe therapeutic environment. Interagency participation is emphasized.

Mental health care

Following thorough assessments, it may be necessary to seek the expertise of the mental health team: psychiatric social workers, psychologists, psychiatrists, community psychiatric nurses. Emotional trauma can cause mental health changes: depressive states, anorexia, withdrawal and social distancing as well as aggression toward authority figures. It has been argued (Neate 1995) that many survivors need psychiatric interventions later in life. Attempting to provide social and psychological help as soon as possible, after a diagnosis of abuse, could reduce negative aftereffects. Horowitz et al (1997) advocate psychotherapy as a method of primary prevention to counteract the negative consequences of abuse, to educate and to provide protection.

In their daily interactions with children, professionals have to cope with parental anger, fears and anxiety. Some mothers may accuse their partners of abusing children, particularly during the process of divorce (Humphreys 1997). Tactful and sensitive assessment of parents' reporting of abuse is necessary. Equally important is the victims' own reporting of what has happened, combined with information from other agencies: e.g. social services and probation service. Clinicians, Hilton and Mezey (1996) emphasized, should be aware of the complex nature of child abuse phenomenon, and that abusers very often are women.

Vulnerable families (parents prone to abusing children) (Appleton 1996) may benefit from the professional support of health visitors. The latter, however, must liaise with the mental health team, to gain a thorough insight of the psychological profile of such families, so that their role in helping parents – in line with official guidelines – can be enhanced. Various methods (reading assignments, videotape vignettes, video feedback and group discussions) have been suggested (Iwaniec 1997) to improve parents' skills and to help them develop insight into their own shortcoming in child-rearing practices.

 Activity 3.4

Make arrangements with the community mental health team to attend their case conferences. Identify the approaches used to communicate information to other agencies.

??? **Question 3.4**

1. It is not easy to interview young abused children. What suggestions can you make to improve the retrieval of information in these cases?
2. Since as many professionals as possible must be involved to counteract the effects of abuse, what do you consider to be the barriers that can impede the process?

PROSTITUTION

If we consider the two previous social phenomena discussed already – marital strife/divorce and child abuse – in the equation of children in need, one finds that prostitution fits in the triangle, or cycle, of abuse. Prostitution does not occur in a vacuum, broad social and psychological forces are at play. Children or adolescent boys and girls do not become prostitutes for no reason. One can argue that these forces find their origins from many sources. First, as pointed out already, marital conflict exerts pressure on children. Secondly, the dysfunctional family is prone to abusing children. Many abused children find no alternative but to run away, and running away from home makes many children homeless. To survive they have to develop strategies.

Since their economic status is very low, their vulnerability to exploitation increases. Furthermore they have a need to be nurtured, cared for and to be loved. When they meet adult strangers who promise them affection and protection, while their defences are fragile, prostitution appears to be the only alternative (Case example 3.4).

Case example 3.4

> Mary ran away from home at the age of 13. She lived with her alcoholic mother who would beat her up frequently; her mother's boyfriend would also molest her. One day she decided to leave home. She took a bus to the city of Glasgow. She wandered the streets for many days, looking for food in the rubbish bins and sleeping in cardboard boxes at night. One day she was approached by a smartly dressed, clean shaven gentleman who took her to his home. He promised her food, security and accommodation, but there was a condition attached: she had to earn her living by prostituting herself.

In order to gain a better understanding of child prostitution, careful consideration should be given to the broader lived social experiences of children, their family environment and the type of neighbourhood they live in (Jesson 1993). Other factors to consider are their economic position, which may compel them to engage in prostitution (McMillan 1995, Reid 1995). Moreover, a link is also made between the type of residential care given to young people and prostitution (Barrett & Becket 1996, O'Neill et al 1995, Thompson 1995b).

When care in children's residential homes fails to provide for their social, psychological and emotional needs, children are known to run away from these homes. Some of these institutions – as frequently reported by the media – have been found to practise child abuse. It is hence understandable that escaping an alien abusive environment is favoured. One can argue, therefore, that some foster homes and children's homes may not be appropriate places for children in need. Social policies (Barrett 1995) that do not tackle the social and welfare problems of chil-

dren's prostitution, can perpetuate the phenomenon. Jesson (1993) argued that other social forces, such as decreased sexual satisfaction in the family, make some men look for alternative sexual gratification, which can be obtained from prostitutes. Commercial sex is hence seen to be part of the normal social structure with specific economic and social management of tension (appeasing the dissatisfied, frustrated person). This view reflects the functionalist perspective, which postulates the positive functions of prostitution in society.

On the other hand, the literature makes frequent reference to the prostitutes' perspective: commercial sex is work, which guarantees some income to help cope with economic adversity. Feminists often interpret prostitution as another expression of male domination over women (Jesson 1993).

In relation to children, however, one is concerned with the exercise of adult power over children whose vulnerability and inclination to seek social, emotional and psychological security force them into prostitution, to gain acceptance and to economically survive. While runaways and homeless children enter a trajectory of prostitution, it must be acknowledged that, to many children still living with their parents, prostitution is already the norm. Grandparents, uncles, aunts and others (mothers, fathers etc.) prostitute their children for sexual and financial gains (Itzin 1996) (Case example 3.5).

Case example 3.5 illustrates the trusting relationship that children have with significant people in their environment, sometimes with disastrous consequences for their well-being. It is

Case example 3.5 Prostitution and pornography

> 'We were taken out where we met strangers and other children. Me and my brother and sister were taken there ... I was taken by my aunt, by uncles, by my grandfather ... It was after one of these sessions – where we'd be in group sex, but without the cameras – that I saw my grandfather buy the pictures, and I knew that he must have been involved in the pornography too ...' (Itzin 1996).

a social problem and interventionary strategies are needed to confront it. Several measures can be taken. These are outlined below.

INTERVENTIONARY STRATEGIES

Interventions become effective only when a thorough awareness and assessment of children's views is developed and understood. A humanistic approach is needed. To achieve this aim, informal, non-stigmatizing interviews must be undertaken with targeted clients. An empathetic approach conducive to establishing a therapeutic relationship becomes necessary. Such measures ensure that the foundation is laid for:

1. encouraging the clients to express their feelings related to their lived experiences
2. assessing and identifying the predisposing and precipitating factors in their social background which channelled them into prostitution
3. encouraging and developing their potential to minimize self-harm and to promote health
4. identifying specific needs so that appropriate agencies can be contacted (e.g. Child Protection Unit; Prostitute Outreach Workers).

MOBILIZING COMMUNITY RESOURCES

A combination of positive initiatives implemented throughout various community health projects aim to counteract the growing problem of child/juvenile prostitution. The role of 'peer empowerment worker' at Prostitute Outreach Workers is one such initiative. Its purpose is to utilize the resources and experiences of teenagers to empower themselves, through discussions, listening to personal problems, advising and guiding as necessary, outreaching other teenagers. The peer worker goes on drug training courses and gains knowledge in sexual health through a Genito-Urinary Medicine Department (O'Neill et al 1995). Other services provided focus on support and counselling, information and education. The philosophy inherent in this type of approach is to integrate health, social and welfare services and voluntary organizations, with the help of women working as prostitutes, in collaboration to promote change and a healthy lifestyle.

Health education and promotion are vital aspects of care. Many juvenile prostitutes are unaware of services available to them. McMillan (1995) made reference to the 'Base 75 Drop-in Centre' in the red light district of Glasgow. It is a health-related care resource centre for local women sex workers. An adaptation of this facility could be organized for juvenile sex workers. The team of health care workers (nurses and medical staff with experience in district nursing, psychiatric nursing etc.) can advise on physical–sexual–mental health matters, while maintaining close liaison with the social work department.

It is, nevertheless, recognized (Reid 1995) that providing health care is not easily achieved. It has been argued that many sex workers do not gain easy access to services. One project aiming to minimize this problem is the 'Safe HIV Outreach Project' in Birmingham. Reid explained that nursing staff at the centre aim to look 'for women working in all areas of the sex industry'. A weekly clinic advising on sexual and reproductive health provides the workers with the necessary information, while preserving confidentiality. According to Barrett and Beckett (1996), accessibility can be improved by the provision of informal drop-in centres, advice lines and mobile services.

In combination with the above, other initiatives that aim to confront the problem of prostitution consist of providing sanctuaries to children by the Children's Society. Moreover, as Thompson (1995a) pointed out, effective measures rely on professionals working across boundaries. In some context, coordinators of sanctuaries such as 'Refuge For Underage Runaways' in London, and the Barnardo's Street and Lanes Project in Bradford, may work with anti-vice units.

Communicating and disseminating information between professionals can help anticipate and prevent problems. For example, strategic planning and implementation of measures by collaborative work between the police, the social services and local children's homes will help identify children prone to go missing, and those likely to be exposed to situations that can be exploitative.

Activity 3.5

Design a model of interagency collaboration work using a labelled diagram.

??? Question 3.5

1. What do you consider to be effective health and social care in relation to child prostitution?
2. In view of the increasing social problem linked to prostitution, what measures can be implemented to combat it?
3. Can child prostitution be prevented? How can this be achieved?

WAR CHILDREN

The abuse of children in different parts of the world can take many forms. To use children as soldiers in national defence demonstrates another extreme of abuse and child exploitation, which reflects one dimension of social ill-fare in some societies. The health consequences are traumatic: psychological trauma, social isolation, criminality (children can kill as early as 7–10 years old), post-traumatic stress disorders which can take many years to treat. Besides, the physical effects are obvious: malnutrition caused by economic deprivation and inadequate food production, worsened by poverty and war (Cliff & Noormahomed 1993). Infectious diseases are the norm, due to lack of sanitation as children and their families live in overcrowded conditions, and where the vaccination and health care facilities have been dismantled.

Child soldiers who are deprived of their childhood (Feeney 1995) are as vulnerable as non-warring children. They become exposed to a life of misery, behaving as 'quasi-adults', taking part in activities severely detrimental to their social and psychological health. Under these circumstances, brutal killing by children as young as 8–10 becomes an accepted behaviour. The penalty for refusing to become child soldiers is physical abuse and death (Carlisle 1998). Children are coerced, as in Uganda and Mozambique in Africa, into participating in atrocities, which may in some cases involve killing their own parents. Girls are abducted to become sexual slaves, or alternatively beaten to death for refusing to join the children's army. Surviving children may be maimed by landmines (Carlisle 1995). In addition they find themselves being cared for in deprived care centres, where conditions are poor and infectious diseases can spread and prove difficult to control (Cliff & Noormahomed 1993, Carlisle 1995, Feeney 1995).

The consequences for children surviving exposure to atrocities and attempting to cope with the adult responsibilities of managing warfare are wide-ranging. For this reason health workers must apply their full potential in managing the rehabilitation process.

REHABILITATION WORK

Child soldiers are abused children. They are the exploited victims of a system which breaks the safety barriers of child protection afforded to other children in peacetime. The realities of war mean that child soldiers become abusers, while being exposed to physical and sexual abuse themselves by their parents, strangers and aid workers (Plunkett & Southall 1997). Rehabilitation must therefore consist of meeting their psychological needs, while attending to their physical need for well-balanced nutritious meals (provided in feeding centres), and control of malarial and sexually transmitted diseases, diarrhoea and respiratory complaints.

Children become displaced from their family surroundings in wartime. Attempts to reunite them should be made. Post-traumatic stress disorder effects can be expected: withdrawal behaviour, loss of appetite, acting out behaviour (aggression), nightmares, convulsions (Carlisle 1998). Other features that may be observed are grief reactions, anxiety disorders, bedwetting and hyperactivity (Turner 1996). Grief and loss reactions related to loss of normal childhood, altered body image (disfigurement, blindness, long-term physical disabilities), in addition to loss of parental support, compound anxiety and feelings of vulnerability. Children also feel physically vulnerable: their immune systems are weakened by infection and they are prone to developing a variety of infectious diseases (Plunkett & Southall 1997).

Rehabilitative measures must encompass provision for counselling: listening and giving emotional support. Turner (1996) recommends the benefits of community-based counselling centres, in addition to the involvement of families in helping to 'heal their children's war-torn minds' within a community-based psychosocial model.

Rehabilitation is, however, a long-term process, with heavy reliance on community support; rallying informal support (families, friends, neighbours) becomes particularly important. The achievement of this objective requires parents and significant others to be educated, and trust to be built between children, families and health workers.

Aid workers must be prepared for children to experience behavioural difficulties and to be disturbed. Where emotional and behavioural disturbance can be observed, local community support under supervised professional expertise is beneficial (Leff 1998).

Some children showing signs of social withdrawal may be helped to express their emotions via the draw-and-write technique. The results can thereafter be analysed by the psychologist and psychiatrist, and the findings used by health workers and welfare agencies to guide their practice.

 Activity 3.6

Write to the World Health Organization in Geneva to obtain some literature related to war children in different parts of the world.

??? Question 3.6

What approach should health workers use to meet the needs of child soldiers and their families?

CHILDREN AS CARERS

Children have, for many years, been the invisible carers of their parents. Many have become their parents' parents because of the amount of care they provide. These children have been invisible to the social welfare agencies and to health care professionals in the community. In many cases, they were not recognized as carers by their own families and by themselves, undertaking tasks such as lifting adults with mobility problems, which would prove detrimental to children's health. Since the NHS and Community Care Act of 1990 – implemented in 1993 – made reference to 'carers' in the community the plight of the latter is being increasingly acknowledged, although the Act does not refer to children as carers.

Over and above these developments, the Carers (Recognition and Services) Act of 1995, as well as the influences of pressure groups such as the Carers National Association (CNA), Action For Carers and Young Carers Project, have added to the debate on awareness raising. Additionally, community care literature has contributed in highlighting the inadequacies and constraints of present social and health care services in meeting the individual needs of child carers.

The needs of all carers are manifold and complex; for children acting as carers, those needs can affect their future. Children caring for their parents have been known to be absent from school and to fail their exams more frequently than non-carers. Their educational needs are therefore not met (Aldridge & Becker 1993a, George 1995, Dearden & Becker 1997) as a result of family needs imposing constraints on them. It is this kinship obligation which ties the young vulnerable carers to the bedside of the sick and disabled parent(s) (Case example 3.6).

Case example 3.6 Tommy

'I am 10 years old. I would like to go to school more often, but I can't. I have to look after my mother who is paralysed in one leg. She has multiple sclerosis. I feel very tired most mornings. Some nights I would stay up for 4 hours because my mother feels very depressed. She cries and asks for my help. I wish my father was around more often. But he works away, and comes home only at the weekend.'

Disabled parents are in a vulnerable position too. Their inability to self-care could mean separation from their home environment and into residential care following decisions from officialdom. To the child carer, it means family breakdown and foster care or care in a children's home, to compensate for parental loss. As Dearden and Becker (1997) point out, their vulnerable position could be exposed by social welfare agencies and health care agencies. It is, however, argued that carers and their sick relatives go to great lengths to maintain the status quo to avoid detection because they fear the personal and social implications.

In addition to educational needs, young carers have a need for information concerning their rights as carers. They need to know to what extent they can extend their caring role. Since they perform intimate tasks (e.g. helping to wash their parents and taking them to the toilet), which in many cases consists of moving and lifting, they are involved in situations with implications for their physical and psychoemotional well-being.

CARING FOR THE CARERS

Support for children carers must be tailored according to individual needs (Cohen 1995b). Assessment of needs should include identifying the age of carers, since some carers could be very young. Secondly, professional awareness must be raised by the provision of training strategies. Training will develop professionals' insight into the complex nature of their work, and increase their sensitivity to the presence of child carers in highly demanding situations of family sickness

Box 3.9 Visit from the district nurse

The district nurse was surprised to find Mrs Smith on her own in the house, considering her frailty, after discharge from the hospital. Her records did not indicate that she had any children. The nurse did, however, still ask her: 'I understand that you do get some help from the children?' Mrs Smith replied she had no children, but her two nieces came sometimes to help. When asked how old the nieces were, Mrs Smith replied '12 and 15'.

and ill-health. During their home visits, questions could be asked about the number of children in the family (Box 3.9).

Discreet observations of children's behaviour in their interactions with parents could be made. Alternatively, direct interactions with the child(ren) present can be instigated, by conversing with them about their feelings concerning their parents' conditions. For example, one can ask: 'How is your mum/dad getting on?'; 'Has your grandad managed to eat his breakfast this morning?' 'How did you help him?'. Open-ended questions may help to broaden the scope of responses, especially when the encounters take place away from the parents.

Carers' needs in regard to leisure time and time for homework can be markedly impaired (Case example 3.7). Their personal worries may include meeting educational deadlines; a difficult objective to achieve when their time is constrained with family obligations. In this context, unless children are able to voice their problems to teachers, they are likely to be perceived as lazy, incompetent and uncooperative. Children have a need to communicate their feelings concerning

Case example 3.7 Mandy's story

'I am 13. Most of my time is spent either helping to move my elderly auntie, with the help of my younger sister, to the bathroom, or cleaning the house. Very often, I am expected to prepare the meals too. When my school friends, who live only six houses down the street, come to ask me to join them in the playground, I have to refuse. I make some excuses, like "I am not feeling well today, or my uncle is visiting us today".'

their living conditions. Opportunities must be provided to them for reflection, away from the caring environment. George (1995) argued for a network of support, involving social services, the youth and community service, health services and the Carers National Association. Support can be provided in the field of education, for example, to ensure children have time for revision, away from caring responsibilities, while receiving support in time and crisis management (George 1995), and to ascertain they have time to manage school homework (Cohen 1995a).

With reference to leisure time – an important aspect in childhood development – the provision of respite care for the disabled parent can provide freedom for the child to interact with children in other relatives' homes, meet friends and go on organized visits to places of interest. Time may also be spent writing, reading and listening to the radio or watching television.

Carers, however, need reassurance and conviction that these initiatives are tailored for their personal needs, and that officials in health care and social services are sensitive to such needs. Cohen (1995b) explained that young carers fear official intervention, and may perceive their efforts (the officials) as intrusive and an attempt to instigate care proceedings. In addition, children may refuse help due to their parents discouraging them. However, Cohen pointed out that non-stigmatizing intervention by the voluntary sector is positively welcomed by young carers. When the children are seen within the school environment, or at a voluntary agency, there is less inhibition.

PROFESSIONALS' ROLE

Professionals have a duty to demonstrate awareness and sensitivity towards young carers. Moreover, their training needs in regard to project initiatives for carers must be developed. In addition, their style of intervention will determine whether parents and their carers will accept their credibility. Cohen (1995b) documented that some families strive to give impressions that they are coping well, to prevent their carers from being removed from the home. Under this framework,

Cohen (1995a) pointed out, training to develop professionals' assessment of needs strategies must be available. In addition, attending conferences and seminars will contribute in assimilating knowledge concerning practices in other health and social care settings. It is important that training encompasses the multiprofessional dimension, while recognizing the need to consider the 'whole family, including parents and children within it' (Cohen 1995a).

While social workers are responsible for evaluating the care needs of sick relatives and the network of carers (George 1997), their assessment tools must be sensitive enough to detect the presence of not only adult carers, but young vulnerable carers as well. Assessment and evaluation of needs must be followed by delivery of services. Welfare agencies must hence help to reduce the impact of consequences of caring on carers by:

1. not perceiving carers on an instrumental basis (i.e. instead of formal statutory provision) (Twigg 1994)
2. mobilizing community resources as effectively as possible to implement care for carers and their families
3. utilizing social and health care personnel's interpersonal skills to develop community-based initiatives
4. aiming to empower vulnerable groups, while recognizing the latter may be operating within specific environmental constraints (Bridges & Lynam 1993)
5. developing an understanding of the possible long-term physical and psychosocial effects of caring on children (Aldridge & Becker 1993b).

In relation to the above, a comprehensive assessment of needs is essential. Professional judgement is exercised in cases when other professionals must be involved, e.g. psychologists and community psychiatric workers, to evaluate the psychological status of carers and their families; paediatricians to assess the physical development aspects; social workers and other community staff to evaluate the socio-economic status of carers and their families.

Findings from an assessment must be collated and made easily available to the network of care professionals. The data will ensure that care implementation meets the targeted group's needs.

Activity 3.7

Write notes in your learning journal on the objectives you have achieved after reading this chapter.

??? Question 3.7

1. To what extent do you think society is responsible for increasing children's vulnerability to exploitation?
2. What examples can you give of situations in community health practice when professionals can demonstrate collaborative approaches in care implementation?

SUMMARY

In this chapter, consideration has been given to the needs of children in a variety of social settings. Their needs, as discussed, have not always been given the attention they deserve. Consequently, children – due to their immaturity, need for affection and need to be nurtured – have been abused and neglected. In many cases, evidence points to a culture, or cycle, of abuse and exploitation. In other situations one finds personal, social and environmental factors, as well as psychological reasons precipitating children toward behavioural changes that are detrimental to their social, psychoemotional well-being; for example, by becoming abusers themselves, by engaging in prostitution or by working as child soldiers. Whatever behaviour is being demonstrated by children, professionals at all levels of clinical practice and across professional boundaries must exercise a non-judgemental and empathetic attitude. In particular, sensitivity toward the wider social context of the child must be shown, while realizing the important functions of families. The latter have needs for support, parental training, counselling and health education.

GLOSSARY

Aetiology   the cause of a disease
Anorexia   loss of appetite that is disease-related
Callus   layers of new bone formed following a fracture
Cerebral palsy   a disorder, which affects movement due to non-progressive damage to the brain
Correlation   the degree to which one phenomenon can be linked with, or can be predicted from, another
Delusion   false beliefs incompatible with one's educational and cultural background
Detached retina   separation of the inner layers of the three tunics of the eyeball
Ghettoization   to be segregated from others
Hallucinatory   characterized by changes in one's senses (i.e. vision, sight, smell, touch, hearing) in the absence of any external stimuli
Hypothermia   below normal body temperature
Identification   in psychology, how an individual comes to think, feel and behave as another person, e.g. sons and daughters identify with their father or mother
Intrafamilial   within the family
Melanasian   inhabitants of Pacific islands (e.g. New Guinea, Solomon Islands etc.)
Personality disorder   an individual's characteristics causing antisocial behaviour, characterized by aggression and violence in some cases

Post-traumatic stress disorder   an anxiety disorder that affects individuals exposed to traumatic events (e.g. war, rape, plane crash). The effects may be delayed and may persist for many years after the trauma
Primarily socialized   in sociological terms, the initial education and training given to children by their parents
Psychosocial   the interactions and relationships of psychological and social factors which may affect an individual (e.g. emotional needs and family support needs)
Psychotherapy   treatment based on psychological principles
Schizophrenia   a mental illness characterized by disorders of thoughts and mood, affecting the sense of self
Social learning   the theory that individuals learn from interactions with their environment
Socio-emotional   factors in the social environment, which trigger emotional responses: e.g. fear, anger, sadness
Sociopathic   antisocial personality disorder
Subjectivity   refers to the feelings of individuals and their perceptions, not perceptible to the senses of another person
Trobrianders   people of the Kiriwina Islands lying off Eastern New Guinea
Urethritis   inflammation of the urethra
Vaginitis   inflammation of the vagina
Vulva   female external genitalia

REFERENCES

Aldridge J, Becker S 1993a Children as carers. Archives of Disease in Childhood 69(4): 459–462

Aldridge J, Becker S 1993b Punishing children for caring: the hidden cost of young carers. Children and Society 7(4): 376–387

Allan A 1995 Effects of parental loss in childhood. Psychiatry in Practice 14(3): 6–8

Appleton J V 1996 Working with vulnerable families: a health visiting perspective. Journal of Advanced Nursing 23(5): 912–918

Axinn W G, Thornton A 1996 The influence of parents' marital dissolutions on children's attitudes toward family formation. Demography 33(1): 66–81

Baldwin C 1996 Munchausen syndrome by proxy: problems of definition, diagnosis and treatment. Health and Social Care in the Community 4(3): 159–165

Baldwin M A 1994 Munchausen syndrome by proxy: neurological manifestations. Journal of Neuroscience Nursing 26(1): 18–23

Barber B L, Eccles J S 1992 Long-term influence of divorce and single parenting on adolescent family- and work-related values, behaviours and aspirations. Psychological Bulletin 111(1): 108–126

Barrett D 1995 Child prostitution. Highlight 135: 1–2

Barrett D, Beckett W 1996 Child prostitution: reaching out to children who sell sex to survive. British Journal of Nursing 5(18): 1120–1125

Beck P, Biank N 1997 Enhancing therapeutic intervention during divorce. Journal of Analytic Social Work 4(3): 63–81

Blumenthal I 1994 Child abuse: a handbook for health care practitioners. Edward Arnold, London, p 10

Bond H 1997 No excuses allowed. Community Care Issue 1179: 23

Bridges J M, Lynam M J 1993 Informal carers: a Marxist analysis of social, political, and economic forces underpinning the role. Advances in Nursing Science 15(3): 33–48

Brown H, Stein J, Turk V 1995 The sexual abuse of adults with learning disabilities: report of a second two-year incidence survey. Mental Handicap Research 8(1): 3–24

Brunngraber L S 1986 Father–daughter incest: immediate and long-term effects of sexual abuse. Advances in Nursing Science 8(4): 15–35

Buchanan A 1996 Cycles of child maltreatment facts, fallacies and interventions. John Wiley, Chichester

Bynum M K, Durm M W 1996 Children of divorce and its effect on their self-esteem. Psychological Reports 79(2): 447–450

Byrne C 1995 A model for supervision. Primary Health Care 5(1): 21–22

Carlisle D 1995 Children of Goma. Nursing Times 91(2): 14–15

Carlisle D 1998 Child soldiers: pulling back from the abyss. Health Visitor 71(1): 8–10

Cashman H, Higgs M, Flynte R 1992 The health consequences of child sexual abuse. Journal of Advances in Health and Nursing Care 2(1): 61–72

Cassin A L 1996 Acute maternal mental illness: infants at risk. A community focus. Psychiatric Care 2(6): 202–205

Clark C 1997 Post-traumatic stress disorder: how to support healing. American Journal of Nursing 97(8): 27–32

Cleaver H, Freeman P 1996 Child abuse which involves wider kin and family friends. In: Bibby P C (ed) Organised abuse: the current debate. Arena, Aldershot, p 231–244

Cliff J, Noormahomed A R 1993 The impact of war on children's health in Mozambique. Social Science Medicine 36(7): 843–848

Cohen P 1995a Rights issue. Community Care 1091: 26

Cohen P 1995b Looking after mum. Community Care 1055: 18–19

Dearden C, Becker S 1997 Protecting young carers: legislative tensions and opportunities in Britain. Journal of Social Welfare and Family Law 19(2): 123–138

Dickson N 1997 Dirty little secrets. Nursing Times 93(45): 22

Dillon P A, Emery R E 1996 Divorce mediation and resolution of child custody disputes: long-term effects. American Journal of Orthopsychiatry 66(1): 131–140

Dubowitz H, King H 1995 Family violence: a child-centered, family-focused approach. Pediatric Clinics of North America 42(1): 153–163

Elliott B J, Richards M P 1991 Children and divorce: educational performance and behaviour before and after parental separation. International Journal of Law and the Family 5(3): 258–276

Emery R E, Coiro M J 1995 Divorce: consequences for children. Paediatrics in Review 16(8): 306–310

Feeney B 1995 Teaching aid. Nursing Times 91(10): 42–44

George M 1995 Campaign: young carers. Community Care 1081: 22

George M 1997 Into the unknown. Community Care 1176: 26–27

Gray O P 1987 Violence and children. Archives of Disease in Childhood 62(4): 428–430

Gulland A 1997 Abuse, spies and videotape. Nursing Times 93(45): 12–13

Hall J M 1996 Geography of childhood sexual abuse: women's narratives of their childhood environments. Advances in Nursing Science 18(4): 29–47

Harold G 1997 Children's perceptions of marital conflict have lasting effects on their development. Childright 139: 8–9

Hartnup T 1996 Divorce and marital strife and their effects on children. Archives of Disease in Childhood 75(1): 1–8

Hilton M R, Mezey G C 1996 Victims and perpetrators of child sexual abuse. British Journal of Psychiatry 169(4): 408–415

Hobbs C J, Heywood P L 1997 Childhood matters: doctors have a vital role of identifying children at risk of abuse. British Medical Journal 314: 622

Hobbs C J, Wynne J M 1990 The sexually abused battered child. Archives of Disease in Childhood 65(4): 423–427

Hobbs C J, Wynne J M 1996 Physical signs of child abuse: a colour atlas. W B Saunders, London, p 103

Horowitz L A, Putnam F W, Noll J G, Trickett P K 1997 Factors affecting utilization of treatment services by sexually abused girls. Child Abuse and Neglect 21(1): 35–48

House A 1997 Damned if you do … Nursing Times 93(46): 38–39

Humphreys C 1997 Child sexual abuse allegations in the context of divorce: issues for mothers. British Journal of Social Work 27(4): 529–544

Itzin C 1996 Pornography and the organisation of child sexual abuse. In: Bibby P C (ed) Organised abuse: the current debate. Arena, Aldershot, p 167–196

Iwaniec D 1997 Evaluating parent training for emotionally abusive and neglectful parents: comparing individual versus individual and group intervention. Research on Social Work Practice 7(3): 329–349

Jesson J 1993 Understanding adolescent female prostitution: a literature review. British Journal of Social Work 23(5): 517–530

Johnson P 1990 Understanding the problem: child abuse. Crowood Press, Marlborough

Kasen S, Cohen P, Brook J S, Hartmark C 1996 A multiple-risk interaction model: effects of temperament and divorce on psychiatric disorders in children. Journal of Abnormal Child Psychology 24(2): 121–150

Kiernan K E 1992 The impact of family disruption in childhood on transitions made in young adult life. Population Studies 46(2): 213–234

Klebes C, Fay S 1995 Munchausen syndrome by proxy: a review, case study and nursing implications. Journal of Paediatric Nursing: Nursing Care of Children and Families 10(2): 93–98

Knight B 1991 Simpson's forensic medicine, 10th edn. Edward Arnold, London, p 197–205

LaFontaine J 1996 Ritual abuse: research findings. In: Bibby P (ed) Organised abuse: the current debate. Arena, Aldershot

Lawrence R A 1997 Child abuse examination enquiry. Journal of Clinical Forensic Medicine 4(2): 73–76

Lee K 1991 The healing way. Community Care 869: p 24–25

Leff S 1998 Disturbed children: local support or specialist referral? Health Visitor 71(1): 19–20

Lynch M A 1992 Physical signs of abuse in children. Archives of Disease in Childhood 67(4): 565–566

McLay W S 1990 Clinical forensic medicine. Pinter, London, p 211–233

McClure A 1997 Opportunity youth: a holistic service for young people. Health Education 5: 175–182

McMillan I 1995 Touching base. Nursing Times 91(33): 27–28

Malinowski B 1987 The sexual life of savages in Northwestern Melanesia. Beacon Press, Boston

Masson H 1995 Children and adolescents who sexually abuse other children: responses to an emergency problem. Journal of Social Welfare and Family Law 17(3): 325–336

Mercer S O, Perdue J D 1993 Munchausen syndrome by proxy: social work's role. Journal of the National Association of Social Workers 38(1): 74–81

Miles M 1991 Implications of The Children Act for paediatricians. Archives of Disease in Childhood 66(4): 457–461

Moncrieff J, Drummond D C, Candy B et al 1996 Sexual abuse in people with alcohol problems: a study of the prevalence of sexual abuse and its relationships to drinking behaviour. British Journal of Psychiatry 169(3): 355–360

Montgomery S M, Bartley M J, Wilkinson R G 1997 Family conflict and slow growth. Archives of Disease in Childhood 77(4): 326–330

Moore J 1991 Child abuse: women can … and do. Community Care 857: 17–18

Mott F L, Kowaleski-Jones L, Menaghan E G 1997 Paternal absence and child behaviour: does a child's gender make a difference? Journal of Marriage and the Family 59(1): 103–118

NCH Action For Children 1994 The hidden victims: children and domestic violence. NCH Action For Children, London

Neale B, Smart C 1997 Experiments with parenthood? Sociology 31(2): 201–219

Neate P 1995 Reflections of the past. Community Care 1057: 25

Neate P, Sone K 1991 Sex, lives and videotape. Community Care 858: 12–15

O'Neill M, Goode N, Hopkins K 1995 Juvenile prostitution: the experience of young women in residential care. Childright 113: 14–16

Payne M 1995 Understanding 'going missing': issues for social work and social services. British Journal of Social Work 25(3): 333–348

Plunkett M C, Southall D P 1997 Children and war. Ambulatory Child Health 3(2): 162–169

Polnay L, Hull D 1993 Community paediatrics, 2nd edn. Churchill Livingstone, Edinburgh, p 262

Powell C 1997 Child protection: the crucial role of the children's nurse. Paediatric Nursing 9(9): 13–16

Pridmore P J, Lansdown R G 1997 Exploring children's perception of health: does drawing really break down barriers? Health Education Journal 56(3): 219–230

Puri B K, Laking P J, Treasaden I H 1996 Textbook of psychiatry. Churchill Livingstone, New York, p 304

Reardon W, Hughes H E, Green S H 1992 Anal abnormalities in childhood myotonic dystrophy: a possible source of confusion in child sexual abuse. Archives of Disease in Childhood 67(4): 527–528

Reid T 1995 A street-wise approach. Nursing Times 91(33): 24–26

Richards N 1997 Paediatric care and child health legislation. Health Visitor 70(10): 385–387

Rogers W S 1989 Introduction. In: Rogers W S, Hevey D, Ash E (eds) Child abuse and neglect. BT Batsford, London

Ross S M 1996 Risk of physical abuse to children of spouse-abusing parents. Child Abuse and Neglect 20(7): 589–598

Sadler C 1997 Child abuse: caught on film. Health Visitor 70(12): 447

Sheeber L, Hops H, Alpert A et al 1997 Family support and conflict: prospective relations to adolescent depression. Journal of Abnormal Child Psychology 25(4): 333–344

Siddall R 1997a Keep them safe. Community Care 1178: 18–19

Siddall R 1997b Child abuse damage limitation. Community Care 1195: 24–25

Speight N 1987 Case conferences for child abuse. Archives of Disease in Childhood 62(10): 1063–1065

Spencer N J 1987 Non-accidental injury and child abuse (battered baby syndrome, Silverman's syndrome, non-organic failure to thrive). In: Black J A (ed) Paediatric emergencies, 2nd edn. Butterworth, London, p 533–537

Stanhope R, Wilks Z, Hamill G 1994 Psychosocial aspects of growth. Failure to grow: lack of food or lack of love? Professional Care of Mother and Child 4(8): 234–237

Stark C, Paterson B, Henderson T et al 1997 Counting the dead. Nursing Times 93(46): 34–37

Stark M M, Rogers D J, Howitt J 1997 Domestic violence: do physicians have a role? Journal of Clinical Forensic Medicine 4(2): 59–63

Taitz L S, King J M 1988 A profile of abuse. Archives of Disease in Childhood 63(9): 1026–1031

Thompson A 1995a Abuse by any other name. Community Care 1091: 16–18

Thompson A 1995b Practice focus: young abusers fresh beginnings. Community Care 1062: 10

Turk V, Brown H 1993 The sexual abuse of adults with learning disabilities: results of a two-year incidence survey. Mental Handicap Research 6(3): 193–216

Turner T 1996 Counselling child victims of war. Health Visitor 69(7): 263–264

Tuttle G 1992 Divorce: how are the children coping? Canadian Nurse 88(11): 13–16

Twigg J 1994 Carers, families, relatives: socio-legal conceptions of caregiving relationships. Journal of Social Welfare and Family Law 16(3): 279–298

Utting D 1995 Family and parenthood supporting families, preventing breakdown. Joseph Rowntree Foundation, York, p 45

Valente S M 1992 The challenge of ritualistic child abuse. Journal of Child and Adolescent Psychiatric and Mental Health Nursing 5(2): 37–46

Volz A G 1995 Nursing interventions in Munchausen syndrome by proxy. Journal of Psychosocial Nursing and Mental Services 33(9): 51–88

Westlake D, Pearson M 1997 Child protection and health promotion: whose responsibility? Journal of Social Welfare and Family Law 19(2): 139–158

Whittaker D K, Aitken M, Burfitt E, Sibert J R 1997 Assessing bite marks in children: working with a forensic dentist. Ambulatory Child Health 3(3): 225–229

Wigglesworth A, Agnew J, Campbell H, Jones J G 1996 The Centre for the Vulnerable Child: a new model for the therapeutic provision for abused children and their families. Public Health 110(6): 373–377

FURTHER READING

Caplan G 1987 Guidance for divorcing parents. Archives of Disease in Childhood 62(7): 752–753

Cooney T M, Smith L A 1996 Young adults' relations with grandparents following recent parental divorce. Journal of Gerontology: Social Sciences 51b(2): s91–s95

Elliott B J, Richards M 1991 Effects of parental divorce on children. Archives of disease in Childhood 66(8): 915–916

Falshaw L, Browne K 1997 Adverse childhood experiences and violent acts of young people in secure accommodation. Journal of Mental Health 6(5): 443–455

Irazuzta J E, McJunkin J E, Danadian K et al 1997 Outcome and cost of child abuse. Child Abuse and Neglect 21(8): 751–757

Linehan T 1997 Insight: lost children: who cares? Nursing Times 93(22): 22–25

Mason J 1997 Insight: care and control. Nursing Times 93(22): 25–26

Naish J 1997 Dangerous assumptions. Nursing Times 93(46): 37–38

Trinder L 1997 Competing constructions of childhood: children's rights and children's wishes in divorce. Journal of Social Welfare and Family Law 19(3): 247–376

Valman B, Chiswick M 1988 Controversy follow-up. Sexual abuse: the final word? Archives of Disease in Childhood 63(4): 446–447

Ward H, Cavanagh J 1997 A descriptive study of the self-perceived needs of carers for dependants with a range of long-term problems. Journal of Public Health Medicine 19(3): 281–287

The needs of the older person in society

The United Kingdom has an ageing population. Between 1961 and 1996, the number of people aged 85 and over trebled to nearly 1.1 million (Central Statistics Office 1998). It is anticipated that during 2030–2039 the numbers of people aged 65 and over will rise to over 15 million. For social scientists, politicians, economists, and health and welfare organizations, this increase has implications for society. In this chapter some major social issues are considered which concern the health needs of older people. Helping the old to maintain a healthy lifestyle is a priority, particularly in the domain of healthy ageing, the prevention of ageism, and its extreme forms, which are becoming regular social problems: violence and abuse. The interplay between the person and the environment is emphasized, and how social circumstances as well as biological factors can impinge on emotional well-being. The role of professionals and informal carers in the field of prevention and care is discussed.

WHAT IS AGEISM?

The concept of ageism can be defined as the expression of negative attitudes towards the aged. The behaviour displayed is discriminatory in nature, denigrating persons on the basis that they are old. The tendency to use stereotypical terms such as 'old bat', 'wrinkly', 'dirty old man' and 'gerries' reflect negative images of old people. Associated with ageism is the term 'stigma'.

Stigma refers to a 'blemish', a negative feature or characteristic of an individual. It is a label that focuses on the deficits of the person (Herrick et al 1997), at the expense of their positive characteristics. The effects on the individual can be damaging, causing lowered self-esteem, emotional and social anxiety (Whitehead 1995) and isolation, leading to group marginalization. Herrick et al commented that menopausal women were once stigmatized, and feminist writers have drawn our attention to the 'psychologization' of women's physical needs and problems (see Chapter 5). Little attention is paid to the fact that older men and women in some societies get categorized in special groups as likely to show dependence on State resources. Older people's increased health care needs, dependence on social services for housing needs, recreational activities etc. and reliance on benefits agencies to support their financial needs are some of the areas with which political parties and pressure groups are concerned.

As old age advances, more physical and psychological problems can be expected: loss of teeth, arthritis, depression, brain failure, visual impairment and so on. Varied disabilities, the consequences of ageing, become classified as the diseases of old age. Stereotypes develop from such classifications.

Generalizations are made (Herrick et al 1997), which subsequently become labels attached to specific features of the old person who, consequently, becomes stigmatized. This is a dehumanizing and devaluative process and shows a lack of respect and sensitivity.

From the above, one can deduce that ageism comprises a pattern of social practices (Newman et al 1997). A conscious effort should be made to realize the importance of socialization influences and social learning in constructing ageist attitudes. Newman et al's research findings show that school-age children's perceptions of older adults and ageing are not as negative as adults tend to conclude. To many children in the study (69%), their grandparents were the oldest people they knew. The latter engaged in a variety of social activities with their grandchildren and were seen

as 'special persons'. Twenty-two per cent of the children reported their parents as the next information sources. Hence, parents and grandparents have an important role to play in creating positive images of old age.

While children are aware that physical changes are linked to old age, their interactions with the elderly in their environment are not negatively affected. More research is needed, however, to identify the stage at which children, teenagers and adults become influenced in developing ageist attitudes. Moreover, the social context of ageist attitude needs to be recognized. In some cultures, for example Mauritius, China, Japan, India and Greece, the old are revered, their wisdom and experience respected, their participation in family management and decision-making sought after and their grandchildren taught the high values attached to being society's elders.

AGEISM AND HEALTH CARE

Concerns have been, and are being, expressed in nursing and medical literature that ageist attitudes are still prevalent today. Additionally, as many writers have pointed out, there is a significant rise in the elderly population – those aged 75 years and over (Slevin 1991). The projected 15% rise of those aged 85 and over, between 1995 and 2019 (Nurse Education Today 1998), and the estimate that by the year 2031 there will be at least 34 000 people aged 100 or over (Greengross et al 1997), give rise to concerns that health and social services, already under-resourced, will be unable to meet the needs of an ageing population.

Ageist beliefs can derail the mobilization of specific resources aimed for the old in society. Moreover, it is argued that ageism as a socially constructed phenomena pervades the nurse educational structure (Haight et al 1994), and that the current Diploma in Nursing Studies, for example, includes only a small component of elderly care (Slevin 1991). In addition to social influences promoting ageism, the biomedical construction of ageing (Koch & Webb 1996) is implicated as well. A review of the literature shows that there is evidence of inequality in health care provision for the aged. Haight et al (1994) have reported that nursing in medicine for the elderly settings is noted to be in crisis not only in the UK, but in the USA too. This is due to the fact that qualifying professionals' areas of interests tend to focus on non-stigmatized specialties. According to the authors, 34% of their study samples chose surgical nursing, 22% paediatrics, 8% community, 4% psychiatry and 2% care of the older person. This has implications for health care practice. Lack of professional resources for this specialized group means staff shortages, causing unequal distribution of care delivery.

It can be argued, hence, that the profession is facing a major problem (Slevin 1991). Slevin's work demonstrates that the fundamental problem resides in society's framework: gender issues which promote caring, nurturing behaviour in girls, while boys are rewarded for their outward, adventuresome and macho behaviour. For this reason, Slevin argued, there are reduced male entrants in nursing. The attitudes and beliefs generated by the educational system promote gender differences and stereotypical behaviour.

Ageism in society is reflected within the profession when nurses show their preference to work in acute settings. This applies to both men and women. Professional socialization has been implicated in the process of influencing beliefs and attitudes, while reinforcing stereotypes. The quality of the experience is responsible in either developing a positive or a negative attitude.

Haight et al's study pointed to the social background experiences of students as predisposing to either a positive or negative attitude. For instance, similar to Newman et al's (1997) study on children's perception of ageing, they commented how 'grandparents had a strong positive influence on student attitudes, and that grandparents were also the most admired older people in the students' lives, even more than parents'.

These studies consolidate the notion that significant older people in the individuals' lives who are good role models, are influential in creating positive attitudes on ageing and towards the aged in society. However, negative experiences in clinical practice and the assimilation of negative values through professional socialization –

and the hidden curriculum – can cause conflicting images, discouraging full commitment in nursing the sick old person.

While it is postulated that the lay person is exposed to the social construction of ageism and its influences, exposure in clinical settings to biomedical models of ageing reinforces the belief. Koch and Webb (1996) found that a 'geriatric style' of nursing compounds the effects of ageist stereotypes (Case example 4.1).

Case example 4.1 'G for geriatric'

'I am old. I am 82, funny enough, but I don't think of myself as an old lady. I mean I found out what the G was in front of the number, I really got a bit vexed, because I didn't really think of myself as geriatric. Well, I think I am young and I am 82. I don't think that I am old at all because … I make things for old people. I was knitting here the other day. One of the nurses and a lady walked past and said what are you knitting? Bed socks I said, for the old ladies at B … and they burst out laughing'. 'Did you hear … she doesn't think that she is an old lady!' (Koch & Webb 1996).

Case example 4.1 highlights several key features pertinent to care delivery and provision:

1. the lady has a positive self-image
2. the term 'geriatric' is distressing to her and is ageist in nature
3. she perceives herself to have a positive function in society; she knits for others
4. the nurse showed unprofessional behaviour and failed to praise her and to promote independence
5. the 'G' on the case note has a negative connotation.

Koch and Webb argued that several factors have contributed to the development of an ethos of ageism:

1. attachment to a traditional and custodial approach to care
2. a mechanistic view of the aged person (the wear and tear theory: the old person is not expected to function once a specific age is attained)

3. the perpetuation of ageism in the wider community (Case example 4.2)
4. professionals in practice can conform to a medically oriented policy of care at the expense of recognizing the whole person.

Case example 4.2 The marathon runner

'My name is Ben. I am 86 years old. I am 5' 11" and weigh 11 stone. I run 3 miles every morning. It is strange really, when I think about the people I encounter on the street, and what they say when they see me running. "Old fool" "Look at him! Who does he think he is!" "Old prune! Get out of my way!" "Watch it old man!" It is interesting to know that children behave differently. One school kid said the other day: "I wish my grandpa could run like you." '

Counteracting ageism in health care demands positive implementation of policies that aim at promoting a positive image of ageing. At the higher levels of society, political parties could use media coverage to promote a purposeful image of old age. Unfortunately, in our society, political organizations (responding to pressure groups' demands) have a tendency to refer to the old during the cold winter months only, when the topic of heating bills and hypothermia is raised.

One cannot dismiss the argument that older people in need have become an economic problem (Crouch 1997). Rationing strategies in varied health care settings, Crouch argued, disable the aged; for example the giving of care priorities and treatment to younger adults. Women aged 45–105 do not have their health needs recognized (Elderly Care 1998); preventative measures to reduce disability among this group would be economically advantageous. Crouch (1997) asserted that the aged in society are socio-economically disadvantaged. The label 'bed blockers' applied to them, she argued, is ageist and derogatory. Such examples further confirm that ageism is evident in society and within health care settings (Behrens 1998).

Kohler (1998a) wrote that too much focus on health and social care services has a negative side-effect: the production of dependence thus discouraging independence. One can debate that the stereotypical view of old age has always been associated with images of social services provision and admission to gerontology wards. In addition, existing conflict and lack of integration between health and social care services due to unclear definition (George 1998), can disturb the balance between dependence and independence. Kohler (1998a) asserted that, since society is ageing, new 'structures' should be in place to help promote active and positive ageing. For instance, older people involved in volunteering as an activity (utilizing voluntary sectors), supported by the Government, will develop a sense of achievement and belonging when undertaking the functions of mentors.

The Government Green Paper on public health (Kohler 1998b) showed signs that initiatives to develop Healthy Neighbourhood Projects through Health Action Zones (alliances between local authority, health authorities and voluntary agencies to promote health) are measures that could promote positive ageing. While the development of positive ageing is recommended, political and social policy forces must be integrated to raise awareness of ageism in society by implementing anti-ageism campaigns. Media reports often make reference to 'racism' and 'discrimination' in connection with minority groups. However, when the aged are mugged, sexually assaulted and murdered, the term 'ageism' is not used. The battered old person is reported as another victim of assault to be added to existing statistics; yet killing the aged is an extreme form of ageism.

In clinical practice, Nazarko (1997) pointed out, under-resourced care within gerontology departments does not make headlines. On the other hand, under-funding in acute care settings would receive immediate media attention. There is a failure to recognize that elderly care is a specialized field (Nazarko 1996).

Ageism is a sensitive and covert issue which emerges to the surface in a variety of practice settings. Professionals have a duty to expose this form of discrimination and to promote ageing as a healthy developmental process.

Activity 4.1

1. Ask children in your neighbourhood to explain the word 'old'. How do they view an old person?
2. Using a sheet of paper, prepare a poster to raise people's awareness of ageism.
3. Ask some 80- to 90-year-old individuals their perceptions of themselves in relation to younger adults.

??? **Question 4.1**

1. How evident is ageism in society?
2. Should the media be using the term 'ageism' in relation to matters which discriminate against the older person?

Ageism and mental health care

Ageist behaviour in the wider community and in care settings can affect the older person's mental health in a negative way. Although ageism can be expressed in subtle ways by one's attitude and non-verbal communication, the old person is still sensitive and conscious of people's behaviour. Even when confusional states are evident, there are brief periods when the individual's conscious awareness is recovered. Similarly, an unconscious patient may still hear conversations, which they will later recall and comment on. When the aged person perceives that others in the environment view their ageing in a negative way, ageism is reinforced, and some may adopt a defeatist attitude (Case example 4.3).

Older people may become passive recipients of a regimen of undervalued comments, which have implications for their mental well-being. Emotional dysfunction: depressed mood and feelings of unworthiness (the result of a lack of social support) have all been linked to increased mortality and morbidity (Grant 1996). An ageist approach to mental health assessment may lead to a failure to identify and/or recognize mental health deterioration due to heavy reliance on the physical symptoms (Grant 1996) and the stereotypical view that the old person's complaints tend to be mainly physical in nature. In addition, Grant noted that the person's self-perception,

Case example 4.3 A losing battle

Since he took early retirement at age 60 due to ill-health, Jim Wintern has constantly been reminded by friends and former workmates that old age has crept on him, and that he should really 'join the old folks down the road for ballroom dancing'. 'You see', they keep telling him, 'if you can't manage it, there is still the day centre in the village. You should go there, it's for people like yourself'.

'I am not that old', he keeps reminding them. 'After all I have only got arthritis in my hands'. 'There you are', his friends responded, 'only old folks get arthritis'.

'Maybe they are right. It must be old age, otherwise they would not keep on the way they do.'

influenced by negative stereotyping and stigma, may develop anxiety states, feelings of hopelessness and depression. Life may be perceived as meaningless. Despite the suicide rate for the elderly population being 50% higher than the younger population (in the USA), care professionals show reluctance to refer them for psychiatric consultation (Grant 1996).

The aged are prone to developing mental ill-health and to suffering from depression (Eliopoulos 1996), which many care professionals may fail to identify during assessment. Eliopoulos felt that it was ageism interfering with effective mental health assessment. Competency in care evaluation is essential to ensure the older adult's needs are met.

A 'seamless service' is, however, still an aspiration, according to the English National Board (1997), with the result that people with psychological dysfunction have unmet needs. Similarly, the Research For Ageing Trust (1997) report, while emphasizing that a whole range of therapies are available, provided evidence that many older people are 'still denied' access to services. Structural constraints, i.e. policy strategies in mental health nursing, have excluded some client groups with dementia (Adams 1996) from obtaining needs-driven services due to inadequate definition of what constitutes 'serious and enduring mental health problems'. Adams (1997) explained that unless organic disorders such as Alzheimer's disease are included within the framework of 'serious and enduring' mental ill-health, in addition to the functional disorders (e.g. schizophrenia, manic depression), the needs of older people may become marginalized. Besides, Adams emphasized, failure to recognize this issue could be interpreted as an expression of ageism.

The literature highlights psychotic and mood disorder illnesses within the definition (Repper & Brooker 1995) which may further reinforce marginalization of older people's needs, while Gournay and Brooking (1994) campaigned for a 'reinvestment' of community psychiatric nursing in meeting the psychosocial needs of schizophrenic patients and their families. They further pointed out that the 'attachment of CPNs (community psychiatric nurses) in primary care and their treatment of people with non-psychotic problems appears to be a case of squandering a precious resource'. If resources are to be redeployed, alternative strategies to meet the needs of the aged with organic disorders must be employed. Service providers, for example, can actively involve clients and their families in the planning, designing and implementation of programmes. Specialized help from professionals with experience in organic disorders can be utilized. A combination of strategies (Box 4.1) is also recommended to combat ageism in mental health care and the wider community.

Box 4.1 The debate of the age

In the 'debate of the age' Westhall (1997) argued that doctors and medical organizations have a duty to participate. Since an ageing population creates multidimensional implications (health, social, economic, demographic, political), Westhall emphasized that communities, and individuals from all walks of life, must contribute to the debate. In particular, she asserts that an exploration of societies' values, beliefs and attitudes towards ageing is needed.

Since many issues can be found at the root of ageism (e.g. that old people have no economic purpose, no intrinsic value) (Stammers 1992), a broad approach is required to deal with the problem. It is therefore suggested – since new challenges in health and social care are manifold – that international cooperation is necessary to halt the existing potential inequalities in health, both within and between countries (Walt 1998). For example, ageism in mental health care can be prevented by utilizing the existing European Network Of Health-Promoting Schools. To make effective use of these schools, avoiding contradictory health messages imparted in society in general must be recognized and resolved (Denman 1998). Parents and children can become agents of change. Their education in informal and formal settings on issues that affect their everyday life can enhance their role in developing healthy values and attitudes in relation to physical and mental well-being (Box 4.2).

Box 4.2 Mental health and children's education

Children show receptiveness and keenness to learn at a very early age. Their understanding of basic concepts is expressed in an unbiased and spontaneous way. Seedhouse (1998) wrote that children are able to explain what is 'good' and what causes 'happiness'. However, he pointed out that this unbiased expression is destroyed over the years, to the extent that in later life, after their A levels, medical education and psychiatric training, many professionals 'are unable to define mental health'. Seedhouse asserted: 'In fact most of them won't understand why you're asking the question'.

Health-promoting schools should build upon children's comprehension of basic concepts. Health-promoting hospitals and training organizations should continue the process of upholding the values taught and learned in early years.

The links between health and old age can be explored. Issues related to ageism can be discussed and analysed. A higher profile is developing on issues of teenage pregnancies and sex education, evident in the national curriculum. Incorporating mental health issues – in conjunction with other pertinent and well recognized health concerns – is a goal to be considered. As Denman (1998) pointed out, at present schools focus on 'sensitive' issues of sex and drug education, which encourage parents to be involved. One should therefore help to develop a high profile concerning health education and promotion in other areas of public health in the early stages of children education; e.g. the promotion of solidarity between generations.

Wright (1995) considered education to be the care professionals' role. In the debate of the age, this area of concern can be analysed and explored with evidence-based knowledge, rather than, as Wright (1995) argued, just providing services based on assumptions of the needs of older people. In addition, critical evaluation of one's own values is required, utilizing clinical supervision as the foundation on which constructive ideas can be formulated.

Combating ageism at every possible angle demands taking responsibilities for one's personal and professional development (Wright 1995). A re-examination of the concept of caring, and the meaning of a patient's charter, can be explored to retrieve the essence of humanistic care. Additionally, the debate can explore issues related to psychosocial interventions (which have empowered the older person) in hospital and community settings, in combination with national and international strategies showing positive results. Cross-fertilization of innovative ideas and new philosophies can thus be encouraged and recognized. Of importance is the Older Person Movement, a movement aimed at 'asserting the economic and political potential' of older people (Wright 1995) to raise awareness of their invaluable role in society, and to stimulate anti-oppressive practice.

Anti-discriminatory practice strategies can be fostered within neighbourhoods. The role of community nurses is invaluable, since health work within such settings is an issue requiring concentrated effort to promote the health needs of older people (Moores 1998). In addition, health-promoting hospital initiatives should aim to maintain continuity of care for those older people who have to leave their home environment for inpatient care (Fig. 4.1). Continuing physical and psychosocial safety in care settings is important. The prevention of abuse is a societal concern and debate on this issue is important. Solutions must be found. Professionals in practice are aware of the existence of abuse (Smith 1998), but positive outcomes can only be achieved through 'constructive debates' and 'ongoing networking'. Furthermore, increased longevity throughout the world requires 'Global Health Watch' and the stimulation of global awareness to prevent an escalation of ageism.

Activity 4.2

Arrange a visit to your local Age Concern office. Discuss with the manager issues concerned with ageism. Make a list of measures Age Concern implement to promote positive images of ageing.

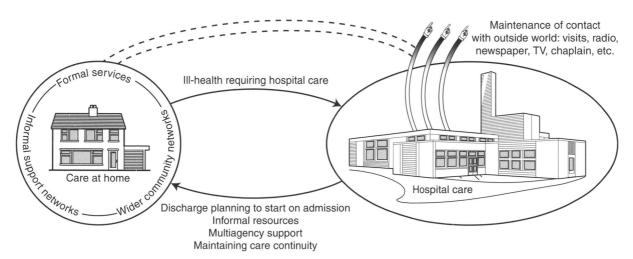

Fig. 4.1 Continuity of care process: from care at home to hospital care and back to the community, with support from multi-agency and informal networks.

? ? ? Question 4.2

1. To what extent will global awareness help to combat ageism?
2. Do you believe that much can be learned from the ways some non-Westernized cultures treat their elders?
3. What considerations should be given to individual responsibility (professional and non-professional) to combat ageism?
4. Sue Smith (1998) argued that nurses in clinical practice who look after older people experience problems in promoting elderly care as a specialized field to their managers. What could be the reasons for this?

Communication and ageism

The impact of speech in promoting negative images of older people has not been studied. Everyday language conveys meanings and expressions that one takes for granted. After all, the words describing a negative message have been used and accepted over a number of years by the people in any culture. Comedians frequently make reference to the old person and their audience responds humorously. Newspapers and television channels communicate ageism in various ways; an insidious and subtle process of which the communicators themselves are unaware. For instance, newspapers publishing advertisements for job opportunities can demonstrate age discrimination; Heath (1989) has made reference to age-based advertisements. Employers who want to make sure that individuals above a certain age do not apply – despite the fact that experience and skills are evident in individual cases – are being discriminatory.

Headlines in newspapers make generalizations that the aged are 'frail', 'dependent' and 'helpless'. Although our society and its health care systems are catering for many old people in need of help, there is evidence that many others in the community are maintaining healthy, independent lives.

A 1998 article in *The Times* newspaper, titled 'My Dad's older than your dad' (Pitman 1998), showed that stereotypic images of the older person are still being produced. Pitman used phrases such

as: 'the antique male shuffling into his eighties'; 'men of this age are settling into their slippers and getting used to a pottering routine of gentling gardening and afternoon naps'; 'an antique father'; and to the effect of ageing: 'the bad backs'; 'stiff joints that make it more difficult to horse around with a football, or catch a child jumping out of a tree'. On the other hand, Pitman's article described some well known personalities' reproductive achievements (Case example 4.4), which to the anti-ageist are examples of positive ageing and confirmation that 'life does not stop at 60'.

Case example 4.4 Age and reproduction

Contrary to the stereotypical belief that reproduction and sexual performance decrease with age, evidence is accumulating in society that men, for example, can still become fathers in old age. Charlie Chaplin had a daughter in his 70s. Anthony Quinn, 84, fathered his 13th child in 1998. Bill Wyman, 58, has three daughters under the age of 5. Jack Nicholson, 62, has children aged 3, 7 and 9. Sir Peter Hall, 69, has six children, the youngest being 5.

When the media transmit such communications their choice of words can convey a negative image, which further supports the belief that old age is accepted as a time of decline. Advertisements focusing on health products usually show young men, women and children. The older person is often seen in an armchair (e.g. Werther's Original Butterscotch sweets adverts), or talking about pensions and insurance policies related to retirement. It is believed that only 'old people' retire. Saving for retirement is considered by many younger adults to be a premature measure.

Written and visual messages can be influential in confirming stereotypes. The power of language, Fuller (1995) observed, should not be underestimated. Speech can exert a destructive effect. When old people interact with the young, there is an accepted defeatist attitude from the former, reflecting a lack of worth. In a small study to observe how 'ageism through speech' is influential, Fuller (1995) commented that evidence exists to prove this notion (Box 4.3).

Box 4.3 Communicating ageist attitudes

A study by Fuller (1995) focused on individuals in non-institutionalized settings (a rural day centre and a shopping centre). Seventy-five per cent of the sample interviewed made a comparison with the days when they were young and how they were spoken to; a current lack of respect shown by young people was a common theme. The findings also disclosed that young people were inclined to be abusive towards them. Fifty-six per cent of the sample showed concern that they were not invited to participate in conversation. The feeling of being society's outcasts was expressed. Forty-four per cent felt they were asked personal questions more than necessary, and 50% felt that their status as valuable members of society had diminished, compared to when they were younger. Eighty-one per cent agreed that they were perceived to be a distinct group. Thirty-one per cent of those interviewed felt uneasy when talking to younger people, yet conversation and interacting with others were considered important to combat isolation, to maintain motivation in life and to meet people.

As shown in Box 4.3, older people appeared 'indoctrinated' into believing that an ageist attitude is to be expected and the only alternative is to be a passive recipient. However, the study also exposed the attitudes of the older persons towards those of similar age. They made reference, for example, to the 'poor geriatrics' and the 'senile folk'.

Language can perpetuate ageism. The aged themselves have set patterns of beliefs that are ageist. A youthful society can show disregard and disrespect towards older individuals by the way they communicate. Unless the older persons in society are prepared to alter their perception of themselves in a positive way, ageism will not be easily eradicated. Moreover, ageism is not a new phenomenon. As Smith (1996) explained, ageism is as old as civilization, and human language contains many adjectives used to denigrate the old. The social construction of ageism through communication has become a powerful force in societies throughout the world.

Human beings formulate concepts according to their perception of behaviour. Meanings are attached to such concepts as 'growing old' and the attributes associated with them based on past learning from parents and significant others. Once associations have been made, inferences are communicated and assumptions made conveyed through language (Case example 4.5).

Case example 4.5 'Old Pop'

Jasper is now 90. He retired 25 years ago. He was a physician, well known and respected by the community. Since he developed a stroke, he has given up his hobbies (gardening and horse betting). He recalls how people's behaviour has changed towards him.

'They used to say, "he looks good for his age". But now it is, "he gets in the way; he is so stubborn and cantankerous; what do you expect at his age; he does not much now. He blames it on his stroke. Was he really a doctor?"

'The other day I asked my grand-daughter to take me to the betting shop in my wheelchair. As she wheeled me in, I overheard comments such as, "what is he doing here? This is not a hospital!"

'The worst thing is being referred to as "Old Pop" and "Poppet". That's what the nurse used to call me until I reminded her that was not my name.'

While the wider community shows evidence of ageism, health care settings are also known as arenas where professionals communicate ageist messages. It is acknowledged that there is an unequal power relationship between the nurse and the patient. The former exercises subtle control, the latter accepts and complies (Hewison 1995). Older people are particularly vulnerable. Control and the exercise of power are subtly camouflaged with 'terms of endearment'. The scenario described in Case example 4.6 is of common occurrence in care settings. Nurses, Hobman (1996) and Hewison (1995) pointed out, are known to treat patients as children. In addition, Jones (1993) explained that nurses' perception of their patients as children increases the patients' dependence in the power struggle relationship.

Case example 4.6 shows a client who has lost control and is disempowered. The language used, although endearing and well meant, is in fact a covert message of social expectation, i.e. the aged can be easily manipulated and their trustworthiness can be exploited to maximize control and persuasion. Hewison (1995) wrote that the unequal power relationship negates collaborative partnerships in care given. One should be

Case example 4.6 A busy 16-bed care of the elderly ward

'Good morning *poppet*. I have come to give you a bed bath.' The nurse pulled the curtain round the bed. 'Now *sweetie*, let's take your nightie off. I would like you to sit up. I mean sit up *sweetheart*, not roll over. *Good girl.*' The nurse called her colleague to give her a hand. 'I think she will be discharged this afternoon', she said to her peer. '*Poppet*, the doctor will come round soon. We have to make sure you are in the day room before he comes *lovy*.'

aware that health professionals are just as prone as the wider community to ageist behaviour, which can be subtly or unconsciously communicated during interactions. Ageism, it is argued, occurs on a wide scale within the health service (Hobman 1996) (Box 4.4).

Oncology and ageism

Cancer patients in care settings also experience the effects of ageism. Social researchers within an American setting exposed social workers' ageist behaviour towards old people with cancer. Such attitudes, Rohan et al (1994) commented, inevitably lead to inequitable health care provision. Rohan et al identified several key issues that can lead to unequal health care provision:

1. The stereotypic view that the old person is suffering from brain failure rather than depression, which may be present.
2. The belief that once old age has been reached, organic changes occur and that health cannot be restored.
3. Since many clients have communication problems and have difficulties in discussing their problems, misdiagnosis is possible.

These factors contribute toward increasing the prevalence of initiating mismatched care, or/and reducing the older person's chances of gaining access to specific care provision.

The implications for the oncology patient in need of social support are varied. Rohan et al described their diverse needs to be:

Box 4.4 Discriminating practice in the NHS and the community

Health care rationing based on chronological age is evident in the following cases. The over 75 are refused treatment by some hospitals; an elderly man a few years ago was refused physiotherapy. Preventive services in the NHS discriminate against women over 65 by not automatically inviting them for breast screening (Hobman 1996) and the cessation of cervical screening at 64, assuming that women are not sexually active at that age (Pashley 1996). Sutton (1997) explained that current health policies ignore the needs of women past the age of 65 who show increasing prevalence of breast cancer.

Many older women live in substandard housing and, similar to men, encounter difficulties in obtaining access to amenities in towns and cities. Courtney (1996) lists cases where health policies in some parts of the country can be restrictive and not standardized. For example, geography and level of dependency are criteria used in decision-making concerning care provision. In contrast, some health authorities make decisions according to bed availability, regardless of dependency or area of residence. Community nursing care is dictated 'by geography rather than need'.

A fragmented service means that the older person's need for care, either in hospital or a community setting, may be inadequately met. In the case of rehabilitation, for example, some authors (Young et al 1998) report that, in spite of literature evidence with regard to national guidance and current practice, uncertainties still exist between acute care hospital and the implementation of rehabilitative care in community trusts. Such uncertainties mean that older people receive inadequate care, and that resources and funding may be deployed to other areas in the health care service.

Activity 4.3

1. Arrange a 1-hour interview with the local hospital Trust manager to discuss progress made in the allocation of resources to meet increasing demands in elderly care.
2. Talk to your community health service manager and find out the measures used to promote healthy ageing.

  Question 4.3

1. In 1998, the Health Minister allocated £500 million for the Health Service. How should a percentage of this sum be spent in elderly care?
2. If demand exceeds supply of scarce resources, what would be the alternative in care provision?

1. reliance on social support
2. support to manage depressive illness
3. access to community resources
4. maintaining independence
5. safeguarding positive family relationships.

In addition, oncology patients have specific needs (Box 4.5), which social workers must recognize to ensure intervention is need-specific. Rohan et al stipulate that oncology patients, in general, benefit from social work intervention.

Box 4.5 The older person with cancer and their needs

Older oncology patients may have a deep sense of personal loss: physical decline due to ageing and disease process, social isolation caused by the loss of loved ones, the effects of hospitalization and the effects caused by disruption of a planned future. Cancer and its treatment are additional dimensions which depress motivation, increase frustrations, disrupt relationships and cause loss of independence, despair and depression. Rohan et al stipulate that oncology patients, in general, benefit from social work intervention. Social workers' professional judgement can empower the clients to cope with their illness. Rohan et al's 1994 research findings, however, indicated evidence of ageism in social work settings (Case example 4.7).

Case example 4.7

Findings from the 1994 study by Rohan et al
A total of 502 adult oncology patients were studied; 60.8% (305) were 18–64 years old; 22.3% (112) were 65–74 years of age; 16.9% (85) were 75 years of age or older. Younger oncology patients received more time and attention from social workers during treatment: 1.8 hours for the 18–64 age group; 1.4 hours for the 65–74 age group; 1.0 hours for the 75 and older age group. Duration of work treatment showed significant differrences: 23.5 days for patients aged 18–64; 15.5 days for patients aged 65–74; 18.0 days for patients aged 75 and older.
Social workers addressed housing problems/medical coverage problems and monetary matters more often with younger patients; the elderly were questioned more about transportation and mobility problems.
Differences in referral sources showed that the elderly were referred by their immediate families, while with younger age groups, it was the social workers who carried out the referral to services.

Social workers' professional judgement can empower the clients to cope with their illness. Rohan et al's 1994 research findings, however, indicated evidence of ageism in social work settings (Case example 4.7).

Rohan et al's study (1994) highlighted inequity in care delivery, which may reflect the covert way ageism can be expressed in oncology care. For care professionals, the implications are that the older person with cancer may not be receiving holistic care. Old people with cancer require multidimensional support: physical support to cope with their ill-health, counselling to help them manage their lives psychosocially and emotionally, while their spiritual needs demand exploration and understanding.

In Britain, trends show that health services in relation to prevention and care of the older person with cancer have aroused critical debates. More elderly women (one-third of cases) in the over 70s are at risk of developing breast cancer (Elwell 1997). Elwell explained that services for older women remain unsatisfactory for the following reasons:

1. compared with younger women their treatment is less rigorous
2. they are 'less likely to be offered breast conserving treatment'
3. there is a tendency for them to receive less informed choice
4. they are not fully encouraged to participate in 'treatment decisions'
5. evidence shows under-representation of older women in trials of breast cancer treatment.

In the main, in spite of evidence that more than 50% of all cancers have been identified in older people (Pendleton & Horan 1997), younger clients are more likely to receive better care and services. Positive changes are required to counteract ageist attitudes in the field of cancer care. New research is needed to observe the effects of advanced cancer therapy on the older person. Besides, treatment and continuing support are major issues to be considered.

Pendleton and Horan (1997) argued for 'multidimensional quality of life measures' in conjunction with effective liaison services to maximize the positive effects of therapy for the older person with multiple pathology. Reducing the impact of morbidity and pathology, however, requires early identification and intervention. The burdens of long-term care can be minimized (Banerjee 1996) by making use of available high-tech resources and sound rehabilitative measures.

Sexuality ageism and the older person

Current media communication constantly fortifies the message that youth, combined with slimness and an active life, is the ideal. Advertisements perpetuate the notion that sex and sexuality are the domains of the young and active. Adverts do not show elderly couples cuddling and kissing each other; films very rarely show older couples having sex. There is, however, a plethora of films and adverts based on the hidden message that a healthy sexual life pertains to the young and attractive.

The older person, in many cases, fearful of disturbing societal view that old age means loss of sexual functioning, attempts to project the image that they have no interest in sexual matters. There is a tendency to be demure, treating sex as a taboo subject. Research findings, nevertheless, present a different picture. Helgason et al (1996) showed that sex is important to elderly men. In their survey of 319 Swedish men, 83% stated that sex was very important. Preservation of sexual functioning and sexuality is significant, and the authors proposed that this dimension should receive adequate consideration in the clinical assessment of elderly men. Clinical assessment should also consider women's sexual needs and problems. Since old age does not necessarily mean loss of sexual interest, and is not a contraindication (Higson 1997), attempts must be made to understand women's sexual needs. Higson wrote that a decreased sex life is linked to the menopause, which can be resolved by using hormone replacement therapy. In addition, where there is evidence of reduced sex drive, women may be helped by medication (e.g. Tibolone) or testosterone supplementation.

The fact that both men and women in old age are interested in sex must not be dismissed by care professionals in clinical practice. The avenues for promoting the maintenance of a healthy sex life are numerous. For instance, Well Men and Well Women Clinics could include sensitive assessment of the older person's sexual functioning and dysfunctioning and counselling services provided as required. Moreover, informed choice can be promoted. Raising older people's awareness of therapeutic products, treatment and support available will enhance their confidence in choosing services specific to individual needs.

Activity 4.4

Design a model of care for older people in relation to their sexuality.

??? Question 4.4

1. What do you consider to be the main foundation for society's attitude towards the sexual needs of the aged?
2. To what extent does the older person perpetuate ageist behaviour in others?

ELDER ABUSE

Elder abuse is not a new social phenomenon. Like child abuse it has existed for many years. Unlike child abuse, and the issues of violence against women and domestic violence, however, it has only just recently been receiving public and professional attention. In fact, North American literature has contributed in stimulating and initiating debate and interest in the subject. It is essential to acknowledge that abuse is not a social problem that occurs in developed countries only (Badrinath & Ramaiah 1998). Similar to child abuse the issue of elder abuse is disturbing and distasteful (Thomas 1996), and professionals in care settings have argued for better guidelines to help them report any malpractice. One argument is concerned with the notion of definition; unclear and inconsistent interpretations may interfere with accurate guidelines and framework for practice.

Elder abuse may be defined as the deliberate and non-deliberate intention to disempower and disable the older person in various ways. Seymour (1997) argued that misjudgements on the part of professionals can cause harm or neglect; in this context the abuse is non-deliberate. A failure to recognize sensitively and professionally issues which have physical, social and psychological implications for the individual are included in this dimension. Actions aiming to injure the person (psychosocially and emotionally), despite professional knowledge and experience that doing so is damaging, are deliberate in nature. The latter is an aspect which current literature makes reference to most frequently.

Elder abuse in care settings

The perpetrators of abuse in care settings are very often professional carers (Shamash 1997). In 25% of cases, according to the pressure group Action on Elder Abuse, nurses are the abusers. They can abuse the old person in various and subtle ways (Box 4.6).

Box 4.6 Methods of abuse

- The exercise of control by overpowering the individual with excessive medications, e.g over-sedation.
- Neglecting the person by not attending to various needs:
  - **physical** – washing, toileting, change of linen, mobility needs etc.
  - **psychosocial** – not responding to the needs for communication, reassurance and interpersonal relationships
  - **emotional** – deliberately not responding to the patient's expression of anxiety, fears, need for affection.
- Purposeful humiliation through sexual gratification (e.g. repeated sexual abuse).
- Stealing and misappropriation of finances.

While institutional settings have been implicated in abuse cases, evidence exists supporting the argument that elder abuse occurs within the older person's own home (Bennett 1997), and occurs in cities and rural areas (Cupitt 1997). Maltreatment as described in Box 4.6 is a common theme. Bennett (1997) further highlighted the practice of theft and financial exploitation which frailty and vulnerability attract. It is argued

(Warren & Bennett 1997) that early primary care intervention can minimize the potential for abuse; the role of General Practitioners (GPs) is not to be underestimated. Their knowledge of the patient's social background can help to identify abuse at an early stage. By making use of local social and health care policies, their preventative strategies can be enhanced. A multidisciplinary team approach is, however, essential. This entails working collaboratively with pressure groups (e.g. Action on Elder Abuse, Age Concern), domestic violence teams, the police, health and social care services. Moreover, the cooperation of family members and primary carers is needed. The links between domestic violence and the continuation of abuse in old age are established (Cupitt 1997). Families can be credible informers in abuse cases. Their participation in prevention is important.

To secure community cooperation and awareness, however, Cupitt argued that a higher profile must be raised on abuse: what it is; what it means; how it can be prevented, and what can be done about abuse when it occurs. She suggests 'mandatory reporting' based on clearcut guidelines to help service managers (Cupitt 1997).

Elder abuse in domestic settings

While elderly people strive to maintain their safety by taking excessive security measures against the possibility of crime (Denham 1993) by minimizing their contact with the outside world, they tend to face bigger crimes perpetrated by their carers against them within the homes. Abuse in domestic settings is well reported in the literature. Manthorpe (1998) made reference to the Hampshire case: Mr Hampshire, a 61-year-old retired teacher, killed his wife, aged 62, in 1994, by stabbing her 300 times. Mr Hampshire was deemed mentally unstable. Although it is argued whether acts of violence due to mental instability (Manthorpe 1998) should constitute abuse, the reality is that it is a form of abuse by proxy. Inadequate recognition by welfare agencies and mental health organizations of violence and abuse by an individual with serious mental ill-health constitutes a form of abuse, perpetrated by professional carers.

Abuse in non-residential home settings, caused by marital discord and living arrangements, has been identified (Wilson 1994). A person who lives alone is less likely to be abused. On the other hand, according to Wilson's (1994) research, where two persons are living together, the incidence of abuse increases. In most cases it is agreed (Wilson 1994) that women are abused more often than men. While family carers can abuse their dependants, the latter, conversely, can abuse their carers too; frustrations, physical and psychological ill-health experienced by the patient can result in explosive behaviour. Retaliation by the carers can then occur.

Compton et al's (1997) study of elder abuse in people with dementia in Northern Ireland showed that, out of 38 interviewed carers, four (10.5%) reported cases of physical abuse; 13 (34%) were verbally abused; and in three cases (8%) verbal and physical abuse co-existed. Abuse in domestic settings by relatives, for whatever reasons, can sometimes lead to murder (Dickson 1993).

Literature on elderly care in the UK, e.g. Bennett et al (1996) on the identification and management of elder abuse; Warren and Bennett (1997) on the role of GPs; Benbow and Haddad (1993) on sexual abuse and the role of professionals; McCreadie and Tinker (1993) on types of abuse and prevention; Homer and Kingston (1992) on preventative screening and the role of the nurse, demonstrates increased awareness of the problem. Many issues addressed relate to the extent of the problem and a failure in its identification due to lack of education and training, as well as a lack of clear protocols to guide professional decision-making.

Research findings in Canada and Australia (Trevitt & Gallagher 1996) show the existence of elder abuse in a variety of settings, including the domestic environment. Under-reporting and failure to detect this social problem only shows the tip of a clinical iceberg. On the other hand, carers themselves, Cupitt (1997) explained, may not perceive their behaviours as abusive. One can argue, too, that the frail elderly person with multiple pathology may not perceive the relationship as abusive. Nurses in Swedish care settings have also identified families to be abusers. A study by Grafström et al (1993) identified the link between the burden of caring and couples living alone with the recurrence of abuse. Deduction can therefore be made that elder abuse is a worldwide phenomenon existing within the context of domestic violence. The causes are varied.

Causes of elder abuse

The frustrations and constraints (e.g. under-funding and lack of resources) attached to caring can disrupt harmonious relationships. Exhaustion and the power imbalance between the caregiver (potential perpetrator) and the dependant (potential abused) can precipitate abusive behaviour (Saveman et al 1993). Other causes are related to the stress and demands associated with physical disabilities and/or psychological ill-health. (Mullan 1995). Frailty and inability to communicate have also been implicated, while other factors such as mental and physical deterioration increase the emotional strain.

Some dependants may be quiet and non-complaining, but the noisiness, shouting, aggressive and vulgar habits of others (Compton et al 1997) have been linked to abuse. The personalities of elderly and mentally ill dependants, in combination with their frailty (Wilson 1994) has a tendency to upset some carers.

Other causes may be linked to geographical location: the isolation of rural living which means that health workers' access may be restricted. This leaves many old people with a lack of social support, exposed to abusive relationships.

Other characteristic causes are:

- inexperience of informal and formal carers
- strained workforce with low morale and burnout coupled with staff pathology (Bennett 1997)
- power abuse and professional misjudgement
- alcohol consumption by staff and lack of restraints.

The experience of depression, financial difficulties and other wide-ranging family commitments can also predispose carers to becoming abusers (Hempel 1993).

Preventative and strategic measures

The protection of elders in society requires a variety of strategies and ideas.

1. The acknowledgement that abuse has no boundaries. Very often the victims are the frail and the aged.

2. Defining the concept of abuse is essential. Abuse literature shows that professionals can be imprecise in its identification.

3. It is argued that the Carers Act (1995) does not acknowledge the needs of carers (Bowskill 1997, Ratcliffe 1998). Consequently, poor and underfunded carer support increases the propensity for abuse to take place. This situation can be prevented by a thorough assessment of the coping ability of carers. Health and social care workers have a duty to inform carers about their rights to be assessed for their ability to care by their local authorities. Remedial action can thus be taken where there is evidence of emotional strain and burnout. Respite care and counselling are possible avenues.

4. Mobilization of primary health care teams, with the involvement of geriatricians (Vernon & Bennett 1995) working collaboratively with other organizations (e.g. Action on Elder Abuse) to disseminate information and promote policy changes. Particularly relevant, too, is the integration of health and social care provision through partnership.

5. The development of screening instruments to include psychosocial and lifestyle assessment. Screening tools must be sensitive enough to detect not only the abused, but also the abusers. Resources should subsequently be deployed according to needs.

6. The feasibility of mandatory reporting should be considered. Whenever abuse is expected, or suspected, professionals should document their observations and disseminate the information.

7. Information gathering by interviewing the older person separately from the carer is important. The carer must be interviewed as well. The aim is to obtain a full picture of the caring relationships. If there is evidence that abuse is taking place there are two possible interventions:

a. discontinuing the carer's involvement with the dependant (Warren & Bennett (1997) suggest legal intervention if necessary)

b. if the dependants are able to communicate their needs and are agreeable, alternative care may be provided. Other family members must be consulted to assess the implications and to identify other alternatives (e.g. self-help groups).

8. Nursing and medical practitioners should frequently review the effects of medication on the person to prevent polypharmacy, to detect depressive features and to initiate social and recreational activities as needed.

9. Carers must develop coping skills. Regular self-help group meetings to discuss the stress and constraints of caring can enhance better awareness. Mandatory training and education in elder abuse should be initiated. Nurses in the community are ideally placed to identify potentially abusive situations. Case conferences can be the avenues to disseminate information.

10. Empowering older people by making them aware of ageism as a malignant force and by listening to their views. Developing the Elder Movement and establishing links with domestic violence teams and Victim Support.

11. It has been found (Davidhizar et al 1997) that frequent home visits by health workers can stop the cycle of abuse. In addition, Homes Watch schemes (Willmott 1997) can be a valuable tool. This requires alliance with police units, with the aim to formulate codes of good practice in cooperation with nursing and residential care managers.

12. A sound educational framework which highlights the links between abuse and quality of life (Kingston & Penhale 1997).

13. Learning from other community health systems and adopting their methods. For example, the elderly in Japan benefit from a model of community-based long-term care named ACC (Around-the-Clock-Care) (Murashima et al 1998). Their philosophy is to provide regular early morning assessment and care, followed by day, evening and night visits by nurses. Visitation frequencies are dependent upon the severity of the client's condition. This system

helps reduce the burden and stress of caregiving, while allowing professionals to prevent health deterioration.

Activity 4.5

1. Contact Age Concern to find out the prevalence of elder abuse in your area.
2. Design a plan of care in relation to the needs of housebound elders.

??? Question 4.5

1. What possible explanations can there be for the trends in elder abuse?
2. Should health care systems develop strategies based on the views of the aged in society?

DEPRESSION IN OLDER PEOPLE

What is depression?

Ageing is a global issue. Early planning is needed by health policy makers and health care organizations in every sphere of the aged person's lifestyle. Failing to plan adequately for the future will increase the negative consequences associated with ageing. Needs identification and specific mechanisms must be in place to address the increase in the aged population (Steel & Maggi 1993). One area requiring attention is related to the prevention of mental ill-health caused by depression.

Depression in the elderly is common. Yet it is not always identified. This may be due to the belief that old age is associated with a general decline of faculties and physical sluggishness. The appearance of the aged person is at the forefront of the observer's field of vision. The psychological appearance takes secondary position, and is often missed. Many elders project their feelings of depression through speech, e.g. talking about their sense of worthlessness, guilt and isolation, and expressing suicidal thoughts. There is an inclination to interpret such behaviour as normal ageing.

While mental sluggishness may be due to impaired memory and lack of concentration – often linked to the ageing process – depressive features may, however, be closely intertwined. It is important to be aware that depression can occur at any age (Armstrong 1998).

Recognizing depression in older people

Since 1992, a campaign called 'Defeat Depression', organized by the Royal College of Practitioners and the Royal College of Psychiatrists, has aimed to promote better public and professional awareness of the existence of depression (Tylee & Katona 1996). The fact that there is a campaign is evidence enough to suggest the importance of detecting this type of mental ill-health affecting the aged. It is argued that ageist attitudes can cause both misunderstanding and misdiagnosis of 'hopelessness and suicidal feelings' as another aspect of ageing (Kirby et al 1997), thus leading to failures in detection.

Other ageist beliefs may consist of professional interpretation that depression is an inevitable consequence of ageing, and that treatment will not improve the situation (Tylee & Katona 1996). These beliefs prevent and discourage diagnosticians from looking beyond the features presented.

The recognition of depression is further hampered by a lack of cultural awareness related to ethnic groups. The Irish, for instance, with strong religious and cultural beliefs, may unwittingly disguise the intensity of their depression and suicidal feelings by disclosing only feelings of 'hopelessness' (Kirby et al 1997). While depression is considered a psychiatric disorder in Western medicine, to the rural population in South Asia, it is perceived through bodily changes: tiredness, lethargy, general malaise, aches and pains (Bhatnagar 1997). Suggesting to a South Asian elder that they are manifesting symptoms of psychological ill-health (mental illness), Bhatnagar explained, will be interpreted as symptoms of 'madness'. Furthermore, South Asians do not present with expressions of altered mood, such as sadness and guilt, but may make reference to the degree of their 'suffering' and ask for ways to end.

The Chinese, on the other hand, according to studies done between 1966 and 1996 (Chen 1998), showed a low prevalence of depression. Chen argued that their social networks may act as buffering mechanisms, reducing the impact of depressive illnesses. In addition, detection rate can be minimized due to failure by the individuals and their families in interpreting their symptoms as depression.

While cultural factors can mask the presence of depression, a purely medical–physical model can impede detection. Evans (1998) asserted that the somatization of disease diverts the clinicians' attention from identifying the real issue. Many older people would refer to their insomnias, loss of appetite and pain, but fail to talk about their moods and feeling. Inability to recognize the meanings attached to their behaviour can trigger a battery of fruitless physical investigations.

Another feature that can obscure the presence of depression is an inability to recall events. Although the ageing process affects short-term memory, while preserving long-term recall, depression can worsen these effects. Lader (1996) explained that 75% of older depressed patients show memory and learning deficits in their performance of tasks learning. Moreover, a clear distinction needs to be made between faculties and behaviour changes in depression, and those of dementia. Lader argued that, in the former, the person exhibits loss of libido and anxiety while retaining good time and direction sense. Medical and nursing practitioners must exercise vigilance during the assessment, remembering the many permutations of depressive symptom manifestations (Table 4.1). Depressive features, as Table 4.1 shows, may be mistaken for dementia, which has implications for treatment and management.

In the field of mental health nursing – within community and psychiatric hospital unit settings – there is a high level of depression among the client population. It is important to acknowledge that, in general nursing practice, there is evidence of depressive features amongst medically ill older patients (Koenig et al 1998). The psychological dimension of care can sometimes receive scant attention at the expense of increased focus on procedures, physical care and reliance on a traditional model of care. While physical ailments can be major causes of depression, isolation, the fear of dying and psychological neglect intensify the depressed moods.

Management and care of the older depressed person

Caring teams should be aware that both men and women are prone to depression in old age, but that women's reasons for depression may be different (Evans & Burgess 1994). Consequently, women need assessing according to their specific needs. Since they live longer than men, Evans and Burgess point out that they are exposed to the grief and loneliness associated with their husbands' deaths. Increased longevity also means susceptibility to long-term disability, which must be remembered in care planning. In spite of disability it is known that many women continue their role as carers. Clinicians have a role in identifying 'caregiver stress in older women' (Cobbs & Ralapati 1998).

Some physical conditions (e.g. chronic obstructive pulmonary disease) are known to cause depression in the elderly (Yohannes et al 1998). This possibility must be borne in mind during treatment regimen, and appropriate action taken (e.g. counselling, medication, occupational therapy).

Team work is essential and care should be coordinated using a multidisciplinary framework. It is recommended (Bentley et al 1998) that a combined service is developed. Within the primary care settings, nurses and/or health visitors are usually the appropriate assessors. Sensitive assessment should comprise the psychological status of the individual, conscious of how social circumstances can impinge on emotional well-being.

Table 4.1   Presentations of depression (From Lader 1996)
Depression without impairment of thought process Depression with features of thought disturbance (pseudo dementia) Dementia with secondary depression augmenting cognitive deficit

To assist community workers in identifying the presence or absence of depressive features, a Geriatric Depression assessment tool should be utilized. Early detection by health workers of people with depressive illness in various settings (hospitals, nursing homes, health clinics, GP surgeries) means that treatment can be initiated early.

Treatment may consist of simple measures, e.g. non-pharmacological interventions: communicating empathetically, active listening, silent companionship and an attempt to identify from the person's perspective their perception of what is wrong. Armstrong (1998) argued that nurses who are adequately trained can guide the patients to find solutions to their problems. Sometimes, however, the only solution to the problem is medical or surgical intervention to prevent disability or to cure a physical illness causing the depression.

When social circumstances are implicated, social support should be mobilized to minimize the impact. The role of the primary care team in this area is emphasized. As Armstrong asserted, where people are experiencing isolation and loneliness caused by inadequate informal support, the care team has the expertise to 'provide information about local sources of self-help'.

Hence, community health teams have a role in promoting dynamic community partnerships with the aim to identify groups of older people who experience health inequalities and are socially excluded because of age. An integrated health and social service approach is demanded (Porter 1998) to ensure the old in society receive care tailored according to needs.

Assumptions, nevertheless, can sometimes misguide professional intervention. Assuming that the older person living in isolation is in need of human contact can be wrong. Non-human contact can be very therapeutic, and for some people pets become the focus of the 'human–animal bond' (Cookman 1996). Cookman suggested that 'ideas and places' also have significance to many people. For example, reminiscing transports the person to places visited in the past which have personal meanings and value. Clinical settings dislocate this bond. Attachment can be preserved by allowing and encouraging the clients and their relatives to keep photographs, ornaments and other personal belongings in their rooms. Pets as visitors should be encouraged.

Helping the person to retain familiar memories and contact with the outside world is a key objective. It is, however, relevant to consider the combination of psychological and social support with pharmacological therapy. The administration of antidepressants can be useful in controlling depression. Prior to drug administration, general observations of the clients are necessary, and the use of a depression rating scale is suggested (Coyle 1996). To defeat depression in the older person, anti-discriminatory practice is a requisite. A re-evaluation of one's ageist attitude is suggested. The focus should be on positive ageing. Changing attitude is not an easy task. Sound education and training can facilitate the process of change. Professionals in all settings must therefore collaborate to prevent the many dimensions of ill-health affecting the aged.

Activity 4.6

List the features of depression in clients you have looked after. Identify their needs. Now prepare a plan of care.

??? Question 4.6

1. Demographic trends show that people are living longer. Consider issues related to social and health care. Do you think that current health care policies are still relevant?
2. Should older people be allowed to work until they are 70–75 years old?

SUMMARY

In this chapter we have considered some key issues in connection with the many dimensions of elderly care in society. It has been discussed that ageism is at the root of society's traditional view of the aged, as applied to varied cultures. Ageism exists in health care, and is evident in the language that we use.

Another issue is concerned with elder abuse. It is a perennial problem in societies throughout the world, and is an issue receiving increased attention by care professionals. The latter have been known to be perpetrators and abuse has been known in care settings.

Depression in the older person is frequent, but is not always identified by carers. This may be because of the attitude that a change of mood is due to normal ageing. Research shows that many factors in the old person's life can cause depression. Care professionals have a role in combining their expertise to combat discrepancies in the care of the aged, and to make use of available resources to meet their many health needs.

GLOSSARY

Alzheimer's disease   a type of pre-senile dementia which tends to occur between ages 40 and 50

Biomedical model   an operational framework founded on biological and medical approaches aimed at curing illnesses

Clinical supervision   a system of working which consists of peer support and feedback on performance

Cognitive deficits   lack of ability to make judgement, to comprehend and to reason

Confusional states   the manifestation of disorientation, thought disturbance and inability to locate oneself in time, space and person

Dementia   organic mental disorder causing social and psychological malfunctioning

Functional disorders   disorders of neurotic origin (without organic disease)

Hidden curriculum   any learning that takes place within an educational setting, apart from the formal policies and guidelines laid down in the formal curriculum

Manic depression   a serious form of mental illness characterized by moods of elation alternating with depression

Morbidity   disease and ill-health incidence

Mortality   death rates

Multidimensional quality of life   the many facets of healthy living to improve standards

Oncology   study of tumours

Organic disorders   disorders affecting the structures of organs and tissues

Polypharmacy   multiple intake of medications

Professional socialization   the attitudes, values and beliefs gained through formal education and training, as distinct from informal education (knowledge gained from family, peers, friends etc.)

Somatization   conversion of psychological symptoms into physical ones (e.g. anxiety causes headaches and palpitations)

REFERENCES

Adams T 1996 The case for breaking through ageism in mental health care. Nursing Times 92(12): 46–47

Adams T 1997 Working in partnership to end ageism in mental health. British Journal of Nursing 6(3): 133

Armstrong E 1998 Clinical update: what is depression? Primary Health Care 8(3): 18–24

Badrinath P, Ramaiah S 1998 Elder abuse should have been discussed in issues on ageing. British Medical Journal 316(7141): 1384–1385

Banerjee A K 1996 Caring for the elderly: problems and priorities. British Journal of Hospital Medicine 56(4): 159–161

Behrens H 1998 Ageism: real or imagined? Elderly Care 10(2): 10–13

Benbow S, Haddad P 1993 Be aware of sexual abuse. Care of the Elderly 5(9): 329 ·

Bennett G 1997 Abuse in care. Geriatric Medicine 27(9): 25–27

Bennett G, McCreadie C, Tinker A 1996 Elder abuse: research to highlight the role of the GP. Geriatric Medicine 26(12): 15

Bentley J, Carter L, Brooks L, Cotter A 1998 Developing a combined service to assess older people's needs. Health Visitor 71(2): 59–61

Bhatnagar K S 1997 Depression in South Asian elders. Geriatric Medicine 27(2): 55–56

Bowskill D 1997 Acknowledging elder abuse. Journal of Community Nursing 11(10): 4–8

Central Statistics Office 1998 Social Trends 28: Population. HMSO, London, p 29

Chen R 1998 East is East? Investigating depression in older people in Europe and Asia. Geriatric Medicine 28(2): 19

Cobbs E L, Ralapati A N 1998 Health of older women. Medical Clinics of North America 82(1): 127–144

Compton S A, Flanagan P, Gregg W 1997 Elder abuse in people with dementia in Northern Ireland: prevalence and predictors in cases referred to a psychiatry of old age service. International Journal of Geriatric Psychiatry 12(6): 632–635

Cookman C A 1996 Older people and attachment to things, places, pets and ideas. Image: Journal of Nursing Scholarship 28(3): 227–231

Courtney M 1996 Last among equals. Nursing Times 92(45): 47

Coyle F 1996 Depression management in primary care. Geriatric Medicine 27(3): 38–41

Crouch S 1997 Bed blocking. Nursing Management 4(5): 24–25

Cupitt M 1997 Identifying and addressing issues of elderly abuse: a rural perspective. Journal of Elder Abuse and Neglect 8(4): 21–30

Davidhizar R, Dowd S B, Durick D 1997 Elder abuse: the American experience. Elderly Care 9(5): 9

Denham M 1993 A crime too many? Care of the Elderly 5(7): 256

Denman S 1998 The Health-Promoting School: reflections on school–parent links. Health Education 98(2): 55–58

Dickson N 1993 Abuse: it's time to tackle one of the last taboos. Care of the Elderly 5(7): 280

Elderly Care 1998 Health needs of older women are neglected. Elderly Care 10(2): 5

Eliopoulos C 1996 The elderly traveller. In: Carson V B, Arnold E N (eds) Mental health nursing: the nurse–patient journey. W B Saunders, Philadelphia, p 645–660

Elwell C 1997 Breast cancer: do not ignore the elderly. Geriatric Medicine 27(10): 13–16

English National Board 1997 Report on practice placement monitoring: mental health nursing, March 1996–February 1997. ENB for Nursing, Midwifery & Health Visiting, London

Evans M 1998 Managing physical illness and depression. Geriatric Medicine 28(4): 49–52

Evans M, Burgess H 1994 Depression in older women. Geriatric Medicine 24(10): 35–39

Fuller D 1995 Challenging ageism through our speech. Nursing Times 91(21): 29–31

George M 1998 Future care needs. Elderly Care 10(2): 8–9

Gournay K, Brooking J 1994 Community psychiatric nurses in primary care. British Journal of Psychiatry 165(2): 231–237

Graftström M, Norberg A, Hagberg B 1993 Relationships between demented elderly people and their families: a follow-up study of caregivers who had previously reported abuse when caring for their spouses and parents. Journal of Advanced Nursing 18(11): 1747–1757

Grant L D 1996 Effects of ageism on individual and healthcare providers' responses to healthy aging. Health and Social Work 21(1): 9–15

Greengross S, Murphy E, Quam L et al 1997 Aging: a subject that must be at the top of the world agendas. British Medical Journal 315(7115): 1029–1030

Haight B K, Christ M A, Dias J K 1994 Does nursing education promote ageism? Journal of Advanced Nursing 20(2): 382–390

Heath H 1989 Old: almost a four-letter word. Nursing Times 85(31): 36–37

Helgason A R, Adolfsson J, Dickman P, Arver S 1996 Sexual desire, erection, orgasm and ejaculatory functions and their importance to elderly Swedish men: a population-based study. Age and Ageing 25(4): 285–291

Hempel S 1993 Abuse of elderly people. Community Outlook 3(2): 26–27

Herrick C A, Pearcey L G, Ross C 1997 Stigma and ageism: compounding influences in making an accurate mental health assessment. Nursing Forum 32(3): 21–26

Hewison A 1995 Power of language in a ward for the care of older people. Nursing Times 91(21): 32–33

Higson N 1997 Continuing sex: helping older people to maintain a healthy sex life. Geriatric Medicine 27(12): 54–55

Hobman D 1996 Second-class treatment. Nursing Times 92(49): 46

Homer A C, Kingston P 1992 Screening by nurse practitioners could prevent abuse. Care of the Elderly 4(5): 220–221

Jones H 1993 Altered images. Nursing Times 89(5): 58–60

Kingston P, Penhale B 1997 Issues in the sphere of elder abuse and neglect: the role of education. Nurse Education Today 17(5): 418–425

Kirby M, Bruce I, Radic A et al 1997 Hopelessness and suicidal feelings among the community dwelling elderly in Dublin Irish. Journal of Psychological Medicine 14(4): 124–127

Koch T, Webb C 1996 The biomedical construction of ageing: implications for nursing care of older people. Journal of Advanced Nursing 23(5): 954–959

Koenig H G, George L K, Peterson B L 1998 Religiosity and remission of depression in medically ill older patients. American Journal of Psychiatry 155(4): 536–542

Kohler M 1998a Don't just sit there. Geriatric Medicine 28(2): 27

Kohler M 1998b Paper tiger? Geriatric Medicine 28(3): 19

Lader M 1996 Depression and cognitive impairment. Geriatric Medicine 26(8): 49–50

Manthorpe J 1998 Learning through inquiry. Journal of Mental Health 7(1): 1–7

McCreadie C, Tinker A 1993 Review: abuse of elderly people in the domestic setting: a UK perspective. Age and Ageing 22(1): 65–69

Moores Y 1998 Nursing the nation better. Nursing Times 94(14): 36–37

Mullan C 1995 'It doesn't happen here … .' Elderly Care 7(4): 36

Murashima S, Zerwekh J V, Yamada M, Tagami Y 1998 Around-the-clock nursing care for the elderly in Japan. Image: Journal of Nursing Scholarship 30(1): 37–41

Nazarko L 1996 Winds of change. Elderly Care 8(6): 37

Nazarko L 1997 Staffing the homes. Nursing Management 4(3): 22–23

Newman S, Faux R, Larimer B 1997 Children's views on aging: their attitudes and values. Gerontologist 37(3): 412–417

Nurse Education Today 1998 Editorial: Education and the continuing care of older people. Nurse Education Today 18(1): 1–2

Pashley G 1996 Older and wiser. Nursing Times 92(30): 58–60

Pendleton N, Horan M 1997 Quality of care: cancer services for the elderly. Geriatric Medicine 27(10): 48–50

Pitman J 1998 My dad's older than your dad. The Times, March 28: 18

Porter R 1998 Centre of attention. Nursing Times 94(16): 16

Ratcliffe P 1998 Not really caring for the carers? Journal of Community Nursing 12(4): 18–25

Research for Ageing Trust 1997 The impact of ageing on acute medical practice. Research for Ageing Trust, London

Repper J, Brooker C 1995 Serious mental health problems: policy changes. Nursing Times 91(25): 29–31

Rohan E A, Berkman B, Walker S, Holmes W 1994 The geriatric oncology patient: ageism in social work practice. Journal of Gerontological Social Work 23(1/2): 201–221

Saveman B, Hallberg I R, Norberg A 1993 Identifying and defining abuse of elderly people as seen by witnesses. Journal of Advanced Nursing 18(9): 1393–1400

Seedhouse D 1998 It's time mental illness took a holiday. Health Matters Issue 32: 45

Seymour J 1997 Lost horizon. Nursing Times 93(13): 43

Shamash J 1997 An abuse of trust. Nursing Standard 11(24): 16

Slevin O 1991 Ageist attitudes among young adults: implications for a caring profession. Journal of Advanced Nursing 16(10): 1197–1205

Smith M 1996 The language of ages. Nursing Times 92(30): 55–60

Smith S 1998 A new look at elderly care. Nursing Times 94(14): 42–43

Stammers T 1992 What is at the root of ageism? Care of the Elderly 4(7): 288–290

Steel K, Maggi S 1993 Ageing as a global issue. Age and Ageing 22(4): 237–239

Sutton G C 1997 Will you still need me, will you still screen me, when I'm past 64? British Medical Journal 315(7115): 1032–1033

Thomas L 1996 Going public on elder abuse. Elderly Care 8(6): 3

Trevitt C, Gallagher E 1996 Elder abuse in Canada and Australia: implications for nurses. International Journal of Nursing Studies 33(6): 651–659

Tylee A, Katona C L 1996 Detecting and managing depression in older people. British Journal of General Practice 46(405): 207–208

Vernon M, Bennett G 1995 'Elder abuse': the case for greater involvement of geriatricians. Age and Ageing 24(3): 177–179

Walt G 1998 Globalisation of international health. The Lancet 351(9100): 434–437

Warren K, Bennett G 1997 Elder abuse: an emerging role for the general practitioner. Geriatric Medicine 27(3): 11–12

Westhall J 1997 The debate of the age. British Medical Journal 315(7115): 1034

Whitehead E 1995 Prejudice in practice. Nursing Times 91(21): 40–41

Willmott J 1997 Home Watch can protect vulnerable residents. Elderly Care 9(5): 36

Wilson G 1994 Abuse of elderly men and women among clients of a community psychogeriatric service. British Journal of Social Work 24(6): 681–700

Wright S 1995 Promoting solidarity between generations: the nurses' role. Nursing Times 91(34): 34–35

Yohannes A M, Roomi J, Baldwin R C, Connolly M J 1998 Depression in elderly outpatients with disabling chronic obstructive pulmonary disease. Age and Ageing 27(2): 155–160

Young J, Robinson J, Dickinson E 1998 Rehabilitation for older people. British Medical Journal 316(7138): 1108–1109

FURTHER READING

Benbow S 1997 Shock waves: using ECT to treat depression. Geriatric Medicine 27(10): 25–28

Burke M M, Walsh M B 1997 Gerontologic nursing: wholistic care of the older adult. Mosby, St Louis, p 140–160

Daniel R 1997 Cancer: the holistic approach to management. Geriatric Medicine 27(1): 29–30

Eagles J M, McLeod I H, Douglas S 1997 Seasonal changes in psychological well-being in an elderly population. British Journal of Psychiatry 171: 53–55

Fradd S 1996 Down in the dumps or depressed? Geriatric Medicine 26(5): 35–36

Pitt B 1997 Defeat depression: a positive outcome. Geriatric Medicine 27(5): 37–40

Reitzes D C, Mutran E J, Fernandez M E 1996 Does retirement hurt wellbeing? Factors influencing self-esteem and depression among retirees and workers. Gerontologist 36(5): 649–656

Women's health and men's health

The health of women and men in society is a topic that attracts the attention of many feminist writers. While there is a plethora of literature findings on women's health, men's health somehow receives scant attention. In this chapter several issues are considered with the bio-psychosocial and sexual dimensions in mind. The main objectives are:

- to raise awareness of key features that affect the lives of men and women
- to discuss how social-environmental influences can affect health
- to identify methods, strategies and interventions which can be implemented by a broad spectrum of professionals in a variety of settings to ensure that their health needs are effectively met.

WOMEN'S HEALTH

HEALTH BELIEFS
Feminist perspective

There is a plethora of literature on women's health. Writings on the subject reflect the cultural diversity and emphasis on health as an important resource for society as a whole. Many feminist writers have contributed to the debate on health education and promotion of health for women. Their views have highlighted perspectives that have enlightened one's understanding that health project initiatives should encompass the individual dimension using the phenomenological perspective – to understand the person's definition of health – before applying health models to practice, thus ensuring needs are efficiently met.

Goudsmit (1994) makes reference to the 'psychologization' of women's physical complaints, whereby professionals in clinical practice fail to diagnose and treat their illnesses, because of the stereotypical view that women are 'hysterical' and 'neurotic'. This view has been extended in the writings of Curtis and Taket (1996) in their analysis of the health concept, when they traced the history of men's perception of women in connection with their mental states. Independent, assertive women were considered to be exhibiting 'hysterical' features of their personality. Similarly, in other instances, women's feelings and mental well-being may be trivialized, in relation to altered body image (Wilkinson & Kitzinger 1994), by inappropriate communication showing lack of insight and sensitivity. With regard to female sexuality and reproductive health, traditional societal values have impeded effective sexual health education (Thomson & Holland 1994). Thomson and Holland pointed out that many approaches have not considered either women's views and perceptions of their sexuality, or the power relationships that exist between women and men. The stereotypical belief is that men show their machismo in sexual relationships, thus increasing women's submissiveness.

In a woman's working environment, moreover, socio-cultural practices indicate that women's health can be negatively affected (Doyal 1994). Since many women in developed and developing countries work in factories, the nature of their work entails their exposure to harmful dusts, predisposing to respiratory illnesses; others are exposed to chemicals that can cause skin conditions. In some parts of the world (e.g. Mauritius, China, India, Africa) female agricultural workers are prone to developing back problems. Constant bending – necessary in rice plantation and tea cultivation – is often the cause. In Westernized work environments women, who form the majority of office workers, are exposed to the harmful effects of electronic equipment, i.e. word processors and computers, which not only can cause eye and hand strains, but can also affect posture.

Feminist approaches toward the position of women in society, as the examples above show, provide us with insight into the degree of inequalities between women's and men's socio-economic status. Feminist perspectives are also expressions of health beliefs as they affect women, since some practices have health implications. When feminist writers express these viewpoints, they are emphasizing their position in regard to health models that have detrimental effects on women. They feel that current practices must be questioned and re-evaluated, and that attitudes should be altered accordingly (Oakley 1990).

For example, one may consider food distribution among families in some cultures, and how it can cause malnutrition in women (Bonvillain 1995), due to the latter receiving parsimonious proportions after they have served their husbands and children. Bonvillain also compared birthing practices in societies, which can adversely affect women's well-being and sense of personal control. She pointed out that the practice of 'dorsal position' in birthing has negative effects on women's physiology: adverse effects on blood pressure and cardiac return. Medical technology is then used to counteract the side-effects of these effects, which minimizes women's control in the birthing process. In comparison, the squatting, kneeling and sitting positions practised by many cultures provide women with some control, increasing their sense of well-being (Bonvillain 1995). Professional and technological intervention can, therefore, interfere with personal control in some circumstances in clinical practice. From a broad sociological perspective, however, it has been pointed out (Naidoo & Wills 1994), that women in society 'have less control over their own lives' in comparison to men. Feminist interpretations of the way a male-dominated society treats women are based on the belief that women's health needs are not being fully met due to oppressive and discriminatory practices. Oakley (1993) believed that women's disadvantaged position in relation to men makes them more vulnerable, and that women are more likely to have their health-related needs unmet due to the relationship being unhealthy and 'exploitative'. Moreover, she pointed out that society is increasingly medicalizing women's distress. Women's health needs, accordingly, are interpreted differently to men's in spite of similarities in clinical features; e.g. women are more likely to receive a psychiatric diagnosis from their general practitioners (Oakley 1993). If this is indeed the case, the implications for health care in relation to women's health needs must be borne in mind (Box 5.1).

Box 5.1 The effects of misinterpreting women's health needs

A psychiatric label will increase the client's distress, particularly when she feels that her complaints are genuinely physical in nature. Misdiagnosing worsens the illness since the treatment does not match the pathology. Besides, ineffective intervention can augment anxiety reactions and worsen any underlying depressive states, leading to the 'self-fulfilling prophecy'; i.e. the client begins to believe that she is mentally ill.

Gender differences are implicated in the way men and women perceive their social world (Ooijen & Charnock 1995). Similarly, one can expect differential understanding in relation to the interpretation of health matters. Ooijen and Charnock argued that, as men and women have differing perceptions about themselves, their communication will be interpreted and understood differently. The expression of feelings and thinking may be interpreted as 'emotional' reactions from a woman; whereas a man is expected to exercise more self-control, suppress feminine reactions, such as being 'tearful' or 'hysterical', and to demonstrate the use of reason and exercise his power. Some authors, however (Krieger & Fee 1994), believe that these patterns of health-related behaviour reflect societal values founded on 'convention', 'discrimination' and 'social order of people'.

When one considers, for example, the cultural convention of female circumcision practised in some countries (Ethiopia, Somalia, Egypt) despite the physical, sexual and psychosocial health implications (Morris 1996, Farooqui 1997,

McConville 1998), there is evidence of subservience to male power. In these circumstances, women's health needs take secondary position to a patriarchal society's values and cultural norms. Clitoral and/or labial excision ensures the perpetuation of men's control and the oppression of women. It is believed that circumcision will control women's sexual appetite, thus ensuring their fidelity. Farooqui (1997) wrote that circumcision has the significance of implying proof of virginity, preventing animosity from in-laws, while maintaining family honour.

Despite the socio-cultural values and the economic benefits entailed (operators must be paid for their work), the side-effects (Box 5.2) can be manifold. While attention is focused on conventional approaches in connection with societies' particular cultural norms and beliefs (Box 5.3) concerning women's sexual and reproductive

---

Box 5.2 Complications of female circumcision

Female circumcision can cause physical and psychological traumas. Physical pain during and after the procedure is common. Psychological pain is experienced through the anticipation of excruciating physical pain, deep anxiety reactions compounded with fear, and the feelings of powerlessness as one is subjugated to the forces of ritualistic practices. Complications of the procedure may include haemorrhage, pelvic and urinary infection, scarring, lack of sexual response, painful intercourse (which can interfere with marital relationships), perineal laceration (which can occur during labour), loss of consciousness and death.

Box 5.3 Socio-cultural rationale for female circumcision

In countries where circumcision is still practised, people believe that clitoral excision will prevent baby death. The argument is that if the baby's head touches the clitoris during birth it will die; in some cases, it is believed to have a strong religious significance. Another reason for circumcision is to ensure the woman's faithfulness to her husband, as well as the prevention of in-laws' accusations that the bride is not a virgin. The practice, therefore, has sexual, marital and social significance. These implications must be borne in mind (see Box 5.4) during encounters between health care professionals from Westernized countries and clients from other cultures.

Box 5.4 Nursing care implications

The practice of female circumcision is an emotive subject. Sometimes, the literature makes reference to 'female genital mutilation', because this is a Westernized society's perception of a practice considered to be barbaric and abusive. It is essential for nurses and allied professions to be non-judgemental, and to approach this complex and challenging practice with tact and sensitivity. Morris (1996) argued that professionals must be educated to confront cultural diversity, while working to 'strike a delicate balance . . . yet promoting change at the same time'.

In addition, a holistic approach to health care is a prerequisite: individuals from other cultures behave the way they do because of ancient rituals and practices which can constrain their behaviour. It is therefore necessary to spend time listening to clients and attempting to gain insight into their cultures.

McConville (1998) pointed out that using the term female genital mutilation is considered an insult to the people of Mali (West Africa). Communication must be tactful, with attention paid to the person's psychological and cultural needs. Changes in attitude and beliefs to prevent adverse physical effects can take a long time. Individuals may seek information from professionals on health matters, and it is during such interactions that medical and nursing practitioners in primary care settings can attempt to alter patients' beliefs (Woloshynowych et al 1998). Patients may ask for advice and look for psychological support to help them cope with their health problems, which may not require pharmacotherapy or investigation.

Professionals in this context must build upon any positive perceptions of health issues that patients have. Since patients' perceptions will affect their attitude in connection with how their health will be affected (Kendall & Lask 1997), the professionals' role is to encourage the individual's positive health lifestyle behaviour, while explaining the adverse effects ensuing from bad practices. While the giving of health information and advice is desirable, it is recommended that a good assessment of the person's socio-economic background is carried out. Failure to do so could cause a mismatch between the health-related advice and the capacity of the person to comply. Defo (1997) noted that the socio-economically disadvantaged status and traditional problems of women in Cameroon have constraining effects on their health-related behaviour. Nevertheless, Defo argued that health education has the advantage of giving women both choices and the knowledge to question current practices, subsequently improving their health status.

---

functions, which have health implications, some authors (Raftos et al 1997) believe female circumcision demonstrates a lack of 'holism' when caring for women.

An exploration of feminist literature indicates the prevalence of a reductionist perspective, that is:

1. women's health literature does not consider the lived experience of women
2. biological–physiological functions in connection with reproductive health are overemphasized at the expense of the mental–spiritual–social dimensions
3. body parts (e.g. uterus, cervix, external genitalia and breast) form the main focus of women's health issues
4. sexual health orientation and motherhood are assumed to be the prevalent concerns of the female.

Researchers emphasize (Raftos et al 1997) the importance of recognizing the context in which women find themselves, to ensure that their personhood is acknowledged and respected. In addition, socio-economic, political and cultural influences are key issues to consider in attempting to understand the health–illness behaviour of women.

The source of health beliefs, one can argue, finds its origin in the family unit, through the transmission of socio-cultural knowledge of society. Tracing the source will help identify other impinging social and psychological factors affecting its trajectory.

An identification of varied social forces will facilitate an understanding of the formation of such health beliefs. Without this awareness, professionals cannot implement health promotional activities (Bright 1997).

Activity 5.1

1. Use CINAHL to examine the literature on women's health from 1996 to 1998, to assess the degree of holism evident in the articles.
2. Contact the Community Health Trust Midwives. Arrange an interview. Prepare a list of questions related to the practice of female circumcision. Write your findings in your reflective practice journal.

??? Question 5.1

1. To what extent have feminists' writings influenced our understanding of women's health?
2. What do you consider to be the most important strategy to use in relation to promoting the health of women?
3. Should Western cultures impose their values on developing countries that have their own traditional health beliefs?

THE NATURE OF WOMEN'S HEALTH NEEDS IN SOCIETY

Domestic violence

Domestic violence refers to acts of aggression occurring within the private confines of the family home. Such acts not only have social and legal implications, but encompass the psycho-emotional and physical effects on the victims. Most often, domestic violence is attributed to the behaviour of the male partner as he acts out physical and verbal aggression towards the female victim: a wife, girlfriend or ex-partner. However, domestic violence should not be restricted to the context just described. As discussed in Chapter 3, domestic violence can take many forms: abusive parental behaviour in relation to vulnerable children who are subjugated to physical, emotional and sexual abuse; siblings abusing their sisters and/or brothers. In addition, one should also bear in mind that domestic violence can occur within the gay and lesbian community.

In this section, attention is focused on adult heterosexual relationships; relationships that follow a life course of continuing violence in the privacy of the home, characterized by physical assault, battering and abuse, and which can end in manslaughter or homicide.

Domestic violence is a sensitive issue. Many victims of home violence either do not report their plight or take a long time before doing so. Fear of reprisal is a common cause: attempts to reveal the situation to the authorities, friends or relatives could lead to further beatings by the husband or boyfriend. Furthermore, some women experience embarrassment in revealing their private lives to others, in particular when there is police intervention, which adds to the stigma of being a battered wife. On the other hand, many women feel that officialdom, as well as informal community networks (relatives, friends, neighbours) will not believe their story. The myth that some women attract violence (Women's Health 1994), in addition to the victim-blaming approach (Lydon 1996), compounds the negative stereotype.

Official figures, however, demonstrate an alarming trend: 43% of all women who died in 1990 were killed by a partner (Parliamentary Home Affairs Committee), while 11% were killed by a stranger (the remaining 46% died from other causes). In 1991, more women in the USA were reported as dying from domestic violence than from rape, muggings and road traffic accidents together (Lydon 1996). The Council on Ethical and Judicial Affairs, American Medical Association (1992) and Keller (1996) all reported similar findings. Moreover, it is estimated (Thobaben 1997) that, in the USA and Britain, in at least five of every 100 marriages, women become the targets of physical violence in the home. Children in the home environment can also be affected, with disastrous consequences. Hampshire (1998) reported the case of a depressed, abusive and violent father who murdered his two children.

Domestic violence is a worldwide phenomenon showing varying degrees of intensity and cutting across cultures of the human race. According to Bignall (1993), New Zealand and Colombia have a 20% rate of domestic violence, while most other countries have a rate of between 30 and 50%. Wife-beating in Southern India, however, is perceived by the community and the victims as a commonplace socio-cultural norm (Rao 1997); indeed the rate for households affected by domestic violence throughout India is 75%. Several factors are attributed to its causation (Rao 1997).

1. Indian society relies strongly on bride dowry: a poor bride with a poor family background is prone to being beaten by her husband, as well as by her in-laws.

2. Alcohol consumption is linked to physical abuse.

3. Female sterilization is the only method of contraception. Consequently, childless women are scorned by their husband's parents, in-laws and their own parents.

4. The number of female children a woman bears increases her likelihood of being beaten. Sons are highly valued in Indian society; more sons could mean fruitful dowries in the future, hence benefiting the whole family. Conversely, female children create economic burdens for families.

5. Education is related to domestic violence. Educated husbands expect a 'larger dowry'. Dowry shortfalls, hence, increase the propensity for violence against wives.

Not surprisingly, as in the USA, homicides and suicides occur in India (Bignall 1993, Rao 1997) following wife abuse.

Box 5.5 relates recent instances of domestic violence in Bangladesh.

Box 5.5 Hot water, hot water

'Hot water' is the name given to concentrated sulphuric acid. Many young women are having acid thrown in their faces by partners or boyfriends, causing severe facial disfigurement. The Dhaka Medical Centre reports many cases. The women victims attempt to put up a brave front. One of the abused women stated: 'I am happy on the outside'. Witnesses believed that the 'girl must have done something'. (Jon Snow, Channel 4 News, 5 February 1998)

Social trends indicate that women are likely to be abused during pregnancy, with consequences for both mother and baby (Flitcraft 1992, McFarlane et al 1992, Newberger et al 1992, Bewley & Gibbs 1994, Richardson & Feder 1996, Mahony 1997, Mezey & Bewley 1997). The physical trauma experienced by battered women affects their mental and emotional well-being. Risk to the unborn baby coerces many women into adopting a passive role, hoping to minimize the violence (Case example 5.1).

The complications of physical assault on the pregnant woman include increased incidence of

Case example 5.1

Narakeshwansimooloo is 6 months pregnant. She has just finished preparing some chappati for her husband who is coming from the sugarcane fields. She is never too sure what mood he will be in. He has been so unpredictable lately. She decides to put her feet up, waiting for his return. She dozes off. Her catnapping is, however, abruptly ended. She receives a blow across the chest and falls to the floor. She knows her husband is back. As he hits her, she raises her hand to protect her face. But she does not make a sound. She is frightened: her baby's safety is foremost in her mind.

stillbirth, miscarriage, preterm labour (Bewley & Gibbs 1994). Some women may present with features of stress-related illnesses (Sugg & Inui 1992), such as insomnia, aches and pains, headaches and anxiety reactions. Physical examinations may reveal bruises on the abdomen, breasts and genitalia.

From a psychological viewpoint the battered woman may show features of low self-esteem, feelings of worthlessness and an inability to communicate clearly her feelings. Full expressions, however, may further jeopardize her relationship with her husband or partner, since disclosure may lead to police intervention. In view of the complex nature of this social phenomenon, a systematic approach in tackling the problem is needed. Several issues must be considered:

1. assessing women's problems and needs
2. setting clear achievable goals or objectives
3. intervening quickly by making use of available resources which are trauma-specific
4. evaluating existing practice and developing training programmes for health care professionals.

Assessment

Literature findings indicate that primary care professionals fail to recognize spouse abuse in a variety of settings, in spite of physical examination evidence that points to its possibility (Council on Ethical and Judicial Affairs, American Medical Association 1992, Council on Scientific Affairs,

American Medical Association 1992, Roberts et al 1997). It is argued that a failure to make effective diagnosis is due to:

- professional barriers, such as lack of training and education
- personal dilemmas caused by fear of intruding into the patients' private lives (Sugg & Inui 1992)
- feelings of powerlessness
- evidence of defence mechanisms such as denial, rationalization and minimization (Filcraft 1992)
- a medically focused model of intervention (Richardson & Feder 1996) relying on objective physical findings, at the expense of the clients' social experiences and problems
- insensitive, non-empathetic attitude (Campbell et al 1994), discouraging abused women from discussing the roots of their problems.

Although the above findings reflect the American experience, Lydon (1996) argued that similarities in professional behaviour have been observed in the UK, with some professionals being guided by beliefs based on stereotypical myths and showing a defeatist attitude. Furthermore, Moelwyn-Hughes (1997) observed that UK general practitioners and health visitors cannot confidently recognize the manifestations of battered women syndrome. While the assessment of physical damage is important, the secondary effects (apprehension, fear, depression, emotional blunting, hopelessness, despair, suicidal tendencies etc.) need attentive identification and acknowledgement.

Practitioners in all health care settings should be conversant with the clinical features that may indicate spouse abuse (Box 5.6).

The assessment procedure in care settings (emergency departments, general practitioners' surgeries, home environment, hospitals) should take place in the privacy of a room, to avoid disruption and to maintain the sufferer's dignity.

Although research findings (Sugg & Inui 1992, Richardson & Feder 1996) indicate that practitioners find assessing victims of domestic violence to be time-consuming, enough time

---

Box 5.6 Features of spouse abuse

Physical assessment
- Injuries to the head, face, upper limbs, breasts and genitalia
- Bruises to the eyes and abdomen
- Scald marks
- Scalp patches, e.g. where hair has been pulled out
- Internal damage, e.g. ruptured spleen and kidneys
- Haematuria
- Weight loss due to loss of appetite (a common feature of depressive illness, worsened by constant fear of impending assault)
- Gastrointestinal changes: 'butterfly' feelings in the stomach, diarrhoea, constipation and ulcer formation.

Psychosocial assessment
- Disturbed emotional state: crying and sobbing, with inability to communicate clearly the reason for the unhappiness (some individuals may emphasize the emotional aspect of their condition in spite of their physical trauma. Roberts and colleagues (1997) postulated that victims find emotional abuse worse than physical abuse)
- Nervousness
- Embarrassment (in the presence of the partner)
- Inconsistent reports of how injuries occurred
- Evidence of alcohol and drug abuse as coping mechanisms
- Depression and anxiety.

Some victims may express the need to move to a place of safety (moving house, looking for new accommodation, women's refuge). In addition, during the interview, if the women's partners are present, they (the abusers) may show a façade of caring and empathetic behaviour toward their victims, monopolizing the conversation and answering questions on their behalf. It has also been known for abusers to fabricate stories prior to the interview, coercing their victims to present them during the assessment. Mahony (1997) observed that the abuser may show a condescending attitude, aimed at minimizing the situation and undermining the woman's integrity.

---

should be allocated to allow the clients to ventilate their feelings. Empathetic listening and an unhurried attitude will encourage victims to talk about their personal experiences at their own pace.

During the interactions, the aim of the assessor is to retrieve detailed information about the individual's home circumstances, so that her specific needs and problems can be identified. It is essential to recognize not only the physical emergency of domestic violence, but the *social emergency* as well. Knowing what to look for is important. The health professional may use specific guidelines related to identifying social chaos, involvement of children (relationships with the abuser), signs of abuse, home safety, plan of safety, factors which precipitate violence etc.). It is, however, advisable to avoid judgemental questioning that is blaming and rejecting in character (Keller 1996), since the client's anxiety could increase, making her feel responsible for what is happening.

Assumptions are often made in clinical practice that abused women are reluctant to divulge evidence of domestic abuse. Research findings show that this is not the case (Grundfeld et al 1994, Keller 1996, Mezey et al 1998), and one survey (Campbell et al 1994) showed that battered women's advocates favoured the idea of formulating specific questions to ask the women. How and what questions to ask is also important, and sensitivity must be exercised (Box 5.7).

Box 5.7 Are you safe at home?

The art of questioning an abused individual demands patience, experience, empathy and perseverance. An open, non-blaming questioning technique should be used. Examples include:

- Do you feel safe at home? If there is a 'no' answer, it can be followed by 'please explain why'. If the answer is 'yes', one can remark: 'You sound as if you are frightened? Do you want to talk about it?'
- In what way do you feel your husband/partner does not understand you?
- Has your husband ever *hurt* you? This question may elicit a defensive protective response. It can, however, be *softly* asked again, followed by *gentle* exploration (Keller 1996).

Keller (1996) argued that a safe environment is more likely to encourage the client to elaborate her answers. Therefore, the context of the clinical interview is important: professional attitude, calm confident behaviour and good time management.

Some clients may not be prepared initially to volunteer sensitive information, due to fear and embarrassment. In these circumstances, it may be useful to give the client the freedom to decide when she is ready to talk, and to support her decision in an empathetic manner (Jezierski 1996). In addition, some women may have illnesses (psychotic confusional states, acute medical or surgical conditions), which make questioning inappropriate.

Activity 5.2

1. Make a list of non-verbal approaches that can be used during interactions with the client.
2. Attempt to role play a mini scenario with your peers, with one acting as the victim and another as a health professional. Describe your experience.

? ? ? Question 5.2

1. If an abused woman is accompanied by her partner, *how* would you relate to him?
2. Can you formulate some questions that you would like to ask him?

Goal setting

Since women's health needs are manifold in the context of domestic violence, goal setting must encompass the holistic dimension:

- attending to the immediate physical needs to restore homeostasis
- helping to regain psycho-emotional well-being
- attending to the patient's social emergencies by developing safety plans and by making alternative social arrangements if needed
- maintaining spiritual integrity.

Care implementation

Prioritization of care is essential. As soon as the physical injuries have been assessed, decisions must be made as to whether surgical interventions or medical measures (e.g. drug treatment for pain relief, or if weight loss and dehydration are severe, hyperalimentation may be instituted) are required.

If haematuria is identified, cystoscopy is needed to investigate the urinary system. The severity of the physical conditions will determine whether hospital care and treatment are advised. In these situations, the giving of adequate information concerning procedures and treatment rationale must be given to the care receiver. The aim is to increase personal mental well-being and comfort, and to mobilize the individual's inner potential to cope with her circumstances. Additionally, her cooperation and understanding are important features in the alleviation of post-traumatic stress and for successful recovery.

Pregnant mothers/women will need specialized support from a nurse midwife. Midwives are at the forefront of tackling abuse of pregnant women due to their frequent interactions with vulnerable individuals. Their assessment of the person's circumstances should be tightly knitted with the intervention process. Their knowledge of organizational policies and guidelines will help in informing their clients of community resources, with the aim of empowering them. The midwife, however, may be influenced by her personal values, beliefs and assumptions, 'which will influence the perception of her role' (King 1996) and the approaches used during intervention. King emphasized the essentiality of a humanistic, objective, non-judgemental care intervention, based on an 'advocacy model' that is woman-centred in nature.

Consistency in approaches coupled with understanding, support and an individual-centred strategy is important so that the community-based resources that are trauma-specific will develop their potential to cope. Consistent health care measures are possible when personnel operate within clear organizational guidelines that are fully accepted and adhered to by all concerned.

Other supportive professional networks may be recruited: police, lawyers, social workers, housing department, education and voluntary groups (e.g. Women's Aids Federation) (Carlisle 1997). The mobilization of community health professionals cannot be overemphasized. Their role in assessment and prevention (through implementation of nursing, psychiatric and health visiting care) can enhance women's health by education and promotion. As Davison (1997) pointed out, nurses' knowledge base in relation to the clinical and social signs of abuse becomes a valuable tool in identifying and meeting their needs. Promoting women's health by empowering them is incomplete without due consideration given to current development in health

promotion strategies. For instance, Benson and Latter (1998) criticize the traditional ways of health promotion based on prescriptive information-giving and directive approaches, at the expense of collaborative, negotiating and individualized strategies. They point out that the integration of interpersonal skills with health promotion practice will empower the client. They label this model the 'new paradigm approach' to health promotion.

In the context of women's health, therefore, victims of domestic violence are not prescribed the action to take, but are made aware of available networks of support and encouraged to use their inner potential to cope. Benson and Latter's new paradigm approach is client-centred, providing the individual with the means 'to choose a course of action' independent from the professional's idea of what is best; this strategy is more likely to empower the client. In addition, the authors assert the importance of considering the 'role of the client', whereas in the past the focus has been on the 'role of the nurse'.

Meaningful interpersonal encounters with women in need will break the barriers imposed by the belief that the professional is the 'expert', aiming to modify behaviour. It is worth emphasizing that professional care does not reside in any one specialized field. Intra-agency involvement – as in child abuse cases – becomes the ethos in domestic violence cases. While medical personnel in the accident and emergency department work as a unit within the wider 'proactive agency' framework, acting as advocates of victims of violence (Shepherd 1995), it is essential for other public health teams (police, Crime Concern, social work division, community mental health, midwifery and district nursing teams etc.) to combine their efforts in care delivery, prevention and protection of vulnerable women and their children.

Morley (1995) warned that women's health needs are usually more adequately met by genuine, empathetic and understanding behaviour from professionals at the initial point of contact in the accident and emergency department. Although she recognized the importance of police work, victims of domestic violence need to have an awareness of community network support services, such as women's refuges.

Since many agencies are involved in cases of home violence, role boundaries may become blurred. Adshead (1995) pointed out that the main responsibilities of care professionals (medical and nursing) are 'victim protection and support'. Crime prevention, Adshead asserted, is within the law boundary, and not the health framework. She explained that implementing protective and supportive measures can be developed by a collaborative partnership between health care providers, medical care organizations, voluntary groups and the Department of Health.

If women are to be empowered to cope, care implementation and support must be initiated as quickly as possible. Furthermore, the wider clinical practice implications should be considered.

WIDER CLINICAL PRACTICE IMPLICATIONS OF WOMEN'S CARE NEEDS

Social emergencies

Care is tailored to meet individual needs. A knowledge of community resources is necessary (e.g. Rape Crisis Line, women's refuges, Women's International Network, Women's and Girls' Network). A plan of safety is designed with the client's collaboration. This may mean making alternative accommodation arrangements by contacting relevant housing associations through local government housing services, or establishing direct correspondence with women's refuges. It is important, however, that the client realizes she has the right to cancel any decisions made. Similarly, she must not feel coerced into moving to a different home or talking to the women at the local refuge (Cody 1996). Cody (1996) pointed out that, in time of family crisis, the family system becomes more secretive and confined. Professionals may hence encounter women who change their minds by reverting their decisions on safety measures, without giving the full reasons. Despite the possibility of failure to uptake services, the full range of procedures should be explained to the client: housing advo-

cacy, referrals for legal and medical care, counselling support groups, with a strong emphasis on the preservation of confidentiality, respect for her decision not to prosecute her abusive partner, and the fact that the police will not be involved without her prior permission. Because the involvement of the police is an issue with strong ethical values, it may create conflict among professionals, a conflict Gillett (1995) identifies as residing between 'respect for autonomy and protection from harm'. In this context, clear-cut local policy guidelines are needed to promote the best course of action, based on the client's personal experiences and professional expertise.

One survey conducted in 230 Canadian hospitals (Hotch et al 1996) indicated that lack of clear policy guidelines engender inadequate care implementation. The importance of local and national policies is recognized in the UK, without which, it is argued (Bewley & Gibbs 1994, Mahony 1997), appropriate support may not be available.

Other factors to be considered are the client's personal belief and value systems. Social, religious and cultural factors can constrain specific groups. Thobaben (1997) provides examples of cultures whose beliefs may prevent them from escaping home violence: Roman Catholics may insist on living with their partners to avoid divorce; Japanese cultures believe in intact marriage and the avoidance of family shame; among some ethnic minorities the mother-in-law is the decision-maker, making it important to include mothers-in-law during decision-making processes.

Financial dependence is another reason that may constrain care implementation, since many victims are reluctant to leave home, as they rely on their partners' financial support to survive (Bewley & Gibbs 1994, Lydon 1996).

In all cases, benefit agencies may be contacted to obtain detailed information on benefits and other social entitlements. In addition, practical assistance may be obtained from voluntary services (e.g. victim support schemes) to advise on monetary matters and legal procedures (Mezey et al 1998).

Associated with financial problems is the

availability of housing to women made homeless through domestic violence. While care professionals may make recommendations and provide contact with agencies, the realities faced by homeless women in the housing market compound their sense of isolation, deprivation and neglect. Malos and Hague's study (1997) reports the inadequacy of housing provision to meet women's and their children's needs:

1. there is delay in providing safe houses for women and their families
2. temporary accommodation provided is sub-standard
3. safety is not guaranteed (ex-partners can still assault them) and lack of privacy is evident
4. many women return to their homes to face more violence
5. some housing officers exhibit hostility towards homeless women applicants
6. these women experience a deep sense of emotional deprivation and social neglect as they attempt to rebuild their lives.

In view of Malos and Hague's findings, professionals have a responsibility to make their clients aware of public policy constraints in meeting their housing needs. Community health personnel must liaise with women's refuge workers, women's aid federations and other community groups, to help reduce the impact of homelessness and the inadequacy of housing on women's psychosocial, emotional and spiritual well-being.

Mental health

A chaotic lifestyle caused by social disruption has mental health implications: a sense of abandonment, suicidal thoughts, depressive illnesses, deliberate social withdrawal. A stressful lifestyle can trigger psychotic symptoms in some individuals: thought disorders, disturbed emotions, altered perceptions and paranoid features. A mental health profile is required to anticipate the person's psychological health needs. The community psychiatric teams, in collaboration with other health and social agencies, must combine their efforts to prevent mental health breakdown and to provide therapeutic interventions,

such as psychotherapy, counselling, support groups, family therapy to enhance clients' coping skills.

An awareness of the aetiology of women's psychological ill-health, in particular the interactions between social–environmental–psychological–biological dimensions, is important. It is argued (Solberg 1989, Jenkins 1990) that women's propensity to develop psychological problems may reside in their individual lifestyle. Socio-economic factors, e.g. poverty, homelessness and unemployment, can predispose to mental ill-health causing behavioural changes (Béphage 1997). In addition, one should be sensitive to the fact that adversity causes individuals to alter their behaviour anyway, to adapt to a new way of life. When mental ill-health occurs, deviant characteristics, i.e. self-harm, drug and alcohol misuse, delinquency etc. can be expected.

Spirituality

Some individuals, when faced with adversity, resort to their spiritual strength: the utilization of one's mental energy to tap into the lived experiences. These experiences may consist of practising one's religious rituals or adopting a philosophical stance: believing that negative life experiences are hurdles that need to be conquered. To others, being spiritual may mean a combination of these two approaches. Spirituality has on occasion been purely related to religion. Caregivers must therefore consider this possibility in their interactions with clients. On the other hand, adversity can destroy spiritual well-being and stability, exhibited by:

- loss of confidence in God(s)
- negative attitude towards other people and about life in general
- loss of faith in people and the structures of society, i.e. the family, the marriage institution, the law and so on.

Since spirituality can be interpreted in many ways, caregivers must remember that spirituality is a very individual matter. The perception and meaning given by people to their idea of the inner spirit (Oldnall 1996) is of utmost importance. Goddard (1995) emphasized that external events, i.e. life-altering events like homelessness, abuse and home violence, which have dramatic effects on a person, are factors that can disturb internal 'harmony'. It, therefore, becomes the professionals' responsibility to restore harmony and mobilize the client's resources in times of personal crisis. Spiritual anxiety or 'spiritual distress' (Oldnall 1995) may not be identified by practitioners if they operate within the narrow framework of a 'bio–psycho–social model'.

Care evaluation

Care evaluation is an ongoing process. Since domestic violence manifests multidimensional characteristics, regular briefing and the collation of data must be done. Clear documentation is essential so that interventions can be compared and altered accordingly. Case conferences become the arenas for discussions and benchmarking. Furthermore, education and training needs for professionals should be identified so that experiences can be shared and clinical skills refined. It has been found (Roberts et al 1997, Varvaro & Gesmond 1997) that personnel in accident and emergency departments respond favourably to training.

Activity 5.3

Use the *Times Index* in your local library to find out the frequency of domestic violence reported over the past 10 years.

??? Question 5.3

1. What do you perceive to be the possible causes affecting professionals' ability to tackle the problem of domestic violence?
2. If you were a victim of domestic violence, would your approach be different in communicating your needs?

SEXUAL AND REPRODUCTIVE HEALTH

Women's reproductive health represents an important area for consideration, and is reflected by:

• the debate that is being stimulated for sex education to be incorporated into the national curriculum (Savage 1997)
• the idea that credence should also be given to the related discipline of family planning (Bigrigg 1997)
• the existence of core services within the community (Baraitser 1997) reflects the need for its promotion
• the realization that sexual problems exist within the community, and that services based on open access within community-based settings (Carr 1997) must be on-going
• the fact that a woman's end of reproductive years are associated with hormonal changes, which have health implications, such as osteoporosis and cardiovascular disease (Wordsworth 1997).

There is a need to ensure that services in a variety of community health settings should be developed according to a quality programme (Bankowska 1997). Women should be made aware of their right to participate in their own care decisions (Jennings 1997), and of the treatment and services available to them.

Although reproductive health is a broad term that includes the recognition of pathology affecting women's reproductive system (e.g. cervical cancer, breast cancer, ovarian pathology etc.), sexual activity without an awareness of its health and social implications can and should be included within its framework.

Young, sexually active women are prone to developing sexually transmitted disease (e.g. genital warts and herpes simplex) (Bigrigg 1997). Beitz (1998) pointed out that specific groups of people are more likely to be affected through unsafe practices:

• young adults who live in poverty
• individuals who have not been socialized into health-oriented sexual teaching programmes

- individuals with a history of sexual abuse
- individuals involved in substance abuse
- people susceptible to the effects of irresponsible media influences (Beitz 1998).

A disciplinarian upbringing combined with strict religious beliefs and practices have been linked with controlled behaviour in regard to sex. However, in the UK there is a high teenage conception rate, which in 1995 showed a similar level to the 1980s, with the rate of pregnancy in girls under 16 rising by 18% (Health Matters 1997). To control the rise in teenage pregnancies, social, political and health care strategies to widen sex and reproductive health programmes and to development research need implementing. Some groups which are difficult to reach (e.g. sex workers, child/adolescent prostitutes, abused children) present challenges to family planning services. Such services may refer teenagers who attend their clinics to other agencies, since their other needs (such as alcohol misuse, drug abuse) require attention. Contraception and pregnancy problems can, in these circumstances, be the tip of the clinical iceberg.

Sexual and reproductive health education are topics many teenagers find hard to discuss with care professionals, not surprising since society's traditional approach has been to treat sex as a taboo subject, to be mentioned only behind closed doors. Many parents still show reluctance to educate their children on sexual matters, leaving the responsibility to sex educators in schools.

In practice settings, many teenagers in their interactions with practice nurses make references to their 'acne, immunizations and weight' (Gregg et al 1998), while avoiding issues such as sexual activities, pregnancy problems, alcohol and smoking. Gregg et al found that many teenagers have a fear that confidentiality on personal matters will be breached. Moreover, they pointed out that many practice nurses lack confidence to discuss sensitive matters in the 'teenage context'.

It can be assumed that if practice staff experience difficulties in relating to teenagers on personal sexual matters, the latter may perceive their behaviour as a reluctance to help. Practice nurses are, however, strategically positioned at the initial point of contact to educate teenagers and to promote sexual health. Their role as agents of change (Baird 1998) must not be underestimated. Avoiding the impulse to *impose* change is a key element in health promotion. Rather, practice nurses' strategic position allows them to *work with* their clients, instilling trust and confidence, being understanding and caring towards their targeted groups (Baird 1998).

Some teenagers may find conventional family planning services inappropriate to their needs (Morrison et al 1997). The provision of sexual health help centres (SHHC) provides an alternative pathway for those who prefer an informal environment with flexible opening times. Several such initiatives are implemented in the UK, giving advice, information, and a wide range of family planning and sexual health services in a non-judgemental and non-threatening environment. In addition, the key issue of confidentiality cannot be overemphasized and is a priority for teenagers (Smart 1997).

Other initiatives to facilitate attendance at clinics are the Young Person's Clinic in Northumberland, which helps sexually active young people to receive practical help and family planning advice integrated with general health issues (Smart 1997), and the Young People's Family Planning Strategic Group, in the Merton and Sutton boroughs of London (Pearson & Gardner 1997). These health clinics are within school proximity. Their aims are to reduce teenage pregnancies and to increase awareness of the 'health and social issues related to pregnancy and childbirth'.

As health and social issues are important features in sexual health education, practice and school nurses can integrate such topics in their programmes. Teaching sexual health is, however, an art. Teaching skills and training are required (Whitmarsh 1997) by school nurses who, according to Whitmarsh, have expressed a need in this area. Furthermore, skills development in promoting health within schools – by extending school nurses' teaching role – supports current health initiatives in connection with the 'Europe-wide initiative aims to develop schools as settings for the promotion of young people's health'

(Healy 1998) (Box 5.8); hospitals could develop similar strategies (Box 5.9).

Box 5.8 Health-Promoting Schools (Rogers et al 1998)

The World Health Organization developed the idea of Health-Promoting Schools in the 1980s. A European collaborative effort, with 37 countries participating in the project, called the European Network of Health-Promoting Schools (ENHPS) has been created. Schools within the network have responsibilities in adopting sound health promotion and education strategies, to include pupils and staff as well as the wider community with the involvement of parents, using a holistic perspective.

Box 5.9 Health-Promoting Hospitals

The role of the nurse in health promotion is widely recognized and accepted. Nurses are in a key position in hospitals to extend their functions beyond 'the narrow borders of acute clinical episodes' (Fielding & Woan 1998) to encompass community settings so that a comprehensive health promotion package can be developed. The World Health Organization is currently piloting a European project with targets to:

- promote human rights and respect for one's socio-cultural beliefs
- improve clients' and professionals' well-being
- develop holistic care
- make efficient use of resources in health care delivery
- promote collaborative partnership in a variety of care settings.

European-wide initiatives as described in Box 5.8 provide avenues for social, health and political organizations to evaluate their own initiatives, by comparing their methods. For example, the Dutch compared with the British system of sexual health education, begin sex education from primary school onwards (Dolby 1998), integrating within their teaching not only the biology of sexual behaviour, but aspects related to wider pertinent issues. The Dutch initiatives include discussions on the concept of 'love', 'relationships', personal attraction, peer pressure and media influences in connection with romanticizing sexual behaviour at the expense of focusing on key health-damaging issues such as sexually transmitted diseases, AIDS, low self-

esteem, dependency on the State and kin support, and the effects of social deprivation. Despite the good intentions of preventative services, in the field of pregnancy reduction and sex education recommended by the Health of the Nation in 1992, one pivotal point in question is to attempt to understand young people (Case example 5.2), so that sophisticated programmes can be designed 'to inform and support reproductive choice' (Weyman & Walsh 1998).

Case example 5.2 Tina's case

'I am 16. I am 3 months pregnant. I don't think my teachers understand me. The other day I overheard them talking about me. Two of them called me a "slag", and that I deserve it. They don't know me and they don't seem to care. If only they could spend some time just to listen to what I have to say. I didn't get pregnant because I wanted to. There is a lot of pressure from my school friends ... those that have done it ... you know ... I wanted to prove to them that I am not a coward, and that I am attractive too ... to the boys, I mean. I am beginning to realize the consequences of my action ... I don't know what to do ...'

An understanding of peoples' social world, its constraints and their perception of their role within it, will enhance professionals' discernment of the socio-psychological dynamics of interpersonal behaviour. To Irwin (1997), traditional approaches that are medically based models and that focus on information-giving, reduce effective sexual health promotion, while a community-centred approach with full awareness of contextual constraints (social, cultural, political and economic factors) will facilitate better health promotion activities.

By looking beyond the traditional boundaries of health promotion, a more effective understanding of the 'diversities within female sexuality' (Few 1997) can be developed. Professionals should also recognize their own traditional values and misconceptions concerning women's sexual and reproductive health needs.

Providing sexual health services to the mentally ill is recommended (Woolf & Jackson 1996), as people with mental health problems have

Table 5.1   Services to meet women's health needs

Family planning and community gynaecology clinics provide:

- contraception, sexual and reproductive health information
- pregnancy counselling
- menopause advice and hormone replacement therapy clinics
- terminations of pregnancy
- treatment of sexually transmitted infections
- sexual problems services
- colposcopy
- services for partners who need vasectomy (Baraitser 1997)
- well woman clinics
- psychosexual counselling
- domicillary services
- services for commercial sex workers
- day care units for the management of high-risk pregnancies (Twaddle 1995)
- abortion counselling (Clark 1997).

sexual health needs that must be met. Sexual health programmes are also of relevance to people with learning disabilities (Vernon 1998). The wide range of services in existence (Table 5.1) should be made accessible to all individuals concerned.

Activity 5.4

Write to the community nursing services to find out the strategies used in raising women's awareness of available services.

??? Question 5.4

Since women tend to live longer than men, what do you consider to be the long-term implications for future services?

SCREENING SERVICES

Cervical screening

Cervical screening is a national programme recognized as an essential component of preventative measures in the detection of cancer of the cervix. The need for vigilance (Willis 1997) is emphasized. There are 4340 new cases per year in the UK, with 1505 deaths (Willis 1997). The rate of screening in 1997 was 3.9 million women between the ages of 25 and 64 (Godfrey 1997). The media have, however, expressed discontent concerning the accuracy of results, and Godfrey (1997) reported an instance when 70 000 women were informed by the Kent & Canterbury hospitals that results could be incorrect. To women affected the situation provokes anxiety. Now, measures are being taken to improve cytology screening standards (Ogden 1998).

Literature findings (Gregory & McKie 1992, Yu & Rymer 1998) indicate that many women experience fear, embarrassment and discomfort when undergoing cervical screening. This has implications for clinical practice because a distressing experience can discourage women from attending future tests (Orbell 1996). A personal and sensitive approach is recommended (Smail & Smail 1989, Yu & Rymer 1998). In addition, an empathetic attitude, coupled with information-giving – through questions and answers, as well as the provision of an environment that will minimize distress – are measures considered necessary.

The procedure itself must be carried out efficiently, to obtain an adequate sample, thus preventing repeat smears, which provoke unnecessary distress in women (Padbury 1997). While the procedure can create anxiety, waiting for the smear result and obtaining a result that shows human papilloma virus, without adequate information, is distressing (Cadman 1998).

Breast screening

Regular breast self-examination is considered to be a primary screening practice in the identification of breast cancer (Foxall et al 1998). Foxall et al's study indicated that nurses lack confidence in breast self-examination, are inconsistent in the technique they use, and demonstrate non-compliance in the frequency of examining their own breasts despite their professional knowledge concerning this important screening procedure.

Breast cancer affects one in 12 women in the Western world (Godfrey 1997), and there are approximately 34 950 new cases a year in the UK (Willis 1997), with 14 080 deaths (Willis 1997, Nursing Standard 1998). In view of these findings, nurses must develop more positive health belief models about themselves, which can subsequently be imparted to non-nurses. Teaching and educating about breast examination is essential.

The preparation of women for more invasive breast screening procedures, e.g. mammography, needle aspiration, needle biopsy and excision biopsy, to prevent psychological breakdown (due to anticipated altered body image) is another crucial aspect of care.

Screening procedures impact on women's lives. Their pre- and postoperative information needs require sensitive management. Accurate information may decrease anxiety and facilitate the promotion of a healthy lifestyle (Deane & Degner 1997). On the other hand, a diagnosis of breast cancer entails preparing women to cope with the threat to their identities posed by the experience of cancer (Lugton 1997). Mobilizing formal (professional) and informal support is desired so that the impact of defeminization is reduced, and the quality of the support is important.

THE MENOPAUSE

To many women in society, the menopause represents another stage in the womanhood trajectory, one which they accept in a positive way. To others, however, the menopause becomes a threat to their general biological functions, in association with altered body image and the development of psychosexual problems (Griffin 1997). Although the menopause is widely accepted to affect women in their 50s, care providers must consider the possibility that a small minority of younger women (from the age of 17 onwards) have been known to develop unexplained premature menopause (Thomas 1997), causing psychoemotional distress.

Many symptoms are associated with the menopause: mood swings, vaginal dryness, hot flushes, bone changes (osteoporosis) and cardiovascular disease. Hormone replacement is a recommended therapy, since it also helps to counteract unpleasant symptoms and is known to reduce osteoporosis and cardiovascular disease (Bilezikian 1994, Scura & Whipple 1997, Hillard 1998).

Hillard (1998) reported that menopausal women may be best helped by giving them choices. Alternative therapies (acupuncture, reflexology, Chinese herbalism) may be offered to individuals who seek non-hormonal treatment. Some women may be influenced by their traditional cultural beliefs and health practices, which may not integrate with Westernized medical and nursing interventions. Approaches must be modified and adapted dependent on individual needs.

Clinicians, nursing practitioners and allied professionals, however, must be prepared to look beyond the menopause, in their assessment of needs to include the social context of women's lives (Woods & Mitchell 1997). For instance, although depression has been linked to the menopause, women may become depressed due to stressful life events; separation, divorce, bereavement and grief are some of these causative factors. Other lifestyle factors, such as over-exercise and excessive dieting, can cause menopausal symptoms (e.g. osteoporosis) among women in their 30s (Hart 1996).

WOMEN'S MENTAL HEALTH

Modern living impacts on women's mental health. It is argued that society's expectations of how women should behave – from birth onwards, through primary and secondary socialization – presents women with obstacles that have negative effects on their mental health (Clinical issues in nursing 1994). Contradictory messages from parents and teachers, for example, predispose women to enhanced stress levels and anxiety. The Royal College of Nursing reports that women are showing an increasing propensity for developing depressive illnesses and to seeking inpatient psychiatric admissions. Many causes are attributed to this prevalence. As pointed out at the beginning of this chapter, women's negative life experiences (domestic violence, history of sexual and physical abuse etc.) are contributory causes. It is also asserted that women's role in society as

Table 5.2 Social issues that can worsen mental ill-health
Homelessness Divorce, separation, home violence Unemployment, redundancy, bankruptcy Stress at work Abuse within the family Drug misuse Children with delinquent behaviour Living with families with a history of mental illness Racism Living in a poor neighbourhood.

child rearers – in particular when there are many children in a family (Ford & Rigby 1998) – predisposes them to high stress levels. However, a combination of other factors (i.e. unemployment, failed relationships, redundancy) can precipitate depressive ill-health (Ford & Rigby 1998).

While organic changes (e.g. brain pathology, electrolyte imbalance and genetic influence) can cause mental ill-health, primary health workers must exercise vigilance in order to detect social issues, which can compound the consequences (Table 5.2).

It is known that there is a growing number of homeless, mentally ill women on the streets (Allen 1996, Hatton 1997). Homelessness can cause mental ill-health. Conversely, severe mental ill-health can cause homelessness (Allen 1996), due to a lack of housing provision for this specific group. While primary care workers are strategically placed to identify needs, Wright (1996) argued that many clients' psychiatric illnesses go unrecognized in general practice. Many patients express their physical needs and problems (e.g. tiredness, exhaustion, headaches, sweating, palpitations), which very often are expressions of psychological problems. Adequate time must be allocated so that the client's history can be pieced together to reach an accurate diagnosis. Services should thereafter be tailored to individual needs.

Postnatal depression

Postnatal depression is common among women soon after birth. It is thought that 10–15% of mothers are likely to be affected. Postnatal depression may be described as altered mood,

characterized by loss of energy and fatigue, feelings of anxiety and irritability, impaired concentration, guilt feelings and loss of self-esteem. Such changes, although noticeable by the women themselves, are still not recognized as features of postnatal depression by the majority of people (Whitton et al 1996). Moreover, Whitton et al emphasize that the condition is not often detected, and remains untreated. Interestingly, women among the higher social class group, they point out, are less likely to recognize their symptoms as being linked to postnatal depression; this has implications for practice. Antenatal classes should include topics on identifying depressive features and postnatal behavioural changes by women and their partners. Moreover, the role of health visitors in education and prevention is well established (Taylor 1997). Their counselling skills can help to minimize the psychological impact of childbirth. Despite childbirth being a positive event to many women (Murray 1997), the pain and distress of labour can create consequences similar to post-traumatic stress disorder among some women postnatally (Charles 1997).

The management of postnatal depression requires a multidisciplinary approach (Hanley 1998). Very often depressive features are associated with relationship problems and how the mother perceives herself to be coping with the baby. Since the causation of postnatal depression is multifactorial, the health visitor has to work very closely with members of the primary care team: the general practitioner, the community psychiatric nurse and the midwife (whose previous knowledge of the mother antenatally is invaluable) in order for issues to be accurately addressed. For example, is the depression caused by a lack of cooperation in child care from the partner? Is the mother experiencing fear and frustrations about the baby? Is she experiencing altered perceptions regarding the baby: that the baby does not meet her expectations? To what extent is she receiving support from informal networks?

Such issues need to be addressed and discussed at team meetings. Above all, mothers postnatally need someone to talk to and who will listen to them. Charles (1997) asserts that listening is a skill providing psychological support. The art of listening is a useful tool (Box 5.10). Many mothers have a need to discuss their views and how they are coping with the birth of the baby. Sensitive support from the health visitor can potentiate the mother's need for empowerment.

Box 5.10 The art of listening

Patience and perseverance are prerequisites to good listening technique. Body posture can indicate whether the person is genuinely listening or not. Listen with the whole body. A mother with a newborn baby wants to tell the world about her experience. Listen. The listener will, from the content of the conversation, identify key areas needing specific attention, i.e. maybe a lack of confidence in breast feeding. Alternatively, the mother may non-verbally break down during interactions, denoting 'hot spots' which will need further exploration.

Empowering women postnatally to cope with their new social experience can be done by involving the father. During depressive phases, postnatal women may misunderstand the father's role. They sometimes experience feelings that husbands are not fully integrated into their status as fathers, feeling they are left to cope on their own. Health visitors have a responsibility to obtain the father's view of the situation. Like mothers, fathers have a need to be listened to and to be understood. Postnatal care philosophy entails family care so that depressive illnesses and family breakdown can be prevented. A comprehensive package of care has to be organized (Box 5.11) to promote mental health.

Box 5.11 Promoting women's mental health

The Royal College of Nursing specifies some key features to be considered in promoting women's mental well-being:

- services tailored with gender issues in mind and accessibility to services improved
- provision for child care arrangements
- formal and informal networks of support for women
- access to counselling, therapy and specific support groups
- appropriate training and development for staff who manage services
- better awareness of women's lives and health inequalities.

Activity 5.5

Prepare a reflective practice journal during your clinical placement on the postnatal ward. In what ways do mothers express depressive features? How would you support them?

??? Question 5.5

1. What measures do you consider should be taken to minimize the impact of postnatal depression?
2. The literature on postnatal depression focuses mainly on the mother and her baby. What can be done to help fathers cope with the anxieties of childbirth?

MEN'S HEALTH

Compared with the plethora of literature on women's health, there is a paucity of information in connection with men's health. A literature search on CINAHL, using the keywords 'battered men', from January 1982 to September 1997, revealed only one article, written in 1994; in the same time period the keywords 'battered women' revealed 97 articles. When the term 'domestic violence' was keyed in, an abundance of papers on the subject referred to women and female children as the victims of male violence; the papers did not indicate in any way whether male partners get assaulted and battered in home violence. In reality, there are some women who will retaliate violently against abuse by their male partners. The victimization of men under these circumstances, although under-reported, can lead to homicide. Women who seek revenge for being regular victims of home violence resort to drastic measures to end their suffering. Also under-reported are cases of women's violence against their innocent male partners.

The literature that makes reference to violence against men focuses on sexual assaults of a homosexual nature. Lipscomb et al (1992) described case stories of sexual assaults committed by men. Their reports, following a study in Tennessee, are based on observations made among sexually assaulted victims from the county penal system. They compared the prevalence of sexual battering between incarcerated men and the non-incarcerated in the community. Their conclusion indicated that the nature of sexual battering is not unique to prisons.

Men in the community encounter similar problems. Their reluctance, however, to reveal their experiences to authorities demonstrate the usual patterns that men are fearful of being misunderstood in relation to their sexual orientation. Lipscomb et al argued that an additional element could be the 'intense embarrassment about being a victim of sexual assault'. They do, however, make reference to a couple of cases when women were the perpetrators.

Health consequences of sexual assault on men

Men, like women, get raped. Unlike female sufferers, men are less willing to report and talk about their rape ordeal. The argument explaining this behaviour rests on the belief that a man's masculinity is likely to be questioned. In a society which places emphasis on the expression of masculine behaviour by men, whose sexual orientation has to be heterosexual in nature, and whose social activities must reflect their manhood in as many ways as possible, serious sexual assault of men is less likely to be disclosed. These attitudes make male victims of sexual assault an unidentified group which is poorly understood and ill-served by health care professionals (Rentoul & Appleboom 1997). Their health needs are diverse. The long-term consequences of being a rape victim of a homosexual nature must be acknowledged and anticipated, so that appropriate preventative measures can be taken.

Rentoul and Appleboom (1997) identified psychological and social reactions by male victims of rape.

Psychological reactions

Psychological reactions may include anxiety, fear, depression and psychosomatic symptoms such as nausea, gastric irritability, altered bowel habits, palpitations, headaches, tension and insomnia. Behavioural changes may lead to feelings of helplessness and submissiveness. The threat to one's masculinity disturbs one's self-image, which creates deep feelings of shame, guilt and humiliation. The individual may develop self-conscious feelings, i.e. that significant others have modified their behaviour towards him in a negative way, perceived to be repulsion. Distress and confusion can be experienced dependent on the nature of the assault. Sexual arousal by the victim, during the assault (which may occur) compounds the psychological distress. Rentoul & Appleboom argued that this type of submission makes the victim of rape feel that he is consenting to what is happening. To the perpetrator(s) it is a strategy that breaks down the defences of the abused.

Social reactions

Social distancing by the victim may interfere with interpersonal relationships. Distrust of male companionship is likely, while sexual relationships with women are dampened. The latter, however, may interpret this lack of interest as a change of sexual orientation, or the possibility of an illicit affair. Unless the survivor is willing to disclose his feelings, and to discuss openly his personal problems, relationships are prone to deterioration.

Therapeutic interventions

The privacy and dignity of the abused must be preserved. Confidentiality is ascertained. Physical care is given; where there is evidence of perineal and genital injuries, appropriate treatment is initiated. Pain relief must be considered. Surgical intervention may be required. Throughout interactions, professionals have a duty to communicate sensitively with the sufferer. Specialized counselling is suggested to prevent the development of psychiatric symptoms. In addition, using the services of self-help groups is recommended. A non-judgemental, empathetic approach will go a long way in gaining the cooperation of the victim.

??? Question 5.6

1. In what ways can society break the barriers preventing men from disclosing rape assault?
2. How important is it for men who have been sexually assaulted to receive psychiatric help?
3. Should male victims be attended by male professionals?

SEXUAL AND REPRODUCTIVE HEALTH

Sex education

We have seen the importance of early sex education for teenage girls to prevent and reduce the rise in teenage pregnancies. Similarly, boys and young men require sound sex education programmes. It is argued, nevertheless (Anderson 1997), that present programmes are inadequate: there is a failure to consider the wider implications of sexuality, such as social values, personal responsibility and interpersonal relationships. Moreover, Anderson pointed out, the stereotypical image of macho men presents a facade that obscures the inadequacies of boys in relation to sexual matters.

Boys' knowledge base is superficial and they have a latent need for support and advice. Anderson asserted that boys – contrary to popular beliefs – are prepared to talk about sexual matters maturely and to explore their feelings, as long as adequate time is allocated to spend with them. Knowledgeable and experienced teachers are preferred to those who lack the necessary skills or who feel embarrassed to talk about sex.

The development of a positive rapport with groups of teenagers, considering their views and needs in regard to sex education, and the type of programmes that suit their needs, will enhance cooperativeness and attentiveness. It is also recommended for educators to recognize positive participation from the groups and to give praise accordingly, when sensitive issues such as homosexuality and lesbianism are discussed, debated and analysed sensibly.

Teachers in schools, however, must work collaboratively with other professionals, e.g. community nurses with specialist training in family planning, in order to design programmes based on identified needs and problems. Additionally, involving the targeted group(s) in the design and evaluation of the programmes (Anderson 1997) will help ensure continuity and credibility, and will encourage attendance. A non-threatening, non-judgemental approach will further promote attendance. The avoidance of imposing one's values and beliefs is important. A Rogerian (humanistic: using Carl Rogers' principles) model to teaching and learning, by providing youngsters with the freedom to explore their thoughts and feelings, will stimulate positive participation. Since sex is a sensitive issue, exploring the reasons *why* it is so, becomes a useful tool. As Davidson (1996) pointed out, one needs to ask specific questions related to what are the main issues for teenage boys: their ways of talking about sex and relationships; cultural, religious and racial influences on their attitudes to sex. An insight into their lives will facilitate an understanding of wider social factors that raise doubts, questions and concerns for them (Davidson 1996).

On the other hand, the powerful influence of parents in shaping their children's attitudes to sexual matters must be recognized. While sex education for teenagers is recommended, it is equally important to make provision for parents to receive support and to be educated so that they can consolidate their children's formal sex education. Blakey and Frankland (1996) suggested workshops be used to enhance parents' sex education skills. Health professionals can also develop projects in their regions with the aim to promote sex education awareness.

Educating parents to become educators should include topics on the psychology of social learning. Since much learning is indirect, incidental and through observation (Hayes 1995), parents can be encouraged to develop self-awareness, so that positive attitudes on sex matters can be imparted to their children in the early years.

Prostate cancer

Prostatic cancer is the third most common cancer

in men (Central Statistics Office 1997). This cancer represents a significant health care problem (Dean 1997), and current trends show that its prevalence is on the increase. In 1991, there were about 14 000 cases diagnosed in England and Wales (Central Statistics Office 1997). It is rare in men under 50, but the incidence increases as the person gets older. Malignant changes have been observed in 95% of men older than 90 years (Dean 1997). Some risk factors have been linked to its occurrence:

- dietary lifestyle: increased fat intake and inadequate uptake of fruit and vegetables
- exposure to chemicals, such as cadmium
- migration from a non-Westernized country to a Westernized one (Peate 1998a).

Other possible causes are a familial history of cancer and promiscuity.

Detection and screening

The early detection of prostate cancer and better awareness programmes will uncover more patients with this condition (Dearnaley 1994). However, unless individuals are prepared to openly discuss urinary outflow problems with their care professionals, the condition may be undetected. Nevertheless, clinicians may increase the detection rate by preventative patient education and information. While well man clinics are well known for their services in blood pressure monitoring, dietary and general lifestyle habits to promote health, extending the services by purposeful monitoring of prostate and testicular cancer will widen their health promotion activities.

Dearnaley (1994) lists three main detection procedures:

1. digital rectal examination, as the prostate can be felt using this approach (Fig. 5.1)
2. prostate-specific antigen estimations (prostatic changes cause release of antigens in the blood)
3. transrectal ultrasound.

In cases where the cancer is suspected to have spread (metastases), other advanced techniques are used: computed tomography and magnetic

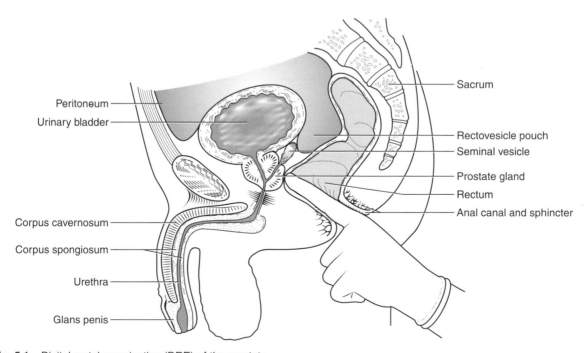

Fig. 5.1 Digital rectal examination (DRE) of the prostate.

Peritoneum

Urinary bladder

Corpus cavernosum

Corpus spongiosum

Urethra

Glans penis

Sacrum

Rectovesicle pouch

Seminal vesicle

Prostate gland

Rectum

Anal canal and sphincter

resonance imaging to detect pelvic nodes enlargement, and bone scanning for analysing cancerous bone deposits.

Client care and needs

The thought of cancer raises fear and panic in an individual. Time should be spent listening to his fears and the expression of personal needs. Available options (Box 5.12) should be carefully explained using diagrams as required. Bone pain due to cancerous deposits can be alleviated by the administration of analgesics in combination with radiotherapy (Dearnaley 1994). Other issues in relation to the person's social background need consideration. The effects of surgery on marital and sexual relationships, the fear of impotence and loss of masculinity can provoke intense personal distress. Sensitive communication is necessary, including significant others in the discussions after seeking the client's approval.

The nurse is ideally placed to be the client's advocate (Peate 1998b). Moreover, the expertise of a multidisciplinary team will ensure the client receives a wide range of pertinent support. Health educators in clinical practice have to give information on the basis that the client's prior knowledge of his reproductive anatomy is minimal and inaccurate. Peate (1998b), for example, pointed out that three out of 40 men were able to identify the prostate gland in a diagram. On the whole 'all of the men labelled the diagram incorrectly'. Explaining the normal structure of the reproductive system should be done prior to giving information on disease process.

Box 5.12 Treatment options for prostatic cancer

- **Transurethral resection of the prostate:**
  - recommended approach when the cancer is small and contained within the prostate. The prostate is resected via a cystoscope using a resectoscope.
- **Surgical removal (Fig. 5.2):**
  - suprapubic approach: the prostate is removed by making an incision through the bladder wall
  - retropubic approach: the surgeon reaches the prostate from behind the pubic region *without* opening the bladder
  - perineal approach: an incision through the perineum, to reach the prostate.
- **Testes removal:**
  - the aim of this surgery is to discontinue the effects of male sex hormones (testosterone) which stimulate tumour growth
  - hormone therapy (anti-testosterone drugs) is given to inhibit testosterone activity.
- **Radiotherapy:**
  - usually in combination with anticancerous medications, this therapy is recommended in cases of advanced prostate cancer.

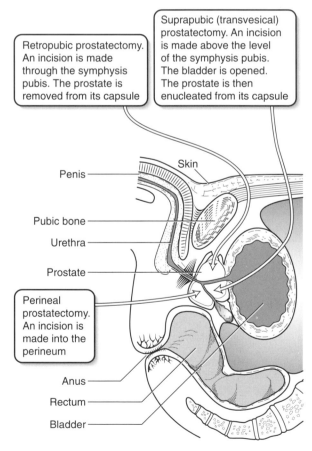

Retropubic prostatectomy. An incision is made through the symphysis pubis. The prostate is removed from its capsule

Suprapubic (transvesical) prostatectomy. An incision is made above the level of the symphysis pubis. The bladder is opened. The prostate is then enucleated from its capsule

Perineal prostatectomy. An incision is made into the perineum

Skin

Penis

Pubic bone

Urethra

Prostate

Anus

Rectum

Bladder

Fig. 5.2 Surgical methods to remove the prostate gland from its capsule.

**Box 5.13 Causes of erectile dysfunction
(From Turner & Wass 1997)**

- Acute and chronic illness
- Ageing
- Respiratory disease: chronic obstructive airway disease, asthma, obstructive sleep apnoea
- Trauma
- Burns
- Heart failure
- Diabetes
- Thyrotoxicosis
- Uraemia
- Chronic renal failure
- Drugs which affect the autonomic system
- Anti-hypertensive medications
- Neurovascular disease
- Cancer
- Psychological factors (not included by Turner & Wass): anxiety, depression, lack of confidence, low self-esteem, poor self-image, fear.

Box 5.14 Treating erectile dysfunction

- **Psychosexual approach:** exploring the client's personal problems and needs through empathetic listening. Directing the individual to identify ways to cope with his problem by exploring aspects of his sexuality, interpersonal relationships and possible inadequacies.
- **Biological approach:** testosterone replacement is known to increase libido. Testosterone patches are popular, since slow release of the hormone through the skin is much preferred to injections. Prostaglandin injections into the penis is the other method used to cause an erection.
- **Vacuum therapy and penile implants:** vacuum therapy consists of increasing penile vascularity by using a pump. Penile implants involve the surgical insertion of a semi-ridged or malleable rod into the corpora cavernosa of the penis.

Erectile dysfunction

Erectile dysfunction is another term for impotence. It can be defined as the inability to maintain penile erection thus making sexual intercourse impossible. It is an emotive subject to many men who experience it, since they perceive the problem as a reflection on their lack of manliness. It occurs secondary to a primary cause(s) which can be linked to physical and/or psychological factors (Duckworth 1997) (Box 5.13). Clinics managed by nurses, according to Duckworth, provide the environment for men who seek advice, treatment and counselling. Their partners are also encouraged to attend. Educational programmes are planned with the aim to raise awareness of pertinent issues, to reassure and to prevent unnecessary anxieties and psychological ill-health.

When men attend such clinics they want to know what can be done to help them. A variety of options are available (Box 5.14). The wide range of treatments allow men and their partners to select specific services to suit their personal needs. The attitude and professional approach of the service providers are criteria which will determine the success rate in increasing attendance. An environment guaranteeing confiden-

tiality and adequate time for discussions will boost the client's confidence. In addition, securing cooperation has the advantage of exposing the individual to other health education and promotion issues. For instance, if the impotence is due to diabetes, the clinician can help to explore self-care and management topics related to this particular health issue. However, referral to a diabetes specialist may be necessary if more indepth problems are identified.

Since erectile dysfunction is not only a biological problem but involves psychological, social, spiritual and sexuality dimensions, care managers in all settings have to implement a holistic perspective in their interactions with clients.

Testicular cancer

Testicular cancer affects men aged between 20 and 34 years, and about 1000 cases are identified yearly, 50% of whom are aged under 35 years (Peate 1997). While women are being encouraged to practise breast self-examination, men on the other hand, have only recently been exposed to health promotion literature encouraging testicular self-examination. Many men are still unsure how to do testicular examination. Additionally, it is a subject that receives scant attention in general practice, until an individual presents with testicular problems. It is this author's observation that professionals are as embarrassed as the client in discussing confidently matters related specifically with the maintenance of healthy testes.

Engaging the patient to talk overtly about his reproductive needs and problems will enhance health promotional strategies. Peate (1997) asserts that individual and public awareness must be raised, by utilizing a wide variety of resources. For example, schools can become the arenas where children can be introduced to healthy practices concerning testicular examination. While other health-damaging issues are at the forefront in school curricular activities: drug addiction, smoking, teenage pregnancies, HIV/AIDS, testicular cancers and their early detection by self-examination are not presented to pupils. Assumptions are often made that children are too young to receive such 'adult' information. It is, however, an example of society's stereotypical belief based on traditional values which remains to be challenged.

Our towns and cities confidently display posters about the dangers of glue sniffing, sexual promiscuity, and promoting the idea of the healthy pregnant mother. Yet, posters promoting testicular self-examination are not evident. In clinical practice, information on testicular examination is not readily available in comparison with breast-feeding, cervical screening, HIV/AIDS, baby care etc.

Men are more reluctant than women to make use of health service facilities. They visit their

Activity 5.6

1. Prepare two unlabelled diagrams: one showing a general plan of the male reproductive system, and the other showing the genitalia and the scrotum and testes. Now, make 50 copies of each diagram. Ask your friends, relatives, neighbours to participate in a small experiment by labelling these diagrams. Collate your findings.
2. Do a similar experiment, this time involving qualified care professionals. Compare the results.
3. Write a conclusion. Reflect upon the findings.

??? Question 5.7

1. If public awareness of men's prostate and testicular cancers is to be raised, what strategies can be used?
2. It is argued that the practice nurse is ideally placed to promote health. How can she be supported in her responsibility?
3. How would you educate the client in practice?
4. Should testicular self-examination be advertised on television?
5. Can you suggest how it should be advertised?

general practitioners less frequently and are less motivated to seek health advice early (Peate 1997). A close partnership between the health education authorities, the media and the health service professional is required so that public awareness of testicular health issues is raised. As soon as men are exposed to a major publicity campaign, related to their general and reproductive health, the likelihood of increased uptake of services is possible.

SUMMARY

There is a diversity of health needs and problems encountered by women and men in society. The topic of domestic violence encompasses not only women as victims and men as the perpetrators, but also the effects of such violence on the social, biological, psychological and spiritual well-being of the person. Moreover, men are also victims of violence: sexual assaults and victimization not only in specific settings such as prisons, but in the wider community as well.

In the field of sexual and reproductive health, screening is considered to be good preventative practice. Breast and cervical screening are recommended for women; men should practise testicular self-examination and utilize health services more, since testicular and prostatic cancers have been more widely identified among men. Sex education is essential for both genders. Sexually active men and women are prone to developing sexually transmitted disease. In addition, effective sex education will help reduce teenage pregnancies.

GLOSSARY

Acupuncture   a Chinese method of healing which uses needles inserted at specific areas on the body to relieve pain etc.

Benchmarking   criterion that can be used for comparison and evaluation

Chinese herbalism   the use of herbs according to Chinese practice and tradition which supports healing

CINAHL   Cumulative Index Nursing and Allied Health Literature

Clitoral excision   surgical removal of the clitoris

Colposcopy   internal examination of the female genitalia (vagina and cervix)

Computed tomography   the production of an image using a computer to show organ structures

Corpora cavernosa   the main body (the dorsum) of the penis which contains erectile tissue

Cystoscopy   bladder examination using a cystoscope

Cytology   the study of cells (e.g. cells of the cervix to detect any cancerous changes)

Defence mechanism   sometimes known as a mental mechanism; strategies used by individuals to cope with their own internal psychological conflict

Defeminization   the loss of one's feminine characteristics

Denial   a defence mechanism which consists of keeping out of consciousness negative experiences

Dowry   in some cultures, a bride's wealth, which is given by her parents to her husband and in-laws

Excision biopsy   the removal of a small sample of tissue (e.g. from the breast) for examination

Genital warts   warts (non-malignant growth of skin tissue) on the genitalia

Haematuria   blood in the urine

Health models   a framework encompassing various perspectives or dimensions of health

Herpes simplex   a virus that causes 'cold sores' and venereal disease

Hormone replacement therapy   a treatment to alleviate postmenopausal symptoms; this entails taking either natural or synthetic hormone preparation

Human papilloma virus   a virus which can cause warts, infections or cancer

Hyperalimentation   increased nutritional intake via artificial means, e.g. intravenously or a nasogastric tube

Hysterical   a term which refers to various physical complaints not caused by physical illness, normally applied to female behaviour

Labial excision   surgical removal of the lips of the female genitalia

Machismo   masculinity

Magnetic resonance imaging   the production of images by using electro-magnetic energy

Mammography   X-ray examination of the breast

Minimization   to reduce the impact of an event by treating it as unimportant or irrelevant

Needle aspiration   drawing out fluid by using a syringe for examination

Neurotics   individuals prone to anxiety attacks, obsessions and phobias

Osteoporosis   a loss of bony tissue causing bones to be brittle and prone to fracture

Paradigm   a model, a framework

Paranoid   a type of delusion with expression of persecution

Phenomenological   in relation to a person's perception of life as a reality

Psychologization   attributing a person's physical changes or ill-health to mental causes

Psychosexual   the interrelationships between mental and emotional attitude and sexuality

Psychotherapy   psychological treatment for mental or emotional problems

Psychotic confusional states   a state of disorientation with features of delusions (false beliefs) and hallucinations (impaired sensory perception)

Psychotic   manifestations of thought impairment, abnormal emotional changes resulting in abnormal behaviour

Rationalization   a defence mechanism which consists of explaining away a behaviour

Reductionist   a way of interpreting phenomena (e.g. social behaviour) by using a micro perspective (e.g. individual action, rather than higher order terms)

Reflexology   a type of treatment and study which focuses on different reflexes of the body

Self-fulfilling prophecy   the realization of an anticipated outcome, following a particular behaviour pattern (e.g. a pupil labelled as a truant becomes one)

Syndrome   a collection of symptoms

Transrectal ultrasound   a scan that aims to detect malignancy or changes in the prostate

Vasectomy   an operation in which the vas deferens are cut to ensure male sterilization

REFERENCES

Adshead G 1995 The psychiatrist's view: preventing violent crime is not a medical role. British Medical Journal 311(7020): 1619–1620

Allen D 1996 Women on the edge. Community Care Issue 1149: 24–25

Anderson S 1997 Sex education and boys: a missed opportunity. Health Visitor 70(10): 390–391

Baird A 1998 Change theory and health promotion. Nursing Standard 12(22): 34–36

Bankowska U 1997 Ensuring a quality service in the community setting. The Diplomate 4(2): 126–127

Baraitser P 1997 Community gynaecology: the diversity of services currently provided. The Diplomate 4(2): 114–119

Beitz J M 1998 Sexual health promotion in adolescents and young adults: primary prevention strategies. Holistic Nursing Practice 12(2): 27–37

Benson A, Latter S 1998 Implementing health promoting

nursing: the integration of interpersonal skills and health promotion. Journal of Advanced Nursing 27(1): 100–107

Béphage G 1997 Social science and healthcare: nursing applications in clinical practice. Mosby, London

Bewley C, Gibbs A 1994 Coping with domestic violence in pregnancy. Nursing Standard 8(50): 25–28

Bignall J 1993 Hidden health burden. Lancet 324(8880): 1169

Bigrigg A 1997 The emergence of the community gynaecologist: mini-symposium. The Diplomate 4(2): 110–112

Bilezikian J P 1994 Major issues regarding estrogen replacement therapy in postmenopausal women. Journal of Women's Health 3(4): 273–282

Blakey V, Frankland J 1996 Sex education for parents. Health Education 5: 9–13

Bonvillain N 1995 Women and men: cultural constructs of gender. Prentice-Hall, Englewood Cliffs, N J

Bright J S 1997 Health promotion in nursing practice. In: Bright J S (ed) Health promotion in clinical practice: targeting the health of the nation. Baillière Tindall, London, p 8

Cadman L 1998 The role of the papillomavirus. Community Nurse 4(1): 32–33

Campbell J C, Pliska M J, Taylor W, Sheridan D 1994 Battered women's experiences in the emergency department. Journal of Emergency Nursing 20(4): 280–288

Carlisle D 1997 Women: domestic violence. A way out. Community Care 1153: 26

Carr S 1997 Sexual problems within the community. The Diplomate 4(2): 120–122

Central Statistics Office 1997 Social Trends 27: Health 7.12. HMSO, London, p 127

Charles C 1997 Post-traumatic stress disorder. Midwives 110(1317): 250–252

Clark A 1997 Sexual problems and pregnancy issues. The Diplomate 4(4): 280–283

Clinical issues in nursing 1994 Promoting mental health in women. Nursing Standard 8(45): 30–31

Cody A 1996 Helping the vulnerable or condoning control within the family: where is nursing? Journal of Advanced Nursing 23(5): 882–886

Council on Ethical and Judicial Affairs, American Medical Association 1992 Physicians and domestic violence: ethical considerations. JAMA 267(23): 3190–3193

Council on Scientific Affairs, American Medical Association 1992 Violence against women: relevance for medical practitioners. JAMA 267(23): 3184–3189

Curtis S, Taket A 1996 Health and society's changing perspectives. Arnold, London, p 46–50

Davidson N 1996 Oh boys! Sex education and young men. Health Education 3: 20–23

Davison J 1997 Domestic violence: the nursing response. Professional Nurse 12(9): 632–634

Dean M 1997 Prostate cancer. Professional Nurse 12(10): 722–724

Deane K A, Degner L F 1997 Determining the information needs of women after breast biopsy procedures. Association of Operating Room Nurses 65(4): 767–776

Dearnaley D P 1994 Cancer of the prostate. British Medical Journal 308(6931): 780–784

Defo B K 1997 Effects of socioeconomic disadvantage and women's status on women's health in Cameroon. Social Science and Medicine 44(7): 1023–1042

Dolby L 1998 Is sex education in The Netherlands better organised than in Britain? British Journal of Midwifery 6(2): 96–100

Doyal L 1994 Waged work and well-being. In: Wilkinson S, Kitzinger C (eds) Women and health: feminist perspectives. Taylor & Francis, London

Duckworth K 1997 Running an erectile dysfunction clinic. Professional Nurse 12(11): 775–778

Farooqui O 1997 Female circumcision: a fair cut for women? The British Journal of Family Planning 23(3): 96–100

Few C 1997 The politics of sex research and constructions of female sexuality: what relevance to sexual health work with young women? Journal of Advanced Nursing 25(3): 615–625

Fielding P, Woan M 1998 In sickness and in health. Nursing Times 94(7): 36–37

Flitcraft A H 1992 Violence, values and gender. JAMA 267(23): 3194–3195

Ford K, Rigby P 1998 Depression and the primary healthcare team. British Journal of Community Nursing 3(2): 97–99

Foxall M J, Barron C R, Houfek J 1998 Ethnic differences in breast self-examination. Journal of Advanced Nursing 27(2): 419–428

Gillett G 1995 The moral philosopher's view: the victim should decide. British Medical Journal 311(7020): 1620

Goddard N C 1995 'Spirituality as integrative energy': a philosophical analysis as requisite precursor to holistic nursing practice. Journal of Advanced Nursing 22(4): 808–815

Godfrey K 1997 Well women. Nursing Times 93(10): 36–38

Goudsmit E M 1994 All in her mind! Stereotypic views and the psychologisation of women's illness. In: Wilkinson S, Kitzinger C (eds) Women and health: feminist perspectives. Taylor & Francis, London, p 7–12

Gregg R, Freeth D, Blackie C 1998 Teenage health and the practice nurse: choice and opportunity for both? British Journal of General Practice 48(426): 909–910

Gregory S, McKie L 1992 Researching cervical cancer: compromises, practices and beliefs. Journal of Advances in Health and Nursing Care 2(1): 73–84

Griffin M 1997 Sexual problems and the menopause. The Diplomate 4(4): 284–288

Grunfeld A F, Ritmiller S, Mackay K et al 1994 Detecting domestic violence against women in the emergency department: a nursing triage model. Journal of Emergency Nursing 20(4): 271–274

Hampshire M 1998 How the law failed Sarah's children. Nursing Standard 12(18): 20–21

Hanley J 1998 Postnatal depression. Nursing Management 4(8): 12–13

Hart L 1996 Risk of osteoporosis in young women. Nurse Prescriber/Community Nurse 2(4): 45

Hatton D C 1997 Managing health problems among homeless women with children in a transitional shelter. Image: Journal of Nursing Scholarship 29(1): 33–37

Hayes I 1995 Sex education in the early years. Health Education 1: 22–27

Health Matters 1997 New moves to reduce teenage pregnancies. Issue 31: 4

Healy C 1998 Health promoting schools: learning from the European project. Health Education 98(1): 21–26

Hillard A 1998 The menopause without HRT. Nurse Prescriber/Community Nurse 4(1): 35–37

Hotch D, Grunfeld A, MacKay K, Ritch L 1996 Research: policy and procedures for domestic violence patients in

Canadian emergency departments: a national survey. Journal of Emergency Nursing 22(4): 278–282

Irwin R 1997 Sexual health promotion and nursing. Journal of Advanced Nursing 25(1): 170–177

Jenkins R 1990 Women and mental illness. In: Pfeffer N, Quick A (eds) Promoting women's health. King's Fund Publishing, London, p 33–43

Jennings R H 1997 The patient advocate: Presidential address. American Journal of Obstetrics and Gynaecology 177(2): 251–255

Jezierski M 1996 Profiles: Annie O'Connor, NP, MS: domestic violence survivor and community advocate. Journal of Emergency Nursing 22(1): 85–89

Keller L E 1996 Invisible victims: battered women in psychiatric and medical emergency rooms. Bulletin of the Menninger Clinic 60(1): 1–21

Kendall S, Lask S 1997 Promoting the health of the nation. Churchill Livingstone, New York, p 63

King M C 1996 Woman abuse: the role of the nurse-midwives in assessment. Journal of Nurse-Midwifery 41(6): 436–441

Krieger N, Fee E 1994 Man-made medicine and women's health: the biopolitics of sex/gender and race/ethnicity. International Journal of Health Services 24(2): 265–283

Lipscomb G H, Muram D, Speck P M, Mercer B M 1992 Male victims of sexual assault. Journal of American Medical Association 267(22): 3064–3066

Lugton J 1997 The nature of social support as experienced by women treated for breast cancer. Journal of Advanced Nursing 25(6): 1184–1191

Lydon C 1996 Too slap happy. Nursing Times 92(45): 48–49

McConville B 1998 A bloody tradition. Nursing Times 94(3): 34–36

McFarlane J, Parker B, Soeken K, Bullock M S 1992 Assessing for abuse during pregnancy. JAMA 267(23): 3176–3178

Mahony C 1997 Babies, bruises and black eyes. Nursing Times 93(51): 14–15

Malos E, Hague G 1997 Women, housing, homelessness and domestic violence. Women's Studies International Forum 20(3): 397–409

Mezey G C, Bewley S 1997 Domestic violence and pregnancy. British Journal of Obstetrics and Gynaecology 104(5): 528–531

Mezey G, King M, MacClintock T 1998 Victims of violence and the general practitioner. British Journal of General Practice 48(426): 906–908

Moelwyn-Hughes A 1997 When home is where the hurt is. Health Matters 31: 10–11

Morley R 1995 The sociologist's view: more convictions won't help victims of domestic violence. British Medical Journal 311(7020): 1618–1619

Morris R 1996 The culture of female circumcision. Advances in Nursing Science 19(2): 43–53

Morrison A, Mackie C M, Elliott L et al 1997 The sexual health help centre: a service for young people. Journal of Public Health Medicine 19(4): 457–463

Murray L 1997 The effect of infants' behaviour on maternal mental health. Health Visitor 70(9): 334–335

Naidoo J, Wills J 1994 Health promotion foundations for practice. Baillière Tindall, London, p 120

Newberger E H, Barkan S E, Lieberman E S et al 1992 Abuse of pregnant women and adverse birth outcome current knowledge and implications for practice. JAMA 267(17): 2370–2372

Nursing Standard 1998 A review of the NHS breast screening programme. Nursing Standard 12(19): 32–33

Oakley A 1990 Who's afraid of the randomized controlled trial? Some dilemmas of the scientific method and 'good' research practice. In: Roberts H (ed) Women's health counts. Routledge, London

Oakley A 1993 Essays on women, medicine and health. Edinburgh University Press, Edinburgh

Ogden J 1998 Screening the screeners. Nursing Standard 12(21): 12

Oldnall A S 1995 On the absence of spirituality in nursing: theories and models. Journal of Advanced Nursing 21(3): 417–418

Oldnall A S 1996 A critical analysis of nursing: meeting the spiritual needs of patients. Journal of Advanced Nursing 23(1): 138–144

Ooijen E L, Charnock A 1995 How men and women view the world: a sexual perspective. Nursing Times 91(28): 38–39

Orbell S 1996 Cognition and affect after cervical screening: the role of previous test outcome and personal obligation in future uptake expectations. Social Science and Medicine 43(8): 1237–1243

Padbury V 1997 Smear taking. Practice Nurse 13(3): 131–132

Parliamentary Home Affairs Committee 1993 Third report on domestic violence. HMSO, London

Pearson J, Gardner G 1997 Improving sexual health among suburban teenagers. Community Nurse 3(4): 20

Peate I 1997 Testicular cancer: the importance of effective health education. British Journal of Nursing 6(6): 311–316

Peate I 1998a Cancer of the prostate. 1: Promoting men's healthcare needs. British Journal of Nursing 7(3): 152–158

Peate I 1998b Cancer of the prostate. 2: The nursing role in health promotion. British Journal of Nursing 7(4): 196–200

Raftos M, Mannix J, Jackson D 1997 More than motherhood? A feminist exploration of 'women's health' in papers indexed by CINAHL 1993–1995. Journal of Advanced Nursing 26(6): 1142–1149

Rao V 1997 Wife-beating in rural South India: a qualitative and econometric analysis. Social Science and Medicine 44(8): 1169–1180

Rentoul L, Appleboom N 1997 Understanding the psychological impact of rape and sexual assault of men: a literature review. Journal of Psychiatric and Mental Health Nursing 4(4): 267–274

Richardson J, Feder G 1996 Domestic violence: a hidden problem for general practice. British Journal of General Practice 46(405): 239–242

Roberts G L, Raphael B, Lawrence J M et al 1997 Impact of an education program about domestic violence on nurses and doctors in an Australian emergency department. Journal of Emergency Nursing 23(3): 220–227

Rogers E, Moon E M, Mullee M A et al 1998 Developing the 'health-promoting school': a national survey of health awards. Public Health 112(1): 37–40

Savage W 1997 Health for women and for all. Health Matters 29: 9

Scura K W, Whipple B 1997 How to provide better care for the post-menopausal woman. American Journal of Nursing 97(4): 36–43

Shepherd J 1995 Towards interagency procedures to protect victims and prevent violence. British Medical Journal 311(7020): 1617–1618

Smail J, Smail S 1989 Making the service suit the patient. Nursing Times 85(8): 49–51

Smart S 1997 A clinic in the countryside. Community Nurse 3(4): 18

Solberg S 1989 Women and their mental health: a reflection of society's expectations and pressures? In: Hardy L K, Randell J (eds) Recent advances in nursing: issues in women's health. Churchill Livingstone, Edinburgh, p 92–109

Sugg N K, Inui T 1992 Primary care physicians response to domestic violence: opening Pandora's box. JAMA 267(23): 3157–3160

Taylor A 1997 Out of the blues. Nursing Times 93(45): 18

Thobaben M 1997 'In every midwife's caseload' … battered women. Midwives 110(1317): 242–244

Thomas S 1997 Tale of the unexpected. Nursing Times 93(45): 30–31

Thomson R, Holland J 1994 Young women and safer (hetero) sex: context, constraints and strategies. In: Wilkinson S, Kitzinger C (eds) Women and health: feminist perspectives. Taylor & Francis, London

Turner H E, Wass J A 1997 Gonadal function in men with chronic illness. Clinical Endocrinology 47(4): 379–403

Twaddle S 1995 Day care for women with high-risk pregnancies. Nursing Times 91(4): 46–47

Varvaro F F, Gesmond S 1997 Emergency department physician house staff response to training on domestic violence. Journal of Emergency Nursing 23(1): 17–22

Vernon L 1998 Access to sexual and reproductive healthcare for people with learning difficulties. Journal of Community Nursing 12(2): 10–16

Weyman A, Walsh J 1998 Family planning: programmes and people. The British Journal of Family Planning 23(4): 111

Whitmarsh J 1997 School nurses' skills in sexual health education. Nursing Standard 11(27): 35–41

Whitton A, Warner R, Appleby L 1996 The pathway to care in post-natal depression: women's attitudes to post-natal depression and its treatment. British Journal of General Practice 46(408): 427–428

Wilkinson S, Kitzinger C 1994 Towards a feminist approach to breast cancer. In: Wilkinson S, Kitzinger C (eds) Women and health: feminist perspectives. Taylor & Francis, London

Willis J 1997 Women's cancers. Nursing Times 93(40): 26–29

Woloshynowych M, Valori R, Salmon P 1998 General practice patients' beliefs about their symptoms. British Journal of General Practice 48(226): 885–889

Women's Health 1994 Nursing Times special publication. MacMillan, London, p 38–43

Woods N F, Mitchell E S 1997 Pathways to depressed mood for midlife women: observations from the Seattle Midlife Women's Health Study. Research in Nursing and Health 20(2): 119–129

Woolf L, Jackson B 1996 'Coffee & condoms': the implementation of a sexual health programme in acute psychiatry in an inner city area. Journal of Advanced Nursing 23(2): 299–304

Wordsworth J 1997 Services for menopausal women in the community. The Diplomate 4(2): 123–125

Wright A F 1996 Unrecognized psychiatric illness in general practice. British Journal of General Practice 46(407): 327–328

Yu C K, Rymer J 1998 Women's attitude to and awareness of smear testing and cervical cancer. The British Journal of Family Planning 23(4): 127–133

FURTHER READING

Amos A 1993 In her own best interests? Women and health education: a review of the last fifty years. Health Education Journal 52(3): 141–150

Anderson K L 1997 Gender, status and domestic violence: an integration of feminist and family violence approaches. Journal of Marriage and the Family 59(3): 655–669

Cowan P J 1996 Women's mental health issues: reflections on past attitudes and present practices. Journal of Psychosocial Nursing 34(4): 20–24

Glover V 1997 Maternal stress or anxiety in pregnancy and emotional development of the child. British Journal of Psychiatry 171: 105–106

Killion C M 1995 Special health care needs of homeless pregnant women. Advances in Nursing Science 18(2): 44–56

Miles A 1991 Women, health and medicine. Open University Press, Buckingham

Rosen I 1991 Self-esteem as a factor in social and domestic violence. British Journal of Psychiatry 158: 18–23

Smith-Warner S A, Spiegelman D, Yaun S et al 1998 Alcohol and breast cancer in women: a pooled analysis of cohort studies. JAMA 279(7): 535–539

Stoter D 1995 Spiritual aspects of care. Mosby, London

Torgerson D J, Gosden T 1997 The national breast screening programme service: is it economically efficient? Quarterly Journal of Medicine 90(6): 423–425

6

Other cultures

Societies throughout the world are undergoing major demographic changes. Improvement in air travel, the pressures of socio-economic development, escape from countries with dictatorial regimes, personal and professional needs are some of the factors which can instigate mass immigration. It is therefore not surprising that many countries, including Britain, have become multi-ethnic. The presence of minority ethnic groups arouses debates at all levels of society, causes controversies, racism and discrimination, and numerous health care and social issues. The aim of this chapter is to:

• address current issues related to ethnic groups
• develop insights into their socio-cultural needs
• discuss strategies that can help minimize health risks specific to ethnicity and race.

DEMOGRAPHIC TRENDS

Britain is becoming more culturally and racially diversified. In 1996–1997, the ethnic minority population of Great Britain comprised 6% of all households, estimated at a total of 3.4 million people (Central Statistics Office 1998). Statistics published for this period show that there is a wide differentiation in ages among ethnic groups. While 16% of the white population were aged 65 and over and 20% were aged under 16, the Pakistani/Bangladeshi population comprised 3% and 39% for the same age groups respectively. Other ethnic minority groups also had a high percentage of young people: 23% of all black Caribbeans were under 16 years old, 30% black Africans and 46% of people within other black groups were under 16. When people within all black groups were averaged together, 29% were shown to be under the age of 16, while only 5% were 65 and over. In addition, 17% of people of Chinese origin were under 16, while only 4% were aged 65 and over; and for groups of mixed origin, the young comprised 44% and the old 2%.

Most ethnic minority groups are located within defined areas of Britain. Results from the 1995 General Household Survey (HMSO 1997) showed that 24% of Indians live in the West Midlands and 37% in Greater London; 13% of the black community are found in the West Midlands and 42% in Greater London. All ethnic groups comprise 16% of the population in the West Midlands and 42% in Greater London.

The survey also revealed differences in household size compared with the white community. The largest household size, averaging 4.53 persons, was found among the Pakistani/Bangladeshi group; the white group had the lowest average household size at 2.39 persons. The Indian group had the second largest mean household size at 3.62 persons, while the black group had a mean 2.56 persons per household.

Some possible reasons for the higher concentration of immigrants in the certain areas have been identified:

- job opportunities are higher in towns and cities, because of industrialization and urbanization
- household size could indicate group solidarity founded on maintaining traditional links with the extended family.

On the other hand, bigger household size could mean shortage of accommodation in the inner cities and deprived areas, and reliance on family support for living arrangements. Overcrowded living conditions can cause ill-health, making it an issue to be considered in ill-health prevention.

RACE AND ETHNICITY

Britain is not only a culturally diversified society, it is also described as multifaith, and is racially as well as multi-ethnically diverse. Since people from other cultures have inhabited the British Isles for at least the past 500 years, the issue of race has been a perennial social problem. Race is considered to be a socio-political construct (Ahmad 1993). Mares et al (1985) believe that the term 'race' is ambiguous: sometimes it refers to groups in society with 'special characteristics', particularly to skin and/or hair colour; thus their external biological features will determine their countries of origin. Race refers to a form of classification; for example, the African race, the British race etc, which denotes one's country of origin.

Ethnicity, on the other hand, relates to one's social identity (Eriksen 1993, Leininger 1995a). Hence cultural practices (e.g. firewalking, totem worship), religious rituals (e.g. church attendance, fasting) and language used, as well as types of food and clothing, add to the distinctive features of the group. Eriksen, nevertheless, pointed out that ethnicity is best interpreted from the groups' viewpoint (i.e. how they perceive their own differentiation in comparison with others) rather than from the observer's interpretation. The latter approach he refers to as 'etic', while the former is called 'emic': what people actually say regarding their ethnicity. The concept of culture, although related to race and ethnicity, is defined as the accumulation of shared learning and values (Leininger 1995a) of a society, and people's 'spiritual factors, kinship, symbols' (Leininger 1995b), as well as their individuality in interpreting their social world and their methods of coping within the environment they live in.

ISSUES RELATED TO RACE AND ETHNICITY

Discrimination and racial harassment have been identified as long-standing problems (Burford 1997). Ethnic minority groups experience discrimination in differing domains of their lives:

they experience greater difficulties than their white counterparts in obtaining houses that meet their needs. Many live in deprived areas and become the targets of racial abuse. In the field of education, black pupils tend to underachieve compared to Asians. Adults encounter discrimination in the workplace, and their career paths are often not smooth. In the National Health Service, for example, white male nurses are more likely to obtain higher and better paid managerial positions than female colleagues with minority ethnic backgrounds (McMillan 1998). Hence gender, ethnicity and race are linked to the cycle of discrimination and racism. It can be said that being Asian, black and female will further block the path to promotion and better wages (McMillan 1998).

Discrimination and racist attitudes can be expressed in other ways, i.e. when colleagues ask clients whether they have any objection to being nursed by a black nurse (Waters 1996). There is an under-representation of black ethnic minority nurses in the health care services (Alderman 1997, Mensah 1997), despite evidence from social surveys that there are many ethnic communities. Alderman emphasized that academics and health policy makers – who are not from ethnic groups – misunderstand sensitive issues related to the latter.

Mayor (1996) reported that black ethnic minority groups can be well motivated to progress in their careers; the discrimination they encounter, however, can leave them despondent, deskilled and disempowered. Very often their occupational position in the hierarchy does not match their experiences and qualifications. Moreover, Mayor described a series of hurdles which stifle the black applicant's motivation to succeed:

- lack of employer support
- restraints in regard to attending courses for personal and professional development
- not receiving information on how to further one's career
- being denied funding when applying for courses.

While a lack of support and encouragement is evident in the workplace, many workers rely on informal networks to maintain their interests and motivation to succeed. Inequality of opportunities can channel minority groups into low status occupations, where they are financially disadvantaged due to low pay (Foolchand 1995). This detrimental consequence of discrimination compounds the negative life experiences of racially harassed individuals who become trapped within a culture of poverty.

As a socio-political construct, the 'race' issue is frequently either deliberately or unconsciously tackled using the concept of 'culture'. There is an over-emphasis on culture and language (Foolchand 1995), which dilutes the true issue of race, racism and discrimination affecting both adults and children (Inman 1998). Racial abuse is a social reality (Foolchand 1995, Inman 1998), and anti-racist strategies must encompass an analysis of the covert ways it is represented. Blaming minority ethnic groups for their disadvantaged position by arguing that language barriers and their ethnocentric attitudes are the main causes show biased and prejudiced views. It is, additionally, an expression of insensitivity.

A lack of sensitive cultural awareness and education have been linked to stereotypical attitudes in regard to minority groups (McGee 1994). This is another issue that has perturbed nurse educators, clinicians and, in particular, the recipients of racial abuse. Concerns are therefore expressed in connection with 'race' and 'culture' factors, in care settings and in conjunction with health promotional activities.

HEALTH PROMOTION, SCREENING AND ETHNIC GROUPS

Services to meet the health needs of ethnic groups have been criticized as inadequate (Chevannes 1990). Health and community services have targeted mainly Asian families and the Afro-Caribbean groups. The latter are well known to suffer from sickle cell disease; the former for their predisposition to have vitamin D deficiencies. In the 1990s when these specific groups were targeted (e.g. the rickets campaign and screening for sickle cell disease), Chevannes pointed out that such measures aroused hostility among these two groups. They perceived these health measures as reinforcing the beliefs that ethnic groups are 'sources of ill-health', and that professionals may develop the attitude that all ethnic group members may experience *similar* forms of ill-health.

Although it is known that black and ethnic minorities are reluctant to make use of available health and social services (Redmond 1993), assumptions have been made regarding the reasons for this. Communication problems are often given as the primary factors; a recurring theme in the literature, with debates on how language barriers can prevent both client and care provider from understanding each other. Research findings, however, give evidence that reasons for non-compliance with screening are not generally related to 'language commitments' (Stone et al 1998).

In Stone et al's analysis of a multi-ethnic community's degree of compliance with screening for infection (in Leicester, UK), the researchers reached the following conclusions:

1. Asians and non-Asians have stated that their non-attendance is due to other factors:
   - stress-related factors in connection with work
   - family pressures
   - appointment times that do not match their needs
   - holidays
   Social commitments were given in 45% (59 out of 131) of cases
2. Seven out of 70 Asians stated not remembering receiving a written notice by post
3. Nine out of 70 said they did not read the letter or had not fully read/understood it
4. Six people forgot the appointment
5. Five were not interested
6. Four responders said they did not have any symptoms to warrant a test.

In relation to language, the researchers found that 86% of those of Indian origin living in England are 'able to speak, and 76% able to read, English'. These findings counteract common assumptions that language problems prevent uptake of services. Besides, where Asians and

others are not able to understand English, interpreters are often available to translate verbal and written communication.

Recognition that other factors are at play in preventing compliance will ensure that professionals redirect their efforts and consider promoting the importance of preventive measures through client education (Stone et al 1998). In addition, education and training for care providers are important. Ethnic awareness will alter the beliefs that Asians are homogeneous groups with similar language, culture, religion and dietary habits. Shah (1997) pointed out that Asians are heterogeneous groups; a fact to remember when health promotion initiatives are implemented. Hindus differ from Moslems, Bangladeshis and Sikhs in their nutritional habits, religious and cultural practices, as well as the language spoken.

A multidimensional approach should also encompass a transcultural perspective. Other cultures have their own individualities, 'identities, values, beliefs and lifeways' (Leininger 1997), which deserve acceptance and understanding. Focusing on health issues (e.g. reducing the incidence of coronary heart disease and diabetes) as they affect the ethnic population is incomplete without due consideration given to wider social influences. The extent of racism and cultural conflicts (Leininger 1997) can affect uptake of services. Additionally, awareness that racism exists among ethnic groups will have implications for health (Box 6.1).

Box 6.1 Effects of racism on health

Racial conflict is a major stressor. It causes tension, triggers depression, can lead to homicide, and has been known to stimulate suicidal behaviour. Fear is generated within communities. Where there is retaliation – physical or verbal – in the form of riots, the social environment suffers. Houses, cars and shopping precincts can be vandalized. People no longer feel safe walking the streets, and the incidence of abuse and rape can increase. Racial tension can also affect the morale of ethnic peacemakers and their relationships with their communities and agents of social control: the police, church leaders and the education system. In addition, physical assaults can cause fatal injuries: ruptured liver, lungs and major blood vessels; head injuries; gun shot wounds and scalp lacerations.

The effects of urbanization on health should be considered for the many Asians, Chinese, Africans and Afro-Caribbeans who come from rural areas in their countries of origin and who may be ill-prepared to cope with the stress of modern city life in a foreign country. Moreover, they are prone to receiving sub-standard care (Shah 1997) because of

- a lack of awareness of their rights to benefits from the health and social services
- inequality of access
- irrelevant and insensitive services that do not match their needs (NHS handbook 1996).

The socio-economic status of a group, and *where* they live (i.e. in rural or city areas) are of significance to health. In one study undertaken in a city in the Shandong province of China (Kaewboonchoo et al 1998), it was found that young people in urban areas experience less hearing impairment (due to better socio-economic status and access to hospitals and services) compared to those living rurally. The findings from this research should help raise our awareness of some key issues, namely:

1. the possibility that some ethnic groups in Britain who live in rural areas may not have access to services available in cities

2. assumptions should not be made that Asians and other groups in cities have easier access to health provision; many may be ill-informed or unaware of what is available, others may only believe in folk medicine

3. better socio-economic status does not necessarily mean that health status is equally good

4. that other factors such as cultural–religious practices and lack of education can impinge negatively on health; for example, the prevalence of iron deficiency is high among Asian children whose parents are both Muslims and uneducated (Lawson et al 1998).

It can be seen from the above that the diversity of issues concerning ethnic groups makes the prevention of ill-health a challenging task, which health educators must tackle in close partnership with ethnic communities. Attentive listening to their views is essential as this approach will enhance the identification of pertinent problems. Hawthorne (1994), in a literature review, pointed out that health education programmes do not always reflect needs. Many South Asians suffer from conditions (e.g. asthma, skin conditions such as eczema which are more prevalent among ethnic groups (Godfrey 1998)) other than rickets and tuberculosis, but these diseases are at the forefront of education. A comprehensive education programme is hence desired congruent with needs.

To promote health, sensitive application of measures based on accurate knowledge of the targeted communities is required. It is suggested that the exploration of ethnic minority groups' health needs may benefit from qualitative research methods (Hennings et al 1996). Although Hennings et al's study was focused on the 'experiences of antenatal care in one health district', in relation to Bangladeshi women, their methods of investigation 'respect cultural diversity' while providing a 'depth of understanding'.

At present several initiatives have been pinpointed (Hawthorne 1994) which reveal the achievement of education programmes for British South Asians in the field of diabetes awareness (Box 6.2).

The role of health care professionals in ethnicity issues

In addition to being conversant with health education and promotion topics, care providers have to broaden their transcultural nursing practice. Transcultural nursing is now reaching the forefront of care delivery, following the initiatives launched by its proponent, Madeleine Leininger, a nurse anthropologist.

As indicated above, while culture care is an intrinsic component of clinical practice, one should nevertheless be conscious that the issues of race, racism and discrimination are a social reality often covertly expressed. Cultural sensitivity is widely being encouraged. Similarly, the issue of racism demands sensitive management.

It is in daily interactions with ethnic groups that clinicians implementing cultural care may uncover repressed feelings of anger, frustration

Box 6.2 Health education initiatives implementation

1. Ethnic working party to collect and disseminate information.
2. Diabetes clinics with trained link workers to help interpret individual client needs.
3. A teacher from the local community whose role is to prompt targeted groups to attend education sessions.
4. An education officer to remind patients of available sessions by telephoning them.
5. Opportunistic advice and education: a method of including information and education during patients' visits to clinics.
6. Education days with tailored programmes according to community needs and demands.
7. Diabetes support group: a social group with informal and formal networks to provide education, support and information on diabetes.
8. 'Dedicated' clinic sessions: specific measures to target groups who have specifically made health workers aware of socio-cultural-churchgoing commitments, e.g. appointment days to be carefully chosen, by avoiding Fridays for example (a holy day).
9. Staff with multilingual and multicultural knowledge of the communities they serve.
10. Coordinated resource centres: to implement education programmes more efficiently, to reach communities in need of support in a well organized manner.

and fear that racist behaviour from others engenders. Sullivan (1998) explains how racism and ethnocentrism perpetuate the problem. It is important to be conscious that ethnocentric behaviour, 'which encourages using oneself as the standard for others' (Sullivan 1998), can be one of the predisposing factors in creating racism. Failure to accept cultural diversity and other people's traditional cultural practices and living patterns erects barriers to effective caregiving. Furthermore, cultural care must encompass the importance of the patient's view of their social world. Approaches should thereafter be innovative (Vehvilainen 1998) and constructed on evidence-based knowledge.

To increase knowledge, research is needed. Exploring other people's cultures, gaining insight into their practices so that independence can be regained will guide nursing practice. Tom-Orme (1998) asserts that the preservation of one's unique caring and spiritual values is a goal to be achieved. This entails recognizing similar aspirations in others, and facilitating their recovery, so that self-care can be optimized.

Integrated cultural and racial care

Expressing cultural sensitivity necessitates more than an awareness of a person's cultural differences. It comprises being responsive to other factors likely to act upon the individual: racial discrimination, socio-economic constraints, geography, genetic influences, religious values and beliefs, communication barriers, ethnocentrism (the individual's and others' ethnocentric behaviour), responses and reactions to unequal power relationships (e.g. doctor–patient, nurse–patient) and gender differences (e.g. men's and women's perceptions of their status and role) which are of significance to them.

While a bio-medical model is relevant to achieve the objective of curing physical complaints, professionals in practice need to be alert to the processes that 'fabricate health and illness within health care organizations' (Mitchell 1996). In particular, an awareness of the perpetuation of traditional practices that exclude the humanistic and cultural dimensions, with a focus on pathology and curative medicine is necessary. This approach has been criticized for being 'uncaring, stigmatizing and disempowering' (Mitchell 1996).

Similarly, cultural care that excludes purposeful attention to issues of race can disempower the ethnic client. It appears that within a constraining financial framework this is likely to happen; a situation caused by the inability to prioritize services, thus making health and anti-racist initiatives exposed to failure (Tate 1996). In addition, until it is accepted that cultural diversity is a social phenomenon, and that ethnic minority groups are heterogeneous (Tate 1996) – with elements of racial and cultural animosity within their milieu (Case example 6.1) – approaches to care delivery are prone to be superficial.

Tate also pointed out that 'race-based animosity' exists between Africans and Afro-Caribbeans, Asians and Afro-Caribbeans, and people whose complexion varies between 'dark brown and light brown'.

Case example 6.1 Warring neighbours

'I don't think the health workers believe us' said Ganesh who came from Uganda in the late 1970s. 'They don't believe that there is conflict between Hindus and Muslims. We are Asians, but we are all different types of Asians. Our cultural beliefs and practices are varied. The types of food we eat are different. Our social lives are not similar. History proves that racial conflict has existed throughout the world between varying Hindu and Muslim groups ... we don't get on with our neighbours across the road who are African Muslims. There is racial tension. A petrol bomb was thrown at our windows last night. We had to call the police.'

Case example 6.2 Jail for parents who kidnapped their daughter

On 6 June 1998, Paul Wilkinson reported in *The Times* the case of an Asian shopkeeper and his wife who kidnapped their daughter to keep her 'away from the evils of drugs'. Although they were genuinely concerned about their daughter's involvement with a drug dealer, it was also obvious that the parents' efforts to bring their daughter up according to Asian tradition were fruitless. As Wilkinson reported, by refusing to accept an 'arranged marriage', which is customary practice in Asian culture, the daughter had actually shown her decision to 'follow a Western way of life'. In an attempt to control her behaviour, the couple drugged their daughter, and tried to put her on a flight to Pakistan, to stay with relatives until 'she had calmed down' sufficiently.

Lack of racial sensitivity among colleagues in professional settings will have implications for nursing practice. The vulnerable ethnic client is likely to suffer. Kelsall (1998) argued that evidence of racial harassment at work clearly shows a deep lack of understanding of the needs of colleagues who are members of ethnic minority groups. Such attitudes discourage recruitment of black and ethnic minority groups into health care organizations. The clients who need care will be further demoralized and disempowered, since a reduction in ethnic group workforce means that their racial and cultural needs may be marginalized. It is also important to fully appreciate the power of traditional practices and socio-cultural beliefs of minority ethnic groups. Sometimes such beliefs compel some individuals to take extreme measures to implement them (Case example 6.2), with the risk of confronting the legal and ethical practices of a majority culture.

Cultural phenomena among ethnic groups have many dimensions. Giger et al (1997) list the following: communication, space, social organization, time, environmental control and biological variations.

Communication

Current literature shows that language barriers are common themes in social interactions involving ethnic groups and whites. To avoid the ill-effects of making assumptions, health profes-sionals must design care strategies with sensitivity. Questions should be asked clearly and concisely, while active listening cannot be over-emphasized. Schott and Henley (1996a) argued that professionals should question without feeling that they ought to know the answers. It is equally important to remember that flexibility during communication should be possible, since identical communication patterns should not be applied to all individuals. A fixed categorization of ethnic groups (Giger et al 1997) augments the problems of misunderstanding (Schott & Henley 1996b).

Many ethnic individuals have communication needs, in particular the needs to express their feelings concerning the racial harassment and discrimination they experience. Sometimes the abuse and violence which heighten their vulnerability may make them less willing to divulge their innermost feelings, particularly when the health worker is white. Perhaps, as discussed above, increasing recruitment of ethnic professionals could help alleviate the problem. While transcultural awareness is accepted as necessary, the psychology of culture-specific behaviour needs to be understood. People communicate more effectively when they feel physically and psychologically safe. Cultural safety must hence be considered too; this is defined as providing care that is culturally and racially sensitive – based on reflective practice and on assessment of one's own 'cultural identity' and how it impacts on care giving (Porter 1998).

The creation of an environment where the expressions of meanings can be shared and understood, by involving significant others (parents, siblings, spouses, neighbours, friends) under the guidance of qualified interpreters can enhance communication.

It has been argued (Jones & Gill 1998) that the NHS has not kept pace with the increasing needs of ethnic groups in connection with language problems, and that there is a lack of interpreters. Very often when interpreters are required as in emergency situations – either in hospitals or community settings – they are not available. Assumptions are also made that families, children and friends of the sick person can act as interpreters. Jones and Gill (1998) warned that informal interpreters can complicate the communication barriers, by failing to translate accurately what is being said, due to lack of vocabulary or insight (Baylav 1996). In addition, there is the cultural barrier associated with disclosure. Personal matters associated with bodily functions, sexuality, sexual relationships and reproduction, for example, are less likely to be revealed to children for translating. Formal interpreters who belong to the client's community may encounter similar problems. Jones and Gill (1998) suggest commercial telephone interpreting when the interpreter is not physically present. This method consists of having a doctor and patient communicating, while a remote interpreter (anonymous to the client and vice versa) translates the conversations. When this system is used, however, the client's non-verbal cues cannot be evaluated by the interpreter.

Murphy and McLeod Clark (1993) identified several communication issues:

1. Nurses lack confidence in communicating with their clients and relatives, which means that psychological care is not fully implemented.
2. Interpreters could not be easily accessed when needed.
3. Nurses relied on relatives to interpret.
4. Since they cannot communicate verbally with the clients, nurses rely on non-verbal communi-

cation most: this reduces the quality of the interactions, and relationship-building suffers.
5. Communication with relatives is not easy as the latter show distancing behaviour.

All these factors prove frustrating and stressful to nurses who have to provide care to ethnic groups. In addition, their perception of clients and their relatives when seen together show how misunderstandings can occur. For example, Murphy and McLeod Clark (1993) observed the nurses' reactions in regard to relatives' behaviour during visiting times (Box 6.3).

Box 6.3 Silent companionship

The relatives, the nurses said, 'would not talk or try to cheer up the client', but would just sit and hardly speak. Silent companionship to many patients and relatives can be as meaningful as verbal interactions. The importance of silence is not to be undermined, but should be respected.

An empathetic attitude is a prerequisite in understanding the situation of the ethnic client. When communication is lacking due to the unpreparedness of health care staff, minority groups in care setting find their sense of alienation, stress and helplessness heightened (Thomas & Dines 1994). Consequently, their (minority groups) inability to communicate, in combination with language barriers, is worsened.

Provision to counteract environmental stressors, and the implementation of on-going staff education and training in the field of socio-cultural care has to be implemented.

Space

Personal space (Giger et al 1997) refers to the area around a person's body. It is inextricably linked to communication. Furthermore, one's personal space is managed according to one's cultural and traditional practice. It is also an individual matter and is dependent on situational factors. Therefore, in some situations (e.g. stressful environment, animosity, fear, anger etc.) the degree of proximity can be intentionally controlled, for one's personal safety. For professionals it is relevant to be aware that multicultural factors can influence some groups' need for space.

Giger et al gave examples of Puerto Ricans and African Americans who have a stronger need to maintain proximity. We have also seen from social trends statistics that Asians from Pakistan and Bangladesh live in close proximity; their dwellings tend to be overcrowded. Very often in clinical settings, one finds numerous visitors around the sick person's bed. This may be explained by their need to uphold close contact with their loved ones. Too many visitors, however, can have health and safety implications. Overcrowding is linked to infection. Tuberculosis, for example, is correlated with a high density of people living in confined areas. Screening and infection control strategies must target these groups.

Social organization

Ethnic groups are socially organized according to their long-standing traditional practices. Social competence in one's own culture is achieved through the process of socialization. The values, attitudes and beliefs instilled from infanthood onward are faithfully adhered to. Migration, however, has the effect of compelling the person to adapt to new social challenges and to re-evaluate the meanings of their social organization. It entails learning new ways of living. It also refers to adapting one's schema of social organization to new social phenomena. A new lifestyle in a foreign country may fragment family networks.

New social constraints can, consequently, precipitate physical and psychological ill-health. Ill-health among minority groups has multifactorial causes (Culley 1996):

1. social environmental conditions:
   • structures in society which perpetuate racism and inequality
   • overcrowding
   • poverty
   • deprivation

2. personal health beliefs:
   • folk medicine and herbal remedies, which contradict Western medicine, being rigidly adhered to in spite of alternatives available

3. social class, age and gender, e.g. women occupy inferior social position in some societies.

Assumptions are often made that minority groups can support themselves by using their extended family networks. A study on race, ethnic and cultural differences in the USA (Connell & Gibson 1997) showed that ethnic groups have a greater need for services and frequently report 'more unmet needs'. In the UK, evidence shows that some women have to cope with racial hostility without family support (Thomas & Dines 1994). There are other instances (e.g. bereavement and divorce) when they feel their needs are unmet. Depression and anxiety are common unrecognized features.

Family fragmentation has other effects. Culture shock can strain relationships and lead to domestic violence (Nesbitt & Lynch 1992). A Western culture which imposes its own values on traditional ethnic practices (e.g female circumcision) can cause dilemmas.

Ethnic groups' social organization (their traditional lifeways) can exert a constraining effect on their behaviour. Adaptation can become a challenging task to many, since it entails integrating into new social structures (health care systems, housing and educational systems and so on) which possess their own ground rules.

Time

Time is an important concept for most people. Western cultures are conscious of the time factor. Our activities are driven by our consciousness that we either have to speed up or slow down to achieve our goals within a specific time allocation. In addition, most of us are aware that the duration of an activity, a habit, will also have an effect on our well-being. For example, most smokers know that years of smoking make them prone to lung cancer, and that heavy drinking and years of sedentary living will have negative health outcomes. We are, therefore, conscious that the time concept is linked to such attributes as the past (what we have been doing), the present (what we are doing) and the future (what is likely to happen). To people in Western societies, time is a reality. When one lives in a culture that is not time-centred it can be disorientating (Box 6.4).

Box 6.4 Time in other cultures

When Madeleine Leininger (1995a) lived with and studied the Gadsup of the Eastern Highlands of New Guinea in the early 1960s, she initially found it disorientating. She recalls: 'there were no clocks or watches in the village, and so no one lived by the clock or kept rigid time schedules. This was very strange for me to adjust to having come from a time-centered culture'.

Giger et al (1997) explained that some ethnic groups (e.g. Native Americans) are *present-oriented*; they emphasize 'current events'. This belief can make health promotion strategies difficult. Since the future has no meaning, they have no expectations. Attempt to explain what is likely to happen as a consequence of present action will have no desired effect.

Western cultures are so used to speed and fast action that we take it for granted. It is a way of life. Nurses in practices, for example, work according to strict time schedule. Ethnic clients whose 'time awareness' may not be similar could respond nonchalantly to emergency situations. This can be frustrating to caregivers. Imposing our time concept on others can, however, develop undesirable effects, such as strained relationships and a misperception of excessive control.

Environmental control

Immigrants have to face new environmental conditions, which can be overpowering. Living in deprived inner city areas, for example, can be daunting. Where there is social deprivation and decay, an individual can experience not only a sense of desolation but a loss of control. Social and health care services can empower the people facing adversity by raising awareness of their human rights to obtain services tailored to specific needs. In order to manage their environment, a degree of adaptation and integration has to be exercised.

The term 'environment' encompasses not only the immediate neighbourhood and workplace areas, but the socio-political, economic, cultural and racial framework as they affect the person. Where there is a language barrier the exercise of control proves more problematic. Many clients in need of health and/or social support can find it hard to negotiate the systems. The problem is further accentuated by racialized inequalities (discussed above).

The environmental context is a meaningful concept that, to the ethnic groups concerned, is commensurate with cultural values and lifestyles, including implications for health. Such influences are wide-ranging, requiring thorough evaluation during interactions with the groups so that care is congruent with identified needs.

Biological variations

The importance of recognizing biological variations in cultural and racial care is well documented. This knowledge can help diagnoticians and health screeners to focus on areas that may otherwise go undetected. For example, there is a high incidence of cardiovascular disease, hepatitis B, tuberculosis and cirrhosis of the liver among Asian Pacific Islanders (Giger et al 1997).

Other variations with implications for care delivery and clinicians' responses are linked to pain experiences. Leininger (1995a) provides insight into the complex interactions between professional behaviour, cultural context and client's perception (Box 6.5).

Since the importance of traditional values can affect the display of pain expressions and reactions to illness and trauma (Calvillo & Flaskerud 1993), professionals influenced by their own cultural beliefs may misinterpret cues. In a study of 60 patients to evaluate the pain response by Mexican-American and Anglo-American women

Box 6.5 Pain management

Health professionals, Leininger argued, make inferences about the degree of pain clients experience. However, their interventions may not be congruent (if pain exists) 'with the perspective of the client'. Sometimes decisions made by the nurse not to provide pain relief are made on inadequate insight into the cultural context of clients' behaviour. Not asking for pain-relieving drugs may be due to:

- fear of addiction (Calvillo & Flaskerud 1993)
- a demonstration of being cooperative, good and strong.

Alternatively, when the person in pain appears quiet and 'utilizes forms of distraction such as reading, watching television or talking with friends or family', professionals are least likely to administer analgesia, since their (the professionals') concept of the pain experience (e.g. crying, writhing in agony, demanding and holding the pain site) is not being expressed by the client.

Some cultures, e.g. Hispanic, promote a stoic attitude. To complain of pain is to admit personal weakness. Leininger thus emphasizes how critical it is for nurses to be conversant with the multidimensional approaches to pain management. In particular, attentive concerns should be shown in regard to the care meanings and expressions which are influenced by the client's world view (Leininger 1995a, Omeri 1997).

and their nurses, Calvillo and Flaskerud reported the following findings:

1. Mexican-American patients moan and complain of pain, since it is an acceptable cultural behaviour.

2. When Mexican-American patients cry it may be a strategy to 'relieve the pain' rather than a way of attracting attention of others for pain relief.

3. Nurses evaluated Anglo-American women's pain as more severe than Mexican-American women's pain. The researchers argue that the higher social class status of the clients (Anglo-American) may predispose them to receiving better pain management than their counterparts.

4. Nurses are prone to potential misinterpretation of the pain felt by their patients due to lack of 'awareness of their (the nurses') own values and perceptions' which can be detrimental to effective pain evaluation.

In the UK, Webster (1997) commented on Asian patients with coronary heart conditions and argued that their illness behaviour shows unique patterns. Compared with non-Asian patients, they are perceived to complain of chest pain more often and to have more physical complaints. While pain experiences are relevant issues for nurses and medical practitioners to consider, other biological variations must be borne in mind during assessment. For example, ethnic differences have been found in the level of risk factors associated with genital human papillomavirus (HPV) infections (Kenney 1996). This virus is linked to cervical cancer. Kenney pointed out that Anglo women – compared with other ethnic groups – are at greater risk of developing HPV. Their tendency to engage in sexual activities at an earlier age and to lead 'risky lifestyle behaviours' increases the prevalence.

Although more research is required to investigate such correlations, for health workers this knowledge is relevant, as an understanding of lifestyle behaviours is connected with biological changes that negate health integrity. Strong personal values, such as giving priority to family needs rather than one's personal health concerns (Sennott-Miller 1994), can prevent some groups (e.g. Hispanic women) from accessing cancer screening services earlier. It therefore leads one to conclude that many Hispanic women may discover cancerous changes too advanced to be effectively treated.

Interest in cultural differences related to biological variations and illness has also been extended to the role of ethnicity in rheumatoid arthritis. Jacono et al (1996), in their epidemiological study of rheumatoid arthritis in Ontario, Canada, concluded that Canadian aboriginals tended to develop the disease earlier than other ethnic groups. Furthermore, it was found that twice as many Finnish Canadians suffer from rheumatoid arthritis as Italian Canadians. Although genetic influences cannot be solely implicated at this stage, other extraneous factors (i.e. lifestyle, socio-economic, environmental, dietary variables) should be included.

Genetic factors are related to differences in body properties (e.g. height differences between Japanese and Africans), while environmental factors (Kelly et al 1997) are considered to be less influential. In their study to compare the growth of Pakistan school children in the UK, Kelly et al found only minor differences compared with indigenous school children. Anecdotally, they argued there has been an inclination to assume that being shorter implies a 'failure to thrive', which would have implications for screening and treatment. As the researchers pointed out, the methods of classification and measurement need careful assessment to ensure accuracy of results.

Sometimes biological factors intermingle with other dimensions: cultural practice, ethnicity, environmental–seasonal variables. One finds such examples in the research findings of Namgung et al (1998) in their investigation of body bone mineral content and bone resorption among Korean newborn infants (Box 6.6).

Box 6.6 Korean winter-born and summer-born newborn infants

Pregnant Korean women are less exposed to sunlight due to their socio-cultural habits. Korean women do not take vitamin D supplements. Lack of vitamin D increases bone resorption, while bone mineralization is lowered. Namgung et al (1998) found Korean babies born in winter had an 8% lower total body bone mineral content compared to summer newborns.

Asian women are prone to vitamin D deficiency. In addition, the prevalence of diabetes is four times higher in people of Asian origin than in whites (Burden 1998). Consequently, Asians are more liable to suffer from renal disease and hypertension. Clients of African descent in Britain and USA and African-Caribbeans are predisposed to a high prevalence of diabetes and diabetic nephropathy (Raleigh 1997).

Very often the presence of these conditions is unknown to the person, caused by a lack of knowledge, professional support and lack of access to diabetes screening services. Primary and community health professionals (Raleigh 1997) have a role in early detection and the implementation of measures to control disease progression.

Explaining to sufferers the importance of self-management, regular physical exercise and obesity control is recommended. However, conscious

effort should be made to understand behavioural variations and the effects of personal health beliefs. Assessment should be sensitive and supported by 'skilful negotiations' (Ghosh 1998) necessary in explaining the nature of diseases and their manifestations.

 Activity 6.1

1. Design a plan of care listing potential needs and problems ethnic clients are likely to have.
2. Organize small group discussions to discuss implementation strategies and methods to evaluate care.

??? Question 6.1

1. What do you consider to be the major constraints preventing ethnic groups from gaining access to health care?
2. How should health workers implement a model of care that is not only culturally sensitive but racially sensitive?
3. It is said that 'racial differentiation in coronary heart disease can be explained by socio-environmental factors' (Papadopoulos & Alleyne 1995) – do you agree?
4. What approaches can be used to combat racism?

ETHNICITY AND REPRODUCTIVE HEALTH

CONTRACEPTION

Women in Britain from ethnic minorities have been identified to have distinct reproductive sexual behaviour and use of contraceptive methods (Raleigh et al 1998). Although reproductive health practice among Pakistani and Bangladeshi women needs further research to obtain additional insight into their behaviour, Raleigh et al emphasize some essential issues relevant to health professionals. Of particular significance is the necessity for family planning, with sensitive support combined with professional counselling and education.

Compared with white women, use of contraception among Asian women was found to be lower: 59% among Pakistani/Bangladeshi women compared with 88% among white women. Attitudes to contraception differ. Minority ethnic women avoid contraceptive measures (e.g. the pill) because they 'dislike it', rather than because of the desire to achieve pregnancy. This attitude may be associated with the belief that artificial methods, in particular the pill (only about 1/3 of Asian women use it), reflect Western values in contrast with their own traditional practices. Out of 671 women, 5% use abstinence, withdrawal and rhythm method.

Asians place a high value on virginity. Unmarried females seeking contraceptive advice will be disfavoured by their communities. When access to health centres is available, the motivation to seek contraceptive advice may be dampened due to fear that personnel may break confidentiality. Losing one's virginity creates family conflict, and the chances of finding a husband are much reduced. Differences in methods used can be found in Table 6.1.

Non-users of contraceptives are prone to becoming pregnant. As the use of condoms is higher among Indians and Pakistani/Bangladeshis, one can anticipate that HIV/AIDS may be less of a threat. In addition, the expression of dislike regarding some methods may mean that some women and their partners may in effect

reduce their opportunities to experiment with other methods. For example, if condoms cause allergic reactions or rupture during intercourse, the pill may suit them. While IUD appears popular among Pakistani/Bangladeshis (12.5%) and Indians (15.2%) the reasons for these choices have not been pinpointed. More research is needed to ascertain that ethnic groups make informed contraceptive decisions. The wide range of devices on the market should be explained, with information on their advantages or disadvantages.

Meeting the family planning needs of ethnic groups demands proactive strategies:

• education and group counselling
• facilitating access to services
• assessing prenatal and postnatal needs
• discussing the implications (social, biological, psychological, economic factor)
• breaking language barriers by making use of interpreters
• participating in ethnic monitoring in collaboration with ethnic and non-ethnic community workers.

CERVICAL SCREENING

The aim of cervical screening is to detect any abnormalities of the cervix such as precancerous changes or established cancerous tumour. It is thus considered an important preventative measure. Uptake of this service by minority groups has been minimal. Several reasons have been given to raise our awareness of this behaviour pattern (Box 1998) (Box 6.7).

Cultural and religious factors are influential in explaining ethnic groups' behaviour (Meehan 1998). These reasons, however, only form part of a complex system conflicting with established ideologies, discouraging uptake of services.

White women show marked differences in their attitude to cervical screening and their doctors. The doctor was perceived to be 'the best person to talk to when they had a problem' (White 1995). Their understanding of cervical smears tended to be generally positive, although the topic of 'embarrassment' and 'distressing' procedures was mentioned.

Table 6.1 Contraceptive methods by ethnic groups (women aged 16–29) (From Raleigh et al 1998)	
IUD	
Pakistani/Bangladeshi	12.5%
Indian	15.2%
African-Caribbean	2.9%
White	3.1%
Condoms	
Pakistani/Bangladeshi	37.5%
Indian	43.5%
African-Caribbean	23.2%
White	24.7%
Non-users of contraception because of 'dislike'	
African-Caribbean	35%
Pakistani/Bangladeshi	25%
Indian	27%
White	12%

Box 6.7 Factors affecting uptake of cervical screening services

- **Personal:**
  - loss of dignity and the embarrassment which ensues when being examined by medical and nursing staff
  - belief that cervical screening is only for a decadent culture where promiscuity is prevalent
  - belief that private body parts should not be seen by strangers, only husbands.
- **Social:**
  - past experiences of hospital procedures
  - the role of families in transmitting a culture of reliance on folk medicine and informal support networks.
- **Psychological:**
  - lack of knowledge, understanding and reassurance from personnel increase the propensity for apprehensive behaviour
  - impersonal and insensitive attitude deepens the lack of confidence in the care delivered.
- **Communication:**
  - in conjunction with language barriers which are perennial themes, the verbal and non-verbal cues of personnel have been implicated in the level of dissatisfaction expressed about the service provided
  - distancing behaviour and avoidance of eye contact (by personnel). When Asian nurses are present, clients have found interactions easier due to their ability to communicate freely.
- **Environmental:**
  - due to misperception of the role and functions of health care centres some women see the environment not to be conducive to cleanliness, believing that they may contract cervical cancer in consulting rooms. This belief can be strong and one woman suggested using 'water to wash it all away'
  - the impersonal and clinical environment creates an atmosphere of distrust and unease.
- **Racial issues:**
  - during screening, a few women interpret the behaviour of those around to be racist
  - opportunities to ask questions were not provided
  - inequality in care delivery indicates potential existence of covert racism.

RITUAL CIRCUMCISION

The Director-General of the World Health Organization, in 1998, Dr Hiroshi Nakajima, accentuated the provision of health care at all stages of community life. Of particular importance, he stressed how necessary it is to encompass care giving with the individual in mind,

rather than focusing solely on social structures. This means achieving the goal in disease prevention and activities control through meaningful dialogue and close multi-sectoral collaboration. Ritual circumcision is practised by many cultures but, similar to any surgical procedures, has health risks (L'archevesque & Goldstein-Lohman 1996). While social structures perpetuate traditional practices, individual cultures possess their own rationale for their behaviour. Nurses and others in the health care field must be aware of this, aiming to maintain the client's autonomy with respect.

According to Jewish faith, baby boys must be circumcised by a Mohel (the person who performs the operation while adhering to strict Jewish religious law) following strict religious ritual (L'archevesque & Goldstein-Lohman 1996). Since the circumcision has deep religious and cultural significance, it departs from the common routine surgical procedure performed by any surgeon in a hospital setting. It can be performed at home, in a synagogue or in a hospital on condition that, in the latter case, the ritual is undertaken by a Mohel. For nurses, this controversial practice has social, biological and ethical implications. The procedure has deep social significance as well as a strong religious connotation. It is an expression of manhood and it confirms one's close tie with the will of God. It is a ceremony that brings the whole family and significant others together.

Biologically, the ritual is associated with the causation of unnecessary pain, the possibility of disfigurement and the predisposition to infection and phimosis (if the foreskin is not adequately removed). The positive effects of circumcision, however, are noted to be reduced incidence of penile cancer and better genital hygiene. L'archevesque & Goldstein-Lohman argued that when parents face the dilemma of whether to have their children circumcised in a synagogue, at home or in a hospital, professionals can intervene to support them, by educating on the benefits associated with the ritual being performed within the operating room of a hospital. In addition, it is an opportunity for both parents and nurses to discuss the issue of personal beliefs and cultural constraints that may impinge on medical/surgical procedures. It becomes a learning situation for both parties. Moreover, parents need reassurance and informed choice. It is a context whereby medical–cultural boundaries can become less distinct.

Ethically, nurses and other health workers may express a judgemental attitude, as the practice may go against the grain of their personal beliefs. In addition, the thought of an innocent newborn being circumcised may cause strong resentment in health care staff.

Despite the possibility of personal conflict regarding such matters, nurses have a duty to educate themselves by 'reviewing the literature' to gain a thorough understanding 'of the religious and medical aspects of the procedure', so that they can be fully supportive towards the parents, in helping them to make an informed choice.

Activity 6.2

Produce a list of benefits and disadvantages in connection with ritual circumcision.

??? Question 6.2

Why is ritual circumcision a controversial subject?

FEMALE CIRCUMCISION (GENITAL MUTILATION)

Empowering women, Nakajima (1998) believed, in all cultures, by using available educational resources for health development, is a desirable goal since it is 'an ethical and technical imperative'. It is worth noting, however, that in sociological and medical literature, the topic of female circumcision has aroused more controversy than male circumcision, to the extent that the former is most frequently referred to as 'female genital mutilation'. It is regarded as evidence of the subjugation of women.

Gibeau (1998) pointed out that female genital mutilation is a more accurate term, first because there is parsimonious evidence that the procedure is similar to male circumcision and secondly, because the practice can be quite extensive. It consists of either clitoridectomies (the removal of prepuce, clitoris and excision of part of the labia minora) or infibulations (which includes removal of two-thirds of the labia majora, labia minora and clitoris).

To feminists and some non-feminists alike, female circumcision is the ultimate exploitation of women. It is considered to be a dangerous practice, with legal, ethical and cultural considerations (Ahmed 1996) as well as biological and psychological implications (McCaffrey 1995).

The practice of female circumcision is not a new social phenomenon. It is estimated that over 80 million women in various countries have undergone circumcision (McCleary 1994). The literature reflects a mainly Western viewpoint of the practice, which may partly explain why the term 'mutilation' is commonly used. Teare (1998) believed that the social and cultural context of female circumcision is misunderstood.

To women entrenched in their culture this custom has deep social significance (Gibeau 1998):

- the rituals are highly prized
- the woman who performs the ritual is venerated
- the custom socializes the woman to the ways of her society
- the custom reaffirms the role of women within family units
- women's sexual and reproductive images are consolidated
- circumcision guarantees them a husband in the future.

Some of the health consequences have been listed as:

- keloid scarring
- anxiety disorders
- depression
- chronic infection
- diminished or lack of sexual sensation

- fistulas
- vaginitis.

Effective medical care for women is exigent.

The role of nurses is to be aware that female circumcision is an offence in the UK, under the Prohibition of Female Circumcision Act 1985, to encourage and/or participate in female circumcision; it is also illegal in most European countries and in the USA (Gordon 1998). Women who have undergone female circumcision should be encouraged to talk freely about their customs. Attempts to understand their rationale should be made. A non-judgemental attitude is recommended.

PREGNANCY AND ETHNICITY

In the midwifery field, concerns are being expressed that negative attitudes toward ethnic groups are jeopardizing their family planning needs and that nurses' skills and knowledge in multicultural care require developing (Papadopoulos & Alleyne 1995). The multi-ethnic needs of minority clients are not fully recognized in midwifery education (Neile 1996). The extension of knowledge applicable to ethnicity issues has the advantage of ensuring that approaches are designed to anticipate potential problems and to meet needs relevant to specific client groups. There is, for example, a wide range of beliefs and practices within every culture (Schott & Henley 1996b). Cultural beliefs in combination with environmental factors impinge on daily activities of living. Assumptions and generalizations must be avoided.

Research undertaken in the USA has shown that ethnicity and substance use – alcohol, illicit drug-taking, smoking – are linked and appear to be prevalent among low-income pregnant mothers (Zambrana & Scrimshaw 1997). Many ethnic groups are socio-economically deprived. The researchers explained that psychosocial factors such as depression, loneliness, single parenthood, poverty and deprived environmental conditions are detrimental to health. For health care providers, the implications are as follows:

1. Conscious effort is necessary to identify the possibility of substance use in pregnant mothers.

2. Education and training should be provided for health workers on the effects of substance use on pregnant mothers, so that the latter can subsequently be educated.

3. The best strategies should be negotiated by involving social and health agencies to institute a programme of prevention and care.

4. The mother needs to be informed of possible side-effects of drugs (e.g. irritability, unresponsiveness) on her child postpartum.

In addition, it is imperative that midwifery teams maintain continuity of carers from antenatal to the postnatal periods (Hemingway et al 1997), to ascertain that both the mother's and child's needs are met adequately. Carer continuity is beneficial in a woman-centred care philosophy (Report by the Standing Nursing and Midwifery Advisory Committee 1998). Some ethnic groups may not be able to negotiate their care needs competently in order to obtain care continuity from their midwives. Explaining that continuity of contact is part of the care package will help alleviate unnecessary anxiety.

Childbirth is a major stressor. Many women are inadvertently disempowered during birthing, which stresses them further. How women exert control over the birth process, despite the medicalization of pregnancy delivery (Scopesi et al 1997), is receiving better consideration. Furthermore, it is pointed out that clients' participation in decision-making in maternity care has positive consequences (Pelkonen et al 1998). The cultural background of the woman is often neglected in regard to her perception of birth, role and needs for support during and after birth. Woollett (1990) argued that these aspects of reproductive psychology are omitted because women and their significant others' cultural practices and beliefs are seen as 'incomprehensible'. Commonplace assumptions are often made based on the notion that they are homogeneous groups, when in fact there is 'considerable variability within a community'.

It is sometimes assumed (Woollett 1990) that Asian fathers are not needed at the bedside of the women in labour. It is, however, well accepted that social ties have protective effects (improved mental well-being and reduced anxiety). Fathers' presence during labour is well accepted by most ethnic women, although exceptions have been found (Scopesi et al 1997), for example, in Genoa, Italy, where in some hospitals fathers' attendance is 'tolerated only'. This may be due to institutional constraints rather than the women's attitude. The aims of obstetric teams are – in view of issues related to ethnicity and labour – to:

- pinpoint the context in which maternity care is delivered
- specify care according to varied needs
- invite partners and significant others (if requested) during childbirth
- reassure and comfort that technology can be integrated with traditional practice.

BREAST-FEEDING: THE CULTURAL CONTEXT

Mothers are encouraged to breast-feed their infants because of its positive biological and psychological effects. Many midwives will promote breast-feeding. While it is well recommended, knowledge concerning the reasons many women choose to avoid breast-feeding is still in its infancy. Hence, the cultural context of breast-feeding becomes an important area to explore. Although culture is influential in guiding social behaviour, one must also include psychological factors. It is argued, for instance, that some women may be sensitive to their husband's or partner's attitude to breast-feeding (Woollett 1987). If fathers express resentment, women may decide to bottle-feed instead, 'to keep the peace'. Woollett gave the example of a father who was jealous of his son being breast-fed. Other reasons could be associated with convenience of bottle-feeding, particularly when there are other children in the family. Family management can thus add strain on mothers' inclination to breast-feed. With bottle-feeding, partners or siblings can help, leaving mothers free to manage the home. In addition, parents may inculcate specific traditional beliefs on their daughters with regard to breast-feeding, i.e. financial considerations: bottle feeds can be costly; breast milk is free.

Mothers, however, may feel a sense of loss of control when attempting to breast-feed. They are unsure about the amount of milk the baby is ingesting, or will argue they are not producing enough milk. Most mothers, nevertheless, show awareness of the psychological and biological importance of breast-feeding.

One can point out that breast-feeding is influenced by the social norms and values of a society (Higginbottom 1998). To a Western mother, breast-feeding may be embarrassing in public or in front of other men. Higginbottom stated that Nigerian women are not self-conscious in this respect. In Somali and Jamaica, breast-feeding is an ongoing process for several months and is socially expected. If a woman abruptly stops breast-feeding, other social pressures come into play: a woman's behaviour may be misinterpreted in the sense that she is thought to 'want to go flirting'. In the West Indies and Caribbean, women are nurtured by their relatives during breast-feeding periods. Higginbottom argued, however, that younger women who have migrated to the UK show a different attitude toward breast-feeding. The social, economical and cultural context in the UK mitigates against breast-feeding. For example, the element of choice (breast-feed vs. bottle-feed) is influential. In addition, the thought of altered body image can discourage young women from breast-feeding, as they feel the need to 'conform to certain body shapes'.

Other issues are related to the institutional racism many women experience in their contact with midwifery teams. Inability to disclose their fears, wishes and needs means that some clients may make wrong choices. Misunderstandings also surround specific 'non-Western' types of behaviour, which are then readily assumed to be another 'belief'. For example, Littler's (1997) study uncovers some pertinent socio-cultural and religious issues concerning why women from Bangladesh only initiate breast-feeding on the third day prior to discharge (Box 6.8). At the time of birth, *colostrum* (a thin, milky liquid containing nutrients, antibodies, specialized proteins and concentrations of vitamins) is secreted by the breasts.

Many Bangladeshi women do not dispute the

Box 6.8 Breast-feeding and beliefs about colostrum

Littler (1997) listed the following reasons which explain Bangladeshi women's attitude to breastfeeding.

1. colostrum is thin and watery; it is not real milk
2. past medical history (e.g. breast abscess) can distort perception of colostrum secretion
3. experience of afterpains would give cramps to breast-fed babies
4. 'sourness' of colostrum, which is unlike real milk
5. the texture of colostrum as 'thin and runny' is equated with diarrhoea
6. since colostrum is not perceived to be immediately essential, the tendency is to wait for the 'thick, full milk'.

value of breast milk. It is, however, necessary to find out their reasons for thinking it is important. Faith in traditional beliefs imparted by mothers-in-law, and in what their religion says have been implicated. For example, the attitude within the Islamic faith (Littler 1997) that the child will reap the biological benefits later on in life. Evidence shows, however, that the women's knowledge base of why breast milk is physiologically essential is weak. Midwifery teams have a role in furthering their clients' knowledge in such a way so that social beliefs and professional knowledge can be usefully integrated.

Activity 6.3

1. Prepare a diagram to be used in client education on the importance of breast milk.
2. Design a model of care to support ethnic pregnant women and their partners.

 Question 6.3

Pregnancy and childbirth are considered to be both stressful and joyful. Do you agree?

ETHNICITY AND CANCER CARE

'Cancer'. In today's society, as the lay person's knowledge of pathology improves via media coverage and health education efforts, the word continues to trigger a multitude of reactions: fear, distress, suicidal thoughts, hopelessness, anxieties and other physiological and psychoemotional responses. But the extent of the impact (Hammick et al 1996) is dependent on many variables: patients' individuality, their families and the degree of support provided, age, gender, sexual orientation, spirituality and, last but not least, concepts of culture and ethnicity have all been linked to the wide-ranging effects that the word cancer stimulates.

As we have already noticed in previous discussions, health and ill-health perceptions vary across cultures. Similarly, ethnicity influences can have an effect on patients' responses to care. With an awareness of ethnicity influences, one has to be conscious that the concept of spirituality can possess different connotations in different cultures.

In connection with cancer care situations, one finds that spirituality assumes a prominent position, in addition to other aspects of care, which merit similar consideration. However, professionals engaged in oncology care must exercise caution; their understanding of spirituality may be markedly different to the ethnic client. One finds, for example, a complex system of interpretations related to perceptions of health, illness and person among Chinese patients (Shih 1996), and to the latent meanings given to spirituality.

To the Chinese, life is dependent on a balanced state – the Yin and Yang – grouped in pairs of opposite, in regard to not only natural phenomena (i.e. night and day, sun and moon), but to social behaviour (Shih 1996), which many Chinese believe to be integrated with this philosophy. This belief is expressed by the taking of herbs or special food according to the season, to maintain the Yin or Yang balance. Other behaviour is related to the confidence in fortune tellers so that the timing for hospitalization may be chosen. Like other ethnic groups, the Chinese are heterogeneous groups, and groups may be affiliated to different philosophies, e.g. Taoist, Buddhist or Confucian. Shih gave the example of Chinese Buddhist behaviour when faced with 'malignant disease': they are inclined to attribute their ill-health to 'their sin', thus blaming themselves. Nevertheless, Buddhists hold a positive image and anticipation of death; to them, after death a better life is found in heaven.

While it is important to know how a client's personhood relates to their perception of health and illness, it is equally imperative to evaluate their understanding of the disease. It is an area that has aroused concerns in both Western and Eastern cultures. Doctors do not make a formal assessment of their patients' knowledge of the disease (Fielding et al 1995). In their Hongkong study of 142 surgeons and radiotherapists who care for Chinese patients with cancer Fielding et al concluded that patients have minimal insight into their conditions due to the paucity of information. This causes distress to cancer patients.

Assuming that patients have already received the required information from others is, in reality, leaving them to manage the fear of the unknown in the dark. Being told the nature of their disease makes it easier for many to confront impending death. Knowing what the future holds helps them to communicate with their families regarding personal and sensitive issues surrounding funeral arrangements, family safety and comfort after death, and the making of a will. In addition, failing to impart information in good time, while the client's rationality is undisturbed, has implications for the Chinese Buddhist. A Buddhist (Nyatanga 1997) will want to die with a 'clear mind'. Nyatanga emphasized that care professionals should consider 'informational care': giving honest information to the client. Equally, relatives' needs for information must be met.

The care culture (hospice, community, hospital settings) should involve relatives in caring for the dying (Andershed & Ternestedt 1998). Conscientious observation is, however, necessary to evaluate the effects of caring for the cancer patients on relatives. Martinson et al (1997), in their study of 89 Chinese families in Guangzhou, China, found marked differences among Chinese parents' reactions to their children with cancer. Chinese families are parent–child-dominated, compared to the 'husband–wife'-dominated culture in Western families. The researchers argued that the strong parent–child bond, and the interdependent nature of family functioning, means that family members are at greater risk when they lose the support system.

Due to social conditioning, the Chinese are known to suppress their emotions. The latter are not dealt with using cognitive strategies, but are translated into somatic symptoms. While in the West, one can say: 'I am depressed', a Chinese person might make reference to the heart and the feelings felt within it. Symbolic meanings, created by tradition, are integrated in such a way with the psychological and the physiological state (emotions and their effects on physiology) that the communication of emotion is stifled (Martinson et al 1997).

The Chinese child with cancer evokes strong emotions in parents, which they feel need to be controlled, but which are expressed in physical symptoms: dizziness, headaches, insomnia, colds etc. In addition, the child relies faithfully on the closeness of parental support. When parents fail to provide support, 'members may feel shame or useless'.

Therefore, family support and closeness need to be encouraged. Quality of life can thereby be enhanced. While socio-cultural sensitivity and support can prevent the pain of social isolation, the effects of cancer pain on quality of life in different ethnic groups need addressing (Gordon 1997). The pain of cancer can be expressed differently in varying groups. Similarly, family reactions to cancer pain are influenced by ethnocultural beliefs: Italian and Jewish people encourage free emotional expressions of pain; English and German people may show a more stoic behaviour; while elderly Filipino patients will mask their pain (Gordon 1997). This type of behaviour is common in societies where 'stoicism and fortitude' are regarded as cultural norms (Smith 1996).

It appears that professionals whose ethnic background is similar to the patients' will perceive the latter as more sensitive to pain. Smith (1996) gave the examples of Japanese and Korean nurses who believed that their patients 'suffered more pain than their American and Hispanic counterparts'.

Caring for ethnic clients with cancer requires knowledge and awareness of their needs (Box 6.9).

Box 6.9 Ethnic cancer patients' personal needs

A great deal of emphasis is placed on cultural sensitivity. However, integrating spirituality within the culture dimension is a requisite. The pain experience can be deeply internalized (culturally and spiritually) by the clients. The intensity of beliefs in community support can buffer the effects of hardship on the sick or dying members.

Ritualized religious practices may not be overtly expressed (e.g. praying, communicating with religious leaders, bible reading etc.), but this does not necessarily mean an absence of faith. This hidden dimension may come to the fore during interactions with the cancer patients. Behind a stoic front, the fear of dying and a painful death may be present. The dying process is a challenge to the faith, spirit and beliefs of the person, whatever the social background.

Many clients may rely on herbal medicine in addition to conventional Western medical treatment; a practice that may become a clinical issue. Therefore, the inclusion of some folk medicine with Westernized practices should be at least considered after thorough discussions with patients and their families.

While the above measures are relevant, preparation should be made for the person nearing death. Harberecht and Prior (1997) explain that the grief accompanying dying and death can create 'spiritual chaos': a state whereby the dying person's psycho-emotional being is disrupted. But the grief process has wide cultural variations. Reactions to loss across cultures show marked differences (Stroebe & Schut 1998). In some cultures crying is encouraged. The Balinese people smile when grieving. The Navajo Native American people grieve for a limited period of four days, during which emotional expression is expected. In Mauritius, Creole families, neighbours and friends unite to express their grief together.

For care workers, these varied manifestations to ill-health may appear confusing. The essential approach is to exert sensitivity and be prepared to understand the meanings associated with the behaviour patterns. Care negotiation with the aid of clients, their relatives and/or community/religious-spiritual leaders is a consideration.

Activity 6.4

Prepare a list of benefits and disadvantages concerning the use of herbal medicine.

??? Question 6.4

Immigrants bring with them their own cultural concepts of health and disease (Chan 1995). How should their holistic needs be met?

ETHNICITY AND PSYCHIATRY

Mental health nurses encounter minority client groups with differing beliefs and perception of their social world and inner selves. Religion and spirituality can very often be the key components of their beliefs; however, beliefs often overlap (George 1998). Immigrants may share aspects of several faiths: Buddhism, Taoism, Christianity, Islam, Hinduism for example. One can expect their communication styles to differ: they may be using a combination of signs and symbols (George 1998), which reflect the communication modes they are used to. East Africans may express feeling depressed by saying they have 'ants in the brain'. A Western-trained psychiatric worker could inadvertently make a diagnosis of somatic hallucination, which has implications for practice.

It is pointed out (George 1998, Yates & Craddock 1998) that there is a high prevalence (62%) of Afro-Caribbean communities in psychiatric hospitals. If health workers in psychiatric nursing settings are unaware of ethnic clients' needs in regard to unconventional communication styles, it is pointed out that their behaviour may be misinterpreted as 'healthy or unhealthy to the uninformed practitioner' (Stolley & Koenig 1997). Failing to assess clients' responses correctly could entail interpreting some behaviour as threatening (Webbe 1998).

Other issues are related to a failure by mental health workers to recognize the effects of social deprivation (e.g. poverty, homelessness), which can exacerbate the relationship between ethnicity and health status (Silveira & Ebrahim 1995). It is estimated that there are many elderly Somali and Bengali people who are prone to anxiety and depression due to impoverished social circumstances. Afro-Caribbeans, on the other hand, according to Bhugra and Bhui (1998) are prone to schizophrenia. Unemployment, social isolation and drug abuse have been linked to mental pathology. Moreover, one has to consider the effects of labelling and stereotyping, which have negative consequences. Jackson (1997) points out that a black Afro-Caribbean person with a psychological problem could easily be diagnosed as 'schizophrenic' with an 'aggressive' personality.

Where there is cultural awareness failure, a person's spiritual self, the driving force behind the behaviour patterns, may be mistaken for mental illness. Jackson argued that *spiritual intervention* may sometimes be the only therapy needed for someone who is emotionally affected, because of belief that the cause is 'an evil spirit' (Case examples 6.3 and 6.4).

Case example 6.3 Spiritual warfare

'Many people given the choice, would ask for some kind of spiritual intervention rather than medication. I can think of one lady who came into the office looking for the Housing Department, which used to be here. She was crying, so I sat her down to talk. We established our origins – me Ghanaian and she Nigerian. She told me she was involved in a spiritual warfare; that spirits were chasing and knew where she lived and she had to be rehoused to get away from them. She said they had already shot her in the spirit. She described what to a white mental health professional would sound just like a visual hallucination, but to her they were spirits and they were real' (Jackson 1997).

Case example 6.4 Obeah

Miss E, a 20-year-old woman who had emigrated to Britain from Trinidad, was compulsorily admitted to hospital after refusing food and drink for several days. She believed that an obeah curse had been placed on her. A diagnosis was made of severe psychotic depression and treatment commenced under the emergency provisions of the Mental Health Act.

Response to treatment was poor, and a traditional healer was consulted, who lifted the curse. She began to eat and drink and showed no other signs of mental illness; she was discharged from hospital two days later (Dein 1997).

One can deduce from the Case examples 6.3 and 6.4 that what constitutes the sick role and illness behaviour to a Westerner may instigate the wrong interventions. Turner (1997) suggests a careful approach is needed, making sure that the ethnic client's illness behaviour is fully understood.

Activity 6.5

If you were admitting the two individuals described above in the examples, would your approach have been different? Describe how you would have communicated with them.

??? Question 6.5

Is it ethical to impose a Western mode of treatment on an ethnic client who believes in the spirit world?

SUMMARY

In this chapter, issues pertinent to minority ethnic groups have been discussed. In many cases their social and health needs differ from their white counterparts. In addition, Western-trained health workers may misunderstand behaviour by ethnic group members and instigate health strategies that may not be culturally sensitive. Moreover, the effects of racism can increase health inequalities. It is also widely accepted that discrimination in health care, and society in general, is common. This means that many ethnic clients may not access services effectively. While cultural sensitivity is recommended, it is equally obligatory to develop sensitive tools to measure the efficacy of interventions.

GLOSSARY

Adhesions   bands of fibrous connective tissues, joining structures or organs following inflammation and damage

Bone resorption   loss of bone caused by physiological or pathological changes

Cirrhosis   a liver disease characterized by a breaking down of the microscopic lobules in the structure

Cognitive strategies   in psychology, using one's faculties

Emic   a person's subjective viewpoint

Epidemiology   a study of disease in relation to people and the environment

Ethnocentrism   centred on one's own culture

Ethnocultural   in relation to cultural practice as it affects ethnic groups

Etic   an external observer's viewpoint

Fire walking   a practice among some cultures (e.g. Tamil culture, Sri-Lanka), which consists of walking over burning coal

Fistulas   an abnormal opening between two internal organs; also applies to an opening from an internal organ to the surface of the body

Folk medicine   traditional use of home remedies

Heterogeneous   diverse features; not having a uniform quality

Homogeneous   of similar nature or characteristics

Intra-uterine device   a plastic or metal coil inserted into the uterus to prevent conception

Keloid scarring   irregularly shaped scar tissues in the skin

Mineralization   deposition of calcium phosphate in bone

Multi-ethnically diverse   varied ethnic communities

Nephropathy   disease of the kidney

Obeah   a form of witchcraft that has elements of Christianity and African religion

Phimosis   opening of foreskin, which narrows over the glans penis

Prejudice   a preconceived view of someone, not based on knowledge

Prepuce   foreskin

Racism   a belief that one race is superior to another, usually applies to act of racial discrimination

Rheumatoid arthritis   a chronic inflammatory disease affecting the joints

Rickets   a condition affecting bone density due to vitamin D deficiency

Sickle-cell disease   a hereditary blood condition with abnormal type of haemoglobin in the red blood cells. The cells take a 'sickle shape' appearance

Socio-political construct   representing something from a social and political viewpoint

Totem worship   objects, plants or animals associated as symbols of the people, with beliefs that they are sacred

REFERENCES

Ahmad W I 1993 Making black people sick: 'race', ideology and health research. In Ahmad W I (ed) 'Race' and health in contemporary Britain. Open University Press, Buckingham, p 14

Ahmed S 1996 Practice: leaving the female body intact. Kai Tiaki: Nursing New Zealand 2(4): 20–21

Alderman C 1997 Delighted to be a role model. Nursing Standard 12(10): 20–21

Andershed B, Ternestedt B M 1998 Involvement of relatives in the care of the dying, in different care cultures: involvement in the dark or in the light? Cancer Nursing 21(2): 106–116

Baylav A 1996 Overcoming culture and language barriers. Practitioner 240(1563): 403–406

Bhugra D, Bhui K 1998 Transcultural psychiatry: do problems persist in the second generation? Hospital Medicine 59(2): 126–129

Box V 1998 Cervical screening: the knowledge and opinions of black and minority women and health advocates in East London. Health Education Journal 57(1): 3–15

Burden M 1998 Approaches to managing diabetes in Asian people. Community Nurse 4(4): 31–34

Burford B 1997 Race to be first: addressing cultural diversity in the NHS. Health Visitor 70(12): 452–454

Calvillo E R, Flaskerud J H 1993 Evaluation of the pain response by Mexican-American and Anglo-American women and their nurses. Journal of Advanced Nursing 18(3): 451–459

Central Statistics Office 1998 Social Trends 28: Population 1.10. HMSO, London, p 34

Chan J Y 1995 Dietary beliefs of Chinese patients. Nursing Standard 9(27): 30–34

Chevannes M 1990 Stamping out inequality. Nursing Times 86(42): 39–40

Connell C M, Gibson G D 1997 Racial, ethnic, and cultural differences in dementia caregiving: review and analysis. Gerontologist 37(3): 355–364

Culley L 1996 A critique of multiculturalism in health care: the challenge for nurse education. Journal of Advanced Nursing 23(3): 564–570

Dein S 1997 Mental health in a multi-ethnic society. British Medical Journal 315(7106): 473–476

Eriksen T H 1993 Ethnicity and nationalism. Pluto Press, London, p 13

Fielding R, Ko L S, Wong L 1995 Inconsistencies between belief and practice: assessment of Chinese cancer patients' knowledge of their disease. Journal of Cancer Care 4(1): 11–15

Foolchand M K 1995 Promoting racial equality in the nursing curriculum. Nurse Education Today 15(2): 101–105

George M 1998 A gulf in understanding. Nursing Standard 12(26): 24–25

Ghosh P 1998 South Asian elders: a special group with special needs. Geriatric Medicine 28(1): 11–15

Gibeau A M 1998 Female genital mutilation: when a cultural practice generates clinical and ethical dilemmas. Journal of Obstetric Gynaecologic and Neonatal Nursing 27(1): 85–91

Giger J N, Davidhizar R, Johnson J Y, Poole V L 1997 Health

promotion among ethnic minorities: the importance of cultural phenomena. Rehabilitation Nursing 22(6): 303–307

Godfrey K 1998 Treating eczema in ethnic minority groups. Community Nurse 4(1): 31

Gordon C 1997 The effect of cancer pain on quality of life in different ethnic groups: a literature review. Nurse Practitioner 8(1): 5–13

Gordon H 1998 Female genital mutilation (female circumcision). Diplomate 5(2): 86–90

Haberecht J, Prior D 1997 Spiritual chaos: an alternative conceptualisation of grief. International Journal of Palliative Nursing 3(4): 209–213

Hammick M, Smith J, Corsini et al 1996 Radiotherapy patients in the United Kingdom: meeting cultural and spiritual needs. Journal of Cancer Care 5(3): 113–115

Hawthorne K 1994 Diabetes health education for British South Asians: a review of aims, difficulties and achievements. Health Education Journal 53(3): 309–321

Hemingway H, Saunders D, Parsons L 1997 Social class, spoken language and pattern of care as determinants of continuity of carer in maternity services in East London. Journal of Public Health Medicine 19(2): 156–161

Hennings J, Williams J, Haque B N 1996 Exploring the health needs of Bangladeshi women: a case study in using qualitative research methods. Health Education Journal 55(1): 11–23

Higginbottom G 1998 Breastfeeding and black women: a UK investigation. Health Visitor 71(1): 12–15

HMSO 1997 Results from the 1995 General Household Survey: living in Britain. HMSO, London, p 16, p 23

Inman K 1998 Everybody hurts … Community Care 1213: 20–21

Jackson C 1997 Worlds apart. Mental Health Care 1(3): 86–87

Jacono J, Jacono B, Cano P et al 1996 An epidemiological study of rheumatoid arthritis in a Northern Ontario clinical practice: the role of ethnicity. Journal of Advanced Nursing 24(1): 31–35

Jones D, Gill P 1998 Breaking down language barriers. British Medical Journal 316(7143): 1476

Kaewboonchoo O, Morioka I, Miyashita K et al 1998 Hearing impairment among young Chinese in an urban area. Public Health 112(3): 143–146

Kelly A M, Shaw N J, Thomas A M et al 1997 Growth of Pakistani children in relation to the 1990 growth standards. Archives of Disease in Childhood 77(5): 401–405

Kelsall B S 1998 Racial harassment in the workplace. RCM Midwives Journal 1(5): 149

Kenney J W 1996 Ethnic differences in risk factors associated with genital human papillomavirus infections. Journal of Advanced Nursing 23(6): 1221–1227

L'archevesque C I, Goldstein-Lohman H 1996 Ritual circumcision: educating parents. Pediatric Nursing 22(3): 228–234

Lawson M S, Thomas M, Hardiman A 1998 Iron status of Asian children aged 2 living in England. Archives of Disease in Childhood 78(5): 420–426

Leininger M 1995a Transcultural nursing: concepts theories, research and practices, 2nd edn. McGraw-Hill, New York, p 63

Leininger M 1995b Teaching transcultural nursing to transform nursing for the 21st century. Journal of Transcultural Nursing 6(2): 2–3

Leininger M 1997 Transcultural nursing: research to transform nursing education and practice: 40 years. Image: Journal of Nursing Scholarship 29(4): 341–347

Littler 1997 Beliefs about colostrum among women from Bangladesh. Midwives 110(1308): 3–7

McCaffrey M 1995 Female genital mutilation: consequences for reproductive and sexual health. Sexual and Marital Therapy 10(2): 189–200

McCleary P H 1994 Female genital mutilation and childbirth: a case report … including commentary by Ohmer-Hashi. Birth: Issues in Perinatal Care and Education 21(4): 221–226

McGee P 1994 Developing a knowledge base for transcultural nursing. British Journal of Nursing 3(11): 544

McMillan I 1998 Discrimination in the NHS. Nursing Standard 12(33): 14

Mares P, Henley A, Baxter C 1985 Health care in multiracial Britain. Health Education Council/National Extension College, Cambridge, p 38

Martinson I M, Liu-Chang C, Yi-Hua L 1997 Distress symptoms and support systems of Chinese parents of children with cancer. Cancer Nursing 20(2): 94–99

Mayor V 1996 Investing in people: personal and professional development of black nurses. Health Visitor 69(1): 20–23

Meehan F 1998 Ending the care lottery. Journal of Community Nursing 12(6)

Mensah J 1997 Positive action. Nursing Standard 12(10): 22–23

Mitchell D P 1996 Postmodernism, health and illness. Journal of Advanced Nursing 23(1): 201–205

Murphy K, McLeod Clark J 1993 Nurses' experiences of caring for ethnic-minority clients. Journal of Advanced Nursing 18(3): 442–450

Nakajima H 1998 Fifty years of making people healthier. World Health 51st Year 2: 3

Namgung R, Tsang R C, Lee C et al 1998 Low total body bone mineral content and high bone resorption in Korean winter-born versus summer-born newborn infants. The Journal of Pediatrics 132(3): 421–425

Neile E 1996 Multicultural education in midwifery. Midwifery Matters 71: 14–17

Nesbitt A, Lynch M A 1992 African children in Britain. Archives of Disease in Childhood 67(11): 1402–1405

NHS handbook 1996 Services for black and minority ethnic people 1996/97, 11th edn. JMH Publishing, Tunbridge Wells, p 216–219

Nyatanga B 1997 Cultural issues in palliative care. International Journal of Palliative Nursing 3(4): 203–208

Omeri A 1997 Culture care of Iranian immigrants in New South Wales, Australia: sharing transcultural nursing knowledge. Journal of Transcultural Nursing 8(2): 5–16

Papadopoulos I, Alleyne J 1995 The need for nursing and midwifery programmes of education to address the health care needs of minority ethnic groups. Nurse Education Today 15(2): 140–144

Pelkonen M, Perälä M, Vehviläinen-Julkunen K 1998 Participation of expectant mothers in decision-making in maternity care: results of a population-based survey. Journal of Advanced Nursing 28(1): 21–29

Porter R 1998 Culture clubbed. Nursing Times 94(6): 34–35

Raleigh V S 1997 Diabetes and hypertension in Britain's ethnic minorities: implications for the future of renal services. British Medical Journal 314(7075): 209–213

Raleigh V S, Almond C, Kiri V 1998 Fertility and contraception among ethnic minority women in Great Britain. Health Trends 29(4): 109–113

Redmond E 1993 Reaching out to the Asian community. Community Outlook 3(7): 13–15

Report by the Standing Nursing and Midwifery Advisory Committee 1998 Midwifery: Delivery Our Future. Department of Health, London, p 12

Schott J, Henley A 1996a Ethnic monitoring: from paper to practice. British Journal of Midwifery 4(2): 61–62

Schott J, Henley A 1996b Meeting individual cultural and religious needs in a multicultural society. British Journal of Midwifery 4(6): 287–289

Scopesi A, Zanobini M, Carossino P 1997 Childbirth in different cultures: psychophysical reactions of women delivering in US, German, French and Italian hospitals. Journal of Reproductive and Infant Psychology. 15(1): 9–30

Sennott-Miller L 1994 Using theory to plan appropriate interventions: cancer prevention for older Hispanic and non-Hispanic white women. Journal of Advanced Nursing 20(5): 809–814

Shah S 1997 Preventing coronary heart disease among people of Asian origin. Health Visitor 70(2): 77–79

Shih F J 1996 Concepts related to Chinese patients' perceptions of health, illness and person: issues of conceptual clarity. Accident And Emergency Nursing 4(4): 208–215

Silveira E, Ebrahim S 1995 Mental health and health status of elderly Bengalis and Somalis in London. Age and Ageing 24(6): 474–480

Smith J W 1996 Cultural and spiritual issues in palliative care. Journal of Cancer Care 5(4): 173–178

Stolley J M, Koenig H 1997 Religion/Spirituality and health among elderly Africans and Hispanics. Journal of Psychosocial Nursing 35(11): 32–38

Stone M A, Patel H, Panja K K et al 1998 Reasons for non-compliance with screening for infection with *Helicobacter pylori* in a multi-ethnic community in Leicester UK. Public Health 112(3): 153–156

Stroebe M, Schut H 1998 Culture and grief. Bereavement Care 17(1): 7–10

Sullivan E J 1998 President's message on … differences what makes us different? Our skin color, our race, our gender. Reflections 24(2): 4

Tate C W 1996 All talk and no action. Nursing Management 3(5): 7

Teare P 1998 Culture shock. Nursing Times 94(27): 34–35

Thomas V, Dines A 1994 The health care needs of ethnic minority groups: are nurses and individuals playing their part? Journal of Advanced Nursing 20(5): 802–808

Tom-Orme L 1998 Waters running deep. Reflections 24(2): 22–23

Turner T 1997 Ethnicity and psychiatry. Practitioner 241(1579): 612–614

Vehvilainen K 1998 Wake up to Finnish nursing. Reflections 24(2): 28–29

Waters J 1996 Nurse vows to fight race law loophole. Nursing Times 92(4): 22

Webbe A 1998 Ethnicity and mental health. Psychiatric Care 5(1): 12–16

Webster R 1997 The experiences and health care needs of Asian coronary patients and their partners: methodological issues and preliminary findings. Nursing in Critical Care 2(5): 215–223

White G E 1995 Older women's attitudes to cervical screening and cervical cancer: a New Zealand experience. Journal of Advanced Nursing 21(4): 659–666

Wilkinson P 1998 Jail for parents who kidnapped their daughter. The Times, 6 June, p 3

Woollett A 1987 Who breastfeeds? The family and cultural context. Journal of Reproductive and Infant Psychology 5(3): 127–131

Woollett A 1990 Multiethnic issues in reproduction. Journal of Reproductive and Infant Psychology 8(4): 230–233

Yates M, Craddock E 1998 Culturally sensitive care in a forensic setting. Nursing Times 94(26): 68–69

Zambrana R E, Scrimshaw S M 1997 Maternal psychosocial factors associated with substance use in Mexican origin and African-Mexican low-income pregnant women. Pediatric Nursing 23(3): 253–259

FURTHER READING

Atri J, Falshaw M, Gregg R et al 1997 Improving uptake of breast screening in multi-ethnic populations: a randomised controlled trial using practice reception staff to contact non-attenders. British Medical Journal 315(7119): 1356–1359

Boyle D M 1998 The cultural context of dying from cancer. International Journal of Palliative Nursing 4(2): 70–83

Briggs L A 1998 Parents' viewpoint on reproductive health and contraceptive practice among sexually active adolescents in the Port Harcourt local government area of Rivers State, Nigeria. Journal of Advanced Nursing 27(2): 261–266

Egan K M, Newcomb P A, Longnecker M P et al 1996 Jewish religion and breast cancer. Lancet 347(9016): 1645–1646

Hewson B 1998 Discrimination and the maternity services. RCM Midwives Journal 1(7): 222–223

Kwast B E 1998 Quality of care in reproductive health programmes: concepts, assessments, barriers and improvements – an overview. Midwifery 14(2): 66–73

Position Paper 1998 Female genital mutilation and the role of the midwife. RCM Midwives Journal 1(7): 218–219

Shih F 1997 Perception of self in the intensive care unit after cardiac surgery among adult Taiwanese and American-Chinese patients. International Journal of Nursing Studies 34(1): 17–26

White C 1998 Giving contraceptive advice. Nursing Times 94(26): 70–71

Wright J 1996 Female genital mutilation: an overview. Journal of Advanced Nursing 24(2): 251–259

2

Organization and delivery of health and social care

In this section consideration is given to the mechanisms policy makers have in place to ensure that individuals in society receive health and social care. The making of policy is explored and its effects on specific social groups investigated. An awareness of the implications of social policy is essential, since it raises questions on issues concerned with the effectiveness of a mixed economy of care.

Introduction to social policy

Social policy and its nature are becoming increasingly the focus of study by students and academics concerned with social issues as they affect individuals in society. Further, the literature on the subject shows that social policy and policy-making do not simply pertain to politicians and their government, but the wider community as well. The characteristics of social policy, which this chapter addresses, indicate that professionals in health and social care practice have a role to play in developing their awareness of social policy issues that impinge on their practice. The aim of this chapter is threefold:

- to discuss the main features of social policy
- to explore the approaches readers can use to study it
- to indicate its relevance to professional practice.

SOCIOLOGY, PSYCHOLOGY AND SOCIAL POLICY

In the previous chapters we have seen how social phenomena can affect the person in society. We have discovered some issues that can threaten the very foundation of the social framework, e.g. the problems of domestic violence, child abuse, elder abuse, racism and discrimination. Although these social problems are topics for debate among sociologists, social policy makers are equally concerned with and involved in such matters.

One can therefore argue that, while social problems affect the functions of society, which is of concern to sociologists, the discipline of social policy cannot be discussed without making reference to sociological findings.

Just as important is the topic of human behaviour – the field of study that concerns psychologists. When social policy writers engage in their subject matter, there is an implicit assumption that social policy, although a distinct subject, is not related to psychology. We can find numerous examples in social life when human behaviour can sway a government and its policy makers. For example, in the summer of 1998, during the football World Cup, hooliganism abroad compelled the Prime Minister and his colleagues to think of strategies to curb this perennial social problem. When the Secretary of State's son was found guilty of illegal drug-taking, the motivation to counteract the problem became more focused. Also during 1998, the case of Steven Lawrence (a black youth murdered in London) aroused public attention to the extent of racism in Britain; the culture of policing, as well as the efficiency of law enforcers, came under close scrutiny. In relation to the nation's health, one finds that complaints about a failing health service pressurized the Health Minister and his team to allocate £500 million to the National Health Service (NHS) in early 1998, and a further £21 billion in the summer of the same year.

Many social issues have a psychological impact on people. For instance, as discussed in Section 1, domestic violence causes not only family breakdown but also mental breakdown. The aim of social policy is to tackle such problems, and to produce welfare reforms to meet needs as they arise.

When individuals in a society are subjected to various bio-psychosocial forces, their personal welfare needs require identification, assessment and provision to meet those needs. Where there is evidence that a person is in need of physical and/or mental health care, the Government has a responsibility to ensure that its *health policies* are adequate to deal with their health problems. To achieve this goal, health and social agencies have to be organized. In Britain, the NHS and the Social Services are considered to be the key components of health policy provision. The latter is said to be concerned with public health: protecting populations from ill-health and the provision of services to individuals (Allsop 1995) in need of health care. The health policy framework entails resource allocation, distribution, management of services and equity of access at the point of delivery. Klein (1995) asserted that health policy measures in regard to NHS resources are complex in nature, since issues of manpower, i.e skilled medical and nursing practitioners, are key features in health policy-making. Where there is a failure of policy (whether social or health), as in cases of increase in unemployment, poverty etc., one can expect an increase in bio-psychosocial ill-health.

Social policy should be considered as a system within other systems (Fig. 7.1). In addition its links with the sciences of sociology and psycho-

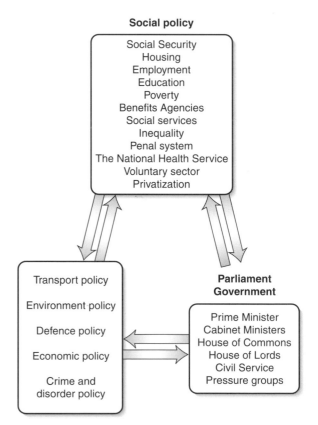

Fig. 7.1 Social policy as a system linked with other systems.

logy show us that it is the human factor that guides social policy. Policies are designed by people within the socio-political arena for all the people of a nation.

The effects of a government action (policy implementation) on its people must always be anticipated, as policies will be judged and assessed for their positive and negative consequences. For social sciences students, the study of social policy should be undertaken with these many dimensions in mind.

THE FEATURES OF SOCIAL POLICY

Various writers have attempted to define social policy. Its attributes are diverse, thus making a clear-cut definition harder. The word 'policy' itself has been interpreted in different ways. Levin (1997) listed the following:

1. policy as a stated intention
2. policy as a current or past action
3. policy as an organizational practice
4. policy as an indicator of the formal or claimed status of a past, present or proposed course of action.

The fluidity of the word 'policy' shows us that its interpretation must be examined within the context in which it is used. For instance, if one looks at the first definition in the list above, one has to identify *whose* intention it is to produce the policy. A Labour Government policy will be interpreted differently by people who support the Conservative party and vice versa, as the perceived implications will be judged differently.

The historical context of policy (current or past) also requires identification. Present policies may be outdated; they may require evaluation and changes made accordingly. On the other hand, a new social problem can drive policy makers to re-examine existing policies, as in July 1998, when Members of Parliament (MPs) called for tighter control in relation to child-minding after Helen Stacey was convicted of murdering the child in her care. A review of existing procedures was undertaken, and people campaigned for the introduction of national standards. A national scheme for registering child-minders was suggested and

the National Child-minding Association called for child-minding training standards as well as standardized and constant police surveillance.

Levin (1997) saw 'policy' as organizational practice in the framework of 'ways in which things are customarily done'. This refers to known practices, e.g. policies to tackle crime, manage the NHS, create jobs and provide education. Practices may, however, be challenged by pressure groups. For example, arranged marriages are common among some Asian communities, but there have been reports (Boggan & Popham 1998) of women being coerced into marriages at home and abroad. This has prompted some women's groups (Southall Black Sisters, Keighley Women's Domestic Violence Forum) to pressurize the Government into allocating finances and to considering the effects of 'forced marriages' on women. Ministers in Parliament may also pressurize government into implementing changes; in particular, MPs in local areas may support their constituents in speeding up changes.

In regard to the statement 'formal or claimed status of a past, present or proposed course of action', the implicit message is that the *Government* is not to be swayed because the policy has been given priority and must therefore be adhered to. During 1998, for example, Gordon Brown, the Labour Chancellor of the Exchequer, repeatedly asserted his position in connection with his monetary policy, aimed at controlling 'boom and bust', despite criticisms of increased interest rates.

In addition to the above, 'policy' may be linked to a government's mission statement and its philosophy. A government's political manifestos in many ways are implicit representations of its philosophy, which will be reflected in future policy implementation.

The term 'policy' can also be attributed to the legal documentation detailing the measures to be executed, including the distribution of responsibilities and the role description of statutory bodies. Moreover, when the Prime Minister and his Cabinet Ministers use the word 'policy' they are re-emphasizing their position as leaders of a political system, as elected by the people, promoting their beliefs that their decisions are the best way forward.

On the other hand, an opposition Party is always ready to disparage the policy(ies) of a Party in power. The adversarial stance of the British political system shows how 'policy' or 'policies' can be used as tools to score points, and to depreciate a Government. Further, one has to be aware of 'policy' as a social-psychological stratagem to influence the electorate and to win votes. The Labour Government – when in opposition – criticized privatization. Once in power, however, Labour was seen to adopt some principles of privatization; for example, by combining private and public 'policy' initiatives, which some critics have argued is *conservative* 'policy' (with a small 'c'). Social policy is to do with initiatives from the Government to meet the welfare needs of its citizens, by providing services (e.g. housing, education, the Health Services etc.) (Ackers & Fordham 1995); social policy necessitates using 'statutory instruments' (Levin 1997) to enforce the decision-making process, thus finalizing the policy-making initiative. This is an action-oriented mechanism to attain specific goals; for example, to control the economy, elevate educational standards, modernize the Health Service, and reduce crime and disorder. Social policy also applies to the complex machinery of the political and administrative context (Moore 1993) which develops proposed initiatives.

Social policy is synonymous with welfare and policy. However, policy – intended, designed and implemented – has to be evaluated. In other words, questions must be asked to find out the effects of policy on consumers/users. Is the health care system malfunctioning? Are lone parents more disadvantaged than couple families? Should the Child Support Agency be re-organized? To what extent is there equalization of opportunities, in regard to disability rights and racial equality?

Social policy affects society as a whole – from the individual to the entire population (Mayston 1996). There is the argument, however, that 'political fervour' generates policies in the absence of clear scientific inquiry. In Section 1, the fact was discussed that despite the Children Act of 1989, evidence shows that children remain a disadvantaged group in society. The Sex Discrimination Act (1975) only receives lip service; inequality of the sexes still prevails. At the time of writing, observers of employment equality argue that, despite the minority of men in the NHS, they are more likely to be promoted to higher posts than their female counterparts. Although Race Discrimination Act has been in place since 1976, racism and discrimination still exist in many spheres of social life. Successive governments have only skimmed the surface of the deep-rooted social problems encountered by minority ethnic groups (Atkin 1996). In addition, one finds that NHS reforms from the 1980s onward have been criticized for deepening health inequalities. Dyson (1999) observed that health policies on genetic screening for haemoglobin disorders – among ethnic minorities – are flawed, due to unclear criteria in the sensitive assessment of what constitutes 'ethnicity'.

In July 1998, the Deputy Prime Minister announced the Government's White Paper to revolutionize the transport system. As a political manoeuvre, it was applauded by environmentalists and pressure groups. Commuters, however, argued that the application of theory to practice will prove challenging, as many practical issues have not been carefully analysed and researched. These examples show that policies, although legislated, have not been subjected to scientific scrutiny. In fact, some critics (Stepney et al 1999), in relation to poverty and exclusion, have argued that the Government policy is drawn from 'discourses' and debates rather than statistical research findings.

Social policy is concerned not only with national welfare but international welfare as well. For example, the emission of radioactive wastes not only affects people and the coastal areas around nuclear power stations but other nations' coasts as well. The Danish Environment Minister, in a Radio 4 interview in 1998, drew attention to the effects of spillage from the Sellafield power station in Britain on Norwegian fishing industries. While nuclear power stations provide employment to many, their long-term consequences on people, nationally and internationally, have not been anticipated.

In 1998, British society saw several successive increased bank lending rates in line with the Bank of England policy to control consumer spending and to restrain inflation. These policy decisions have national and international economic implications. Critics were quick to point out that the strong Pound was curbing exports, as buyers abroad could not afford British products. In Britain, industrialists and economic analysts point to industries facing job losses, reduced production and recession.

Social policy must, therefore, be analysed by considering it from both a micro and macro perspective, i.e. nationally and globally. Hill (1997) argued that social policy is 'interconnected' with 'economic policies'; he refers to this aspect as the 'redistributive' elements in economic terms. For example, one should consider how £3.5 billion, which the Labour Government wants to spend on housing, will alleviate the problems of social exclusion. The redistributive functions in relation to this sum of money require assessing. One can also argue to what extent will a new education policy help to develop the economy of a country. Similarly, while a new transport policy may help reduce pollution, economists will question its economic implications.

Social policy is a bureaucratic process. The implementation of policy is seen to be *bureaucratic* in nature, compared with the *democratic* policy-making aspect of the State (Alcock 1996). Legislation must be adhered to. Control is exercised in many areas of policy implementation. For example, the arm of the law extends to voluntary charitable organizations, specifying their roles, functions and relationships with statutory organizations. Equally, social security claimants are subjected to clearly defined guidelines regarding their eligibility to claim benefits.

Benefits provision has always been judged to be the hallmark of welfare policy. It should, however, be remembered that welfare philosophy finds its origin from Fabianism. Fabians (i.e. its founders, who were Bernard Shaw, Beatrice Webb and others) believed in State intervention to counteract social problems. Their writings, based on socialist ideas, have been influential in shaping the ethos of State Welfare. Welfare policy has, nonetheless, undergone many changes since its inception in response to social change. As it happens, individual responsibility is now encouraged in many spheres of social life. We find, for example, that individuals are instigated to make private pension provision for their retirement; in the health field, private health insurance is now becoming more common; home ownership is another concept that is now widely acknowledged.

Social policy is related to political sociology. Social change and new social pressures can instigate a government to implement policy changes. It is a two-way process (Bilton et al 1996); radical changes require cooperation of key ministers, civil servants, pressure groups etc., before policies can be finalized. Failure to seek approval could jeopardize a government ethos of democratic decision-making.

To conclude, social policy is not just a government-oriented action. There are consequences and issues that accompany any political decision. Social policy is a socio-political process, and is considered to be an eclectic field (David & Groves 1995). In other words, it vacillates across other academic disciplines (e.g. social economics, sociology, psychology etc.). David and Groves argued that it is in many ways an interdisciplinary subject. One should, however, be conscious of the fact that social policies develop within not only a national framework, but also an international one. The many features of policy contribute in making it a subject students of social policy may find very complex.

STUDYING SOCIAL POLICY

A rich source of approaches is at the disposal of the reader or student of social policy. The diversity of the subject means that the reader may choose to focus on the policy-making machinery of government. Alternatively, one may consider the implementation of policies and their evaluation. For example, the Benefits Agency, which is an area familiar to many social policy students, could be studied in relation to its functional nature in tackling income inequalities. On the other hand, the focus could be on comparing and contrasting successive governments' attitude to specific areas of social policy. This may entail a review of their philosophy, methods of grappling with social and economic problems, priorities and their relationships with the civil service and pressure groups.

It is equally important to encompass in one's study the 'welfare dynamics'. Welfare dynamics refer to the on-going social change and personal circumstances of an individual over a period of time. This may be illustrated by exploring how a specific group can be 'welfare dependent' over time. Noble et al (1998) made evident the 'dependency culture' of British lone parents. Their research findings show how lone parents – subject to changes in personal circumstances – can move in and out of their welfare dependency states: a new, stable relationship will affect their benefits dependence. The effect is that some lone parents may no longer be eligible for state support. Alternatively, they may only require partial income support.

The term 'welfare dynamics' can also be applied to the process of government decision-making as it faces fluctuations in the economy, life pressures and reactions of the electorate at large, and its influences in stimulating change.

A comparative approach can also be used in studying social policy. Noble et al (1998) compared British lone parent claimants with those in the USA. By extending one's method of studying social policy – in a transcultural way – one is able to be more critical of how social policy is being managed. Social policy provides insights into other governments' methods of dealing with similar social economic problems, and encourages a forum for critical evaluations of one's own policy strategies.

It has been argued (Deakin 1993) that cross-fertilization of ideas is beneficial to a country. Deakin made particular reference to the idea of 'policy-making process' as a comparative dimension. He provides examples of how lessons can be learned not only from the USA, but from the experiences gained in the rest of Europe. One may, for example, compare implementation of crime and disorder control policies between Britain, France and Holland. However, students of social policy should be aware that the adoption of foreign policy initiatives is not always possible; adaptation, nevertheless, could be an alternative option. On the other hand, ethnocentric beliefs could impede the implementation of certain foreign policy measures.

Policy studies can also be done by investigating issues concerned with social identity. In Section 1 the concepts of ethnicity, race and cultural variations and how they create a sense of belonging and group identity were discussed. Of relevance to social policy makers and social policy is the extent to which the latter has a role 'in the process of identity formation' (Taylor 1998). This approach shows a different facet to the standard 'welfare provision' and 'benefits oriented' ethos of social policy. Taylor suggests that social policy debates within the political arena often centre on identified communities; i.e. groups with specific identities, demanding welfare support, such as lone parents or the gay community.

To receive benefits entitlements, groups with 'different identities' have to persuade social and health agencies that denying them a 'fair redistribution of resources' is a demonstration of injustice and inequality. In 1998, the Prime Minister and his Cabinet had to rethink their policy of curbing lone parent benefits because of the strong feelings of injustice it stimulated.

The perspective of re-looking at social policy, Taylor pointed out, helps to compare:

1. the practical aspects of social policy (i.e. policy as provision)
2. the 'social' aspects of policy (i.e. insight into the social position of individuals in society, their circumstances, the level of inequalities they experience and their relationships with the welfare state.

The welfare state can perpetuate 'group identities'; i.e. by confirming that 'lone mothers' are perennial users of welfare benefits system. The research by Noble et al (1998) contradicts this argument.

The realism of social policy implementation is a field worthy of study. Any shortcoming or inadequacy can be assessed. Section 1 highlighted the many informal carers in the community; however, although the NHS and Community Care Act (1990) does make reference to informal carers, one finds that policies do not reflect the real constraints, pressures and personal difficulties affecting service providers, informal carers and the cared-for person.

Twigg and Atkin (1995) explored the factors that cause providers of service to fail in assessing and meeting needs positively. Additionally, the authors discovered that the characteristics of carers, the person cared for and the wider kin network can all have a part in either 'blocking' implementation of services, or seeking professional help as required. For example, some carers believe it their duty to support their disabled relatives without seeking professional help. It was found that some cared-for individuals would go to great lengths to hide the true nature of their illnesses from their carers to avoid social care agency intervention.

Other factors relate to issues of gender, race and age. Care provision may not be aggressive if it is found that the carers are female, but male carers are better able to make use of services (Twigg & Atkin 1995). With reference to age, younger carers believed that service providers are more inclined to support older carers. Race issues are connected with the inaccessibility and unsuitability of some community service provision for black people. Studies could be conducted to investigate how discrimination and racism are being combatted. Of particular importance and relevance is the investigation of how European social policy guidelines translate into action. It is argued (Royal College of Nursing 1998) that the issue of race and other forms of discrimination should be reflected in the new European Treaty (the Amsterdam Treaty). As ethnic groups are likely to work and live in European countries, their protection against race discrimination has been proposed by the European Commission's new social programme.

These issues clearly show the complexity of the policy process. To gain better awareness of the process, social policy should be studied not only theoretically but at a critical and pragmatic level. Some authors have even suggested researching the policy process (Pollitt et al 1990). This entails using an ethnographic approach, similar to anthropologists' methods of study. However, one must be aware that Government departments may not be willing to expose their procedures to analytical scrutiny by independent researchers. Pollitt et al (1990) raised awareness of resistance met by scholarly investigators of 'sensitive policy issues'. In Britain, Meerabeau (1996) explained, policy makers and practitioners need to be persuaded of the benefits of research. She argued that policy makers in the USA are more open to research and that they have an impressive record of research material related to health services. While the nursing and medical literature in Britain show that evidence-based practice should be the norm, Government departments and their policy-making machinery could be studied to evaluate the level of evidence-based policy development.

??? Question 7.1

1. What are the implications of allowing independent researchers to research the Government's policy process?
2. How can social scientists and students of social policy use other disciplines to complement their work?

Studying the interdisciplinary nature of social policy

Can social policy be studied without a knowledge of sociology? Although many will argue that it can be done, a study of social policy without the integration of sociology in its framework will border on superficiality. A failure to link and understand the complex and dynamic processes of human conditions will only prevent one from contextualizing social policy.

Bilton et al (1996) have written that the discipline of sociology aims at making us aware of people as social beings, stimulating us to question what we take for granted. As discussed in Section 1, functionalists perceive societies as social systems with specific functions: to maintain social homeostasis, to prevent disorganization and disequilibrium, to control deviancy and so on. To attain these goals, group leaders in society have to devise policies to help manage more efficiently human and material resources. Since a society is not problem-free, decisions are required to tackle social problems as they arise. The aim of social policy is hence to control and prevent socio-economic and health problems, and to make society a more comfortable place by attending to needs.

Social problems are varied: homelessness, unemployment, racism, discrimination and poverty are some examples. A social problem can also develop into a health problem (Case example 7.1). Conversely, a health problem can undermine one's social health. Sickness can cause social isolation, disrupting interpersonal relationships and fragmenting valuable social networks.

Case example 7.1 The homeless person

Many homeless people in Britain spend their days and nights on the streets seeking shelters. Many live in cardboard boxes. Others, however, may be seen huddled on the floor by the front entrance of a shop.

Robert, aged 35, has been homeless for the past five years. He has chronic bronchitis and he suffers from malnutrition. In addition he is exposed to violence from other vagrants: he was assaulted one night as he entered a disused building to settle for the night.

Health problems that concern not only the individual but the Department of Health, e.g. outbreaks of *E. coli* poisoning, can instigate Ministers into developing research strategies to help tackle the problems. In these instances, current legislation needs to be re-examined and social policies designed to confront issues.

Wellard (1998) explained how a government initiative to deal with problems of homelessness will reduce mental health and drug/alcohol problems. Policies to develop the role of local authorities in coordinating interventions are hence necessary. In addition, Wellard points out the intention of the Government to set up a new body for London, headed by a 'streets tsar' who

will manage finances allocated and who will help to control the number of rough sleepers.

In the above example, the way in which social problems trigger reactions and action within a community, instigating statutory bodies to promote health initiatives, is discussed. On the other hand, students of social policy may wish to investigate the nature of sociological issues and how local government formulates local policies (within the directives of central government) to meet needs at a grassroots level. Additionally, the role of voluntary services can be explored and their relationships with statutory services analysed.

The social context of social policy can be a complex field of study. Social stability is dependent on sound policies and it is important to prevent implementation failures.

A critical approach to social policy is another avenue of research to consider: one could focus on the perennial issue of children in care services and how the state of services is constantly being deplored for a 'catalogue of mistakes, mismanagement and downright incompetence' (Hunter 1998) (Boxes 7.1 and 7.2).

Box 7.1 Policy implementation failures in society

'In London, Hackney Council was heavily criticised by the SSI (Social Services Inspectorate) for its staff vetting procedures, its lack of a central record for unallocated children and inadequate care plans' (Hunter 1998). Other councils show a lack of sound selection procedures, inadequate record-keeping and lack of contact with children in care. Vulnerable children do not always receive services tailored to needs. Others are found to be accommodated in bed-and-breakfast that has not been designed to meet their special needs.

Boxes 7.1 and 7.2 show some pertinent sociological issues, as well as the extent of social problems confronting policy makers. Using a sociological perspective one can note that:

1. social order is threatened
2. there is a lack of integration between agencies concerned in implementing policies
3. there are differences in values: deviant subculture values and the values of policy makers (the former can be the child abusers,

Box 7.2 Avalanche of negative reports

Concerns are expressed regarding the integrity of the British child care system. Reports from the National Children's Bureau residential care unit identify a lack of insight into how the service works. A lack of strategic planning by managers of services, who are reactive rather than proactive, is one of a series of factors, which explains loopholes in the system.

Rickford (1998) lists a succession of policy implementation failures that sustain society's problems of managing the needs of young people:

1. delayed annual report on the Children Act (1989) by the Department of Health
2. 75% of children in care do not meet educational standards
3. lack of care continuity, which induces failure in diagnosing chronic health conditions (e.g. eyesight, hearing problems)
4. high prevalence of mental health problems among young people in care
5. long waiting periods for an appointment with a psychiatrist.

the latter formulate policies for law enforcers).

There are other examples in social life proving the interconnections between sociology and social policy. Haralambos and Holborn (1995) point out that government policies 'have always had an impact on family life':

- monetary policies can affect many families who have mortgages
- education policies that reduce bursaries and grants could mean more families having to contribute financially to their child's education
- policies that concern employment (e.g. encouraging more women to work) have implications for child care.

Haralambos and Holborn argued that single parent benefits have contributed to the elevation in taxation. The implication is that 'many wives with young children are forced to take paid employment to make ends meet'.

In the health sector, some policies aimed at controlling expenditure can constrain strategies to combat health inequalities:

- reduced access to services in some deprived inner city areas
- increased crime rates

- homelessness
- drug misuse.

Burgess (1996) believed that social policy principles are based within a broad framework, encompassing *culture*, the *environment*, the *economy* and *health*.

Freeman (1996) further illustrated the interrelationship between sociology and social policy. He wrote that policy makers may misperceive the reality as experienced by families and community; i.e. that political definitions of self-sufficiency will have an impact on policy-making, which the community will ultimately experience. Policies may subsequently enable or disable a person's social condition. To achieve social justice, new research and policy agendas, in order to integrate policy development into clinical and community practice, are prerequisites.

On the whole, government social policy agendas reflect an awareness of how a socio-economically disadvantaged environment can affect health; e.g. when the Secretary of State for Health remarks that 'poverty, poor housing, low wages, unemployment, air pollution, crime and disorder can all make people ill in both body and mind' (Kingman 1998).

While the study of sociology broadens the context of social issues facing communities, the study of social policy with its sociological underpinnings exposes the deep socio-political and economic issues as they concern whole communities at various levels of society. Peillon (1998) makes reference to a 'sociology of welfare'; the notion that social forces drive the welfare system. Further, there are interactions between agencies and their clients. In addition, Peillon argued that such interactions between 'social policy agencies' and the people they serve have not been researched in 'any depth'. As society develops, social needs increase and social problems intensify. Policy makers have to refine their policy-making machinery in line with social change. For students of social policy, the integration of other disciplines – by using an eclectic approach – opens the way to a better understanding of key factors as they affect not only the individual in society, but major corporations. One should

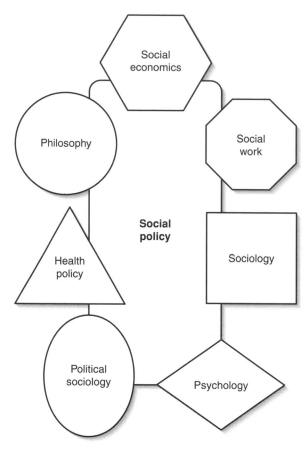

Fig. 7.2 Interdisciplinary nature of social policy.

Activity 7.1

1. Talk to your local MP. How are local social issues dealt with? To what extent do social policy initiatives reflect local demands (e.g. safety needs, crime rate reduction, homelessness, domestic violence, poverty, employment)?
2. Write down a list of sociological issues that students of social policy have to consider.
3. Prepare a timetable containing some key issues currently being discussed by politicians. Note the days/months when these issues are raised. Compare the perspectives of the political parties. Write down the measures suggested to tackle such issues. Six months later compare and contrast the arguments raised on similar issues. Note any changes. Now discuss in small groups the content of these social issues and how successfully the problems have been solved.

??? **Question 7.2**

1. It is argued that sociology cannot be separated from social policy. What do you consider to be the reasons for this argument?
2. Do you agree that social policy concerns every individual in society and not just the government?
3. There are many forces in society that help shape social policy. Can you name them?
4. Do you think that social policies have their limitations in eradicating some social problems?
5. What approaches should students of social policy develop when situating the context of social policy?
6. Is social policy purely a political and academic subject?
7. In what ways can a knowledge of social policy help social and health care professionals to undertake their functions?

therefore be flexible enough to utilize a model that encompasses some pivotal disciplines as they relate to the study of social policy (Fig. 7.2). Of relevance too, is the utilization of a case study approach, with interviews and group discussions. One may select case stories from real life, which describe the positive as well as the negative consequences of social policy initiatives. Social issues can thereafter be examined in depth by comparing and contrasting past experiences with new welfare developments.

SOCIAL WORK AND SOCIAL POLICY

The relationships between social work and social policy have over the years been intensely scrutinized, possibly due to the enduring debates that social services, social workers and the nature of social work are continually accused of poor performance. Their practice frequently makes headlines. In 1998 a new White Paper, which enshrined 'Best Value', aimed to make it the duty of councils 'to promote the well-being of communities' (Community Care 1998a). The same journal reported how some social services failed to support a mother and her son escaping domestic violence. This case reinforced the attitude that the child care system provides sub-standard services (Hunter 1998).

While the translation of policies into practice is a complex process, the study of policy can be approached by investigating the nature of social work, the constraints service providers experience and how social policy can impact on practice. This entails a critical evaluation of social policy, to assess how its formulation and implementation are congruent with social reality.

Despite a plethora of literature on ethnicity, race and multiculturalism, evidence still shows that social services and social work practice do not reflect multicultural sensitivity. Weaver (1998) asserted that indigenous groups in a multicultural society present unique social and health issues for human services. What are the issues which concern ethnic groups so that they do not access services? What prevents social work practitioners from implementing social policy initiatives? Should research be done to elucidate the obstacles preventing policy implementation, *before* policy making? The possibility that research findings in social work can influence practice and policy is acknowledged (Bradley 1997). Further, scientific analysis and evaluation of social care outcomes remain underdeveloped. There are situations that prompt quick changes in policy and become legislation. Stanley and Manthorpe (1997) made reference to 'tragedies' relating to mentally ill individuals and the wider community that produced the implementation of the Mental Health (Patients in the Community) Act 1995. Although it is argued (Dziegielewski 1998) that it is a 'social work tradition' to help clients achieve optimal levels of health functioning, evidence shows that policy and social work practice can be incongruent.

An empirical study (Colton et al 1997) to assess the extent of stigma-producing services, showed that the climate under which social services providers operate can reinforce the power of stigma. The latter, the researchers argued, still carries the negative connotations that have always been attached to the characteristics of service users, service providers and the fashion in which service providers interact with families, and the type of action service providers take. Several of Colton et al's findings (Box 7.3), with implications for policy and the practice of social work, are discussed.

It is evident from the findings described in

Box 7.3 Social work and stigma

Stigmatized services have been an issue since Elizabethan times. It is a topic which in many ways concerns contemporary service users. Social workers are conscious that their presence can exert negative reactions from some users of services.

Social workers can feel stigmatized because of the nature of their work, i.e. contact with the socially excluded in society; drug users, abusers of children, petty criminals, delinquents, the homeless, the unemployed etc. Sometimes 'particular services may be organized and delivered' with the aim to increase feelings of embarrassment 'or shame which amount to stigma'. If service providers' attitudes convey the implicit message that the poor, unemployed and homeless are not deserving of social support, this may explain why policy directives can be difficult to implement. In addition, contemporary practice can show that the malpractice evident during the 'Poor Law' periods has not been totally eradicated.

Colton et al (1997) discovered that users of services felt less stigma attached to health-related services, whereas social problems (disturbed family situations, domestic violence, behavioural problems, delinquency) were perceived to be more stigmatized. Seeking the help of social workers and establishing contact with probation officers mean exposure to a stigma-prone organization; this is a stereotypical view shared by social workers themselves, who consider their work to carry a stigma. Both providers and users expressed the view that the public holds a negative perception of those who are in need of foster care and residential care. When asked about the integrity of the services they provide, providers pointed out the following:

1. access to services and benefits is not easy
2. material help and money provision can be hard to obtain
3. service provision does not match government rhetoric
4. services are under-resourced
5. less than 10% of workers in the study feel that the services they provide are non-stigmatizing
6. 75% agreed that child and family services have a stigmatizing effect on recipients. This may be due to the beliefs and experiences of people that social workers' traditional role has been to remove children from their homes and place them in statutory care
7. local authority uses deterrence to reduce the number of claimants of services
8. stigma helps the process by 'discouraging dependency'.

Box 7.3 which factors can lead to policy failure. Perhaps students of social policy should analyse 'policy implementation', implementation failures and successes, as well as a critical evaluation of how and why centrally designed policies could fail in practice. As suggested already, researching

the policy process could help minimize implementation failures. Colton et al (1997) discovered
that government action in relation to policies is
not perceived by service providers to be caring.
The bureaucratic nature of policy-making and
service provision could be blamed. Nevertheless
one should also consider the attitudes, beliefs
and experiences of social service providers
toward social policy and its implementation; the
views of users are equally relevant. For Corrigan
and Bishop (1997), children and families are
at the hub of contemporary society. They suggest
that the nature of 'family-centred, community-
based, integrated service systems' make it
imperative to utilize family participation, in the
training of a 'new generation of interprofession-
ally oriented service providers in education,
social work and health'. Their collaboration
and contribution can become an integral feature
of professional leadership. Additionally, service
providers' participation in decision-making could
help combat the stigma attached to statutory
provision of social support.

Attempts to combat learned helplessness, which
an under-resourced work setting can promote, is
an issue to consider. Latting and Blanchard
(1997) suggested ways to empower staff and to
develop 'visionary goal setting', thus contributing to the prevention of institutionalized
oppression. Similarly, Cohen and Austin (1997)
explained that the empowerment of social workers
in the workplace is in need of attention to meet
the challenges human services organizations are
facing.

Social work and the practice of implementation can perhaps be boosted in a positive way by
the application of a 'communitarian philosophy'
(Boettcher 1997) when working with families
and communities; the latter have empowerment
needs too. Social policy, however, may have a
constraining effect on communities' freedom to
empower themselves. Freeman (1996) postulates
that the family and community 'self-sufficiency'
can be misunderstood due to policy makers'
'biased definitions of self-sufficiency'. To prevent
unnecessary barriers being erected, which
discourage self-empowerment, Freeman argued
that several measures can be taken:

1. Social workers to exert influence on policy-
   making by sharpening their insight into the
   'world views' and 'values' internalized by
   politicians.
2. Community research to identify support
   needs.
3. Re-evaluation of social work practice and
   education to empower service providers so
   that they can have a stronger influence on
   social policy.
4. New research and policy initiatives to attain
   social justice goal, and to apply policy
   measures to clinical and community practice.

In addition to the above, evaluation of social
work practice should include a critical analysis
of traditional approaches in interpreting clients'
social needs and problems. The methods of social
policy development, Chapin (1995) explained,
have been inclined to be 'problem-focused' and
'pathology-oriented'. Chapin emphasized the
need to concentrate on the *positive* characteristics
of the individual; in other words, focus should be
on the 'strengths perspective'. This methodology
has the advantage of identifying and mobilizing
people's strengths and resources and what their
environment can offer. The helping ethos and
credibility of social work can thus be preserved.
In addition, Chapin asserted that social policy
development can be positively maximized in the
process. Thus new 'tools' can be developed to
interpret social needs and problems, aiming to
potentiate individuals toward self-empowerment.

SOCIAL ECONOMICS AND SOCIAL POLICY

Social economists are concerned with social
issues and problems as they affect individuals in
society (Box 7.4). The relationship between social
economics and social policy is inextricable. Social
economics issues as described in Box 7.4 cannot
be extruded from social policy-making and
implementation. For students of social policy,
social economics provides another area of fruitful
investigation into the social issues social policy
makers grapple with, while simultaneously
balancing the economic implications their public
policies might generate.

Box 7.4 Social economics

As far back as the early 1980s social economists were debating the nature of social economics which, McKee (1984) argued, encompasses the 'social areas of economic enquiry while incorporating humanistic values'. The emphasis is also placed on the role of community forces (social groups) which relate to the economy. Thus, McCain (1984) focused his argument on the 'human individual' as much unlike a robot, but a creature with feelings and 'creativity'. The value of the individual is hence at the hub of social economics.

When one refers to poverty, homelessness, unemployment, domestic violence and cases of abuse, the economics of social deprivation – as they concern the disadvantaged groups in society – become the affairs of governments and policy makers who aim to promote welfare rights.

The field of social economics not only raises our awareness of socio-economic issues, but explains how such problems impinge on the economic infrastructure of a society. When the Labour Government announced in 1998 its strategy to boost education, health and welfare by allocating £57 billion to its New Deal for Communities programme, it was not only a political decision, but a social economics one too. For example, the poor need social support; the Inland Revenue has to use its taxation system to support benefits agencies. The homeless rely on local authorities and private agencies to provide housing, and the unemployed rely on social security systems to meet their financial needs. Cases of community violence and abuse in homes impinge on the scarce resources available in community and hospital settings. Fair redistribution of social and health care resources can be a difficult goal to attain.

The Amsterdam Declaration was signed on 10 June 1997. Walker (1998) explained that the aim was to 'remind' communities in Europe (citizens, politicians, social scientists, social economists, policy makers etc.) that the Western European model of development is a unique feature. The argument given is that its philosophy consists of several features:

- economic growth
- competitiveness
- social justice.

It aims to improve the quality of life of its citizens. The concept of social equality is promoted. To achieve this objective, it is asserted that citizens should have the freedom to participate in the 'social and economic life of their communities'. However, conditions must be created for them to self-actualize, by developing their potential.

Social quality, however, Walker argued, is reliant on some key components:

- economic security
- the degree of social inclusion
- social cohesion/solidarity
- autonomy and empowerment.

The Amsterdam Declaration was making allusion to those groups in society who are in a position of inequality and are socio-economically disadvantaged. Poverty in Britain and the rest of Europe and the world runs parallel with social, economic and political implications. Social pressures are also caused when the market economy fails to satisfy the housing and employment needs of others. When social policies fail to meet their objectives, one finds that issues connected with social and health care can be compounded. People with low socio-economic status are more prone to ill-health; where community health systems are under-resourced the problems can be exacerbated.

In the late 1990s one finds that, as a result of social change and development in Europe the effects of social economics on the lives of citizens are receiving higher recognition. Although present policies aim to counteract social exclusion, critics argue that the socio-economically disadvantaged remain excluded.

The inclination to link social services with the traditional concept of care provision is now being scrutinized in regard to its relevance to *social action* (Box 7.5).

Box 7.5 Social action

Although the term 'social action' includes measures taken by statutory departments to meet the needs of citizens, the Portuguese (Madeira 1998) interpret the concept to include action that purposefully aims to increase social inclusion; services aiming to improve quality of life are therefore included. Also, initiatives to develop programmes and projects, which concern the well-being of families, groups and organizations are considered to be 'social action-oriented'.

The social and economic needs of groups (children, the aged, individuals with learning disabilities or mental ill-health etc.) are assessed, and policies at a local and national level (based on European principles) are formulated. Social protection becomes the focus of social action: protecting the vulnerable in society, by encouraging active participation of society's members.

In Britain, service providers are now referred to as *enablers*, or facilitators (Wistow et al 1996). Their objectives are nonetheless similar to the Portuguese and other European communities: to address social exclusion. One finds in Britain, for example, the social economics of policies which consist of Communities Regeneration. The Labour Government announced in July 1998 their objective to confront social deprivation on some of the worst estates in the country. Their New Deal for Communities Programme was allocated £800 million. While financial injection to counteract the negative life circumstances of being socially excluded is commended with the goal to 'enable local groups in deprived areas to play a fuller part in society' (Holman 1998), lack of resources have constrained development in this area. Holman cited Scotland as an example where the Social Exclusion Network is failing in its role to improve inclusion (Box 7.6).

Box 7.6 A failing social exclusion network

'In practice though, the network is timid rather than bold. It has no resources and concentrates on better coordination of existing programmes; it specifies no figures as to how many people will be taken out of poverty; it has no plans to fund locally controlled projects; its decision-making membership is confined to civil servants and representatives of the Benefits Agency, with Lord Sewell as its chairperson' (Holman 1998).

Holman wrote that membership of these committees are exclusive, while the *socially excluded* are not included in the decision-making processes that affect their lives. Constraints on resources (financial and human) can minimize the life chances of the socially deprived. Policies on expenditure and the ideal of combatting social inequalities can be conflictual: a dilemma facing a government that wants 'a major assault on social exclusion – and a tight control on public expenditure' (Fletcher 1998). Social economists may argue that the 'redistributive' function of the welfare state does not match the rhetoric of social policies. The role of market economics in swaying policy implementation designed to confront social problems is not to be underestimated. The

inclusion of a social economics perspective in the debate on the nature of social policy permits social policy students to explore complex social issues and how they relate to the economics of policies.

Students may be interested in the socio-economic issues of European migration, and the responses of policy makers to the problems. While some may argue that migrants can cause negative consequences in the labour market (e.g. reducing the employment chances of the indigenous population), Zimmermann (1995) pointed out that immigration 'may help erode institutional constraints' by increasing competitiveness in the employment market. Immigrants can contribute to economic growth. Policy makers nonetheless have to be sensitive to the socio-economic implications of immigration:

- strains on an already constrained housing market
- misappropriation of social security funds
- issues of citizenships and voting rights
- the perennial problems of racism and discrimination, which have legal and economic repercussions.

The study of social policy and social economics can also include some other perspectives (Box 7.7).

Box 7.7 Study options: social experimentation

Social experimentation refers to randomized field trials with the aim of obtaining data on the effectiveness of programmes. Burtless (1995) sees this research tool as a strategy to influence policy-making by informing policy makers on issues affecting human behaviour, so that they are better informed on 'policy effectiveness'. Linton (1998), on the other hand, pointed out that the application of research findings in policy-making is an underdeveloped area. Thus the utilization of social scientists' research reports by politicians (Ware 1998) to refine socio-economic decisions and policy-making processes is a field that requires scrutiny.

FEMINISM AND SOCIAL POLICY

Feminists have explored social issues concerning the effects of social policy in marginalizing the role of women in society. According to feminist writers, many women are socio-economically disadvantaged. Two studies (Glendinning & Millar 1991, Millar & Glendinning 1992) have referred to the invisibility of women's poverty in Britain. Their arguments are founded on the belief that there is a failure to acknowledge how gender can be related to poverty. Women in society are stereotyped, and assumptions are made that most women *share* the financial position of the men they live with, but it is known that women who are married or living with partners experience poverty. Other issues concern the inadequacy of policy in ensuring women's accessibility to employment, family and leisure activities (Beuret 1991). The impact of unemployment on women (Callender 1992) does not receive similar attention compared with men.

In addition, these problematic social issues are compounded when sensitive and pervasive problems such as racism and ethnic minorities groups are combined. Social policies in this context may not be a true reflection of the negative life experiences of women that belong to differing statuses (i.e. lone parents, cohabitees, single, married, non-heterosexual relationships). Feminists will hence add to their arguments that women's 'maternal identity' is *oppressive* to them, in the home and in the employment market (Lawler 1996).

SOCIAL EXCLUSION AND MENTAL HEALTH

In 1997 the British Government set up the Social Exclusion Unit. Its objective is to promote social inclusion and to consider the needs of those who are socially disadvantaged. It is contended, however, that Government policy and service delivery are incongruent with the needs of those individuals who are mentally ill (White 1998). Policy implementation, according to White, lacks sensitivity while failing to recognize the 'stigma and issues' mentally ill people have to encounter daily. Moreover, Sayce (1998) professed that the goal should be to challenge and combat discrimination, which in combination with exclusion disempower the individual with mental ill-health. She stated that an agenda of 'policy development

and advocacy' is needed. Community workers, clients and informal carers can unite with pressure groups to influence policy initiatives in government. Further, policy development should take into account local strategies to help homeless children and families with mental health problems to secure safe accommodation and social support (Vostanis et al 1998). Issues concerning long-term support to prevent increasing isolation caused by mental ill-health (Quilgars 1998) should also be on the policy agenda. Social exclusion concerns social and health care workers who may also suffer mental health problems. Steele (1998) reported that workers who experience psychological ill-health fear dismissal due to the stigma associated with mental ill-health. Although there is legal provision under the Disability Discrimination Act 1995, to prevent employers from treating job applicants less favourably, evidence points to the existing 'taboo' surrounding mental illness.

SOCIAL POLICY AND NURSING

Some authors have drawn attention to the 'current invisibility' of nursing in regard to policy development (Maslin-Prothero & Masterson 1998) in Britain, and to parsimonious reference to policymaking in the literature and nurse education in the USA (Digaudio 1993). Maslin-Prothero and Masterson (1998) put forward that the health care role as applied to nursing is often neglected by social scientists and government. The issue, they emphasize, applies to continuing care settings, the nursing role and other care delivery arenas. Nursing, compared to medicine and the medical profession, stands on the margin of social policymaking. Maslin-Prothero and Masterson feel that full involvement is required by the nursing profession and that nurses can become effective pressure groups to 'effect' change for themselves or their clients. It is important for health care professionals to gain insight into the nature of social policy: its processes; the machinery of central and local government; how policies can be shaped, developed and put into practice.

To develop their confidence in policy participation, the role of nurses is to have an awareness that they function within a broad policy frame-

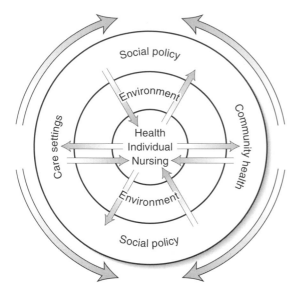

Fig. 7.3 Dynamic process of social policy interactions with the individual–health–environment–nursing.

work (Fig. 7.3). Rowden (1998), for example, acknowledged the valuable contribution nurses can make to influencing decisions in the mental health policy context.

SOCIAL POLICY AND PSYCHOLOGY

Society's survival is dependent on human motivation. How society is organized is reliant on many psychological factors. When sociologists make reference to the 'functional' nature of society, they are also making allusion to

1. human groups and their leaders, who are 'driven' by the needs to cope and survive.
2. the imperative needs to develop policies by resorting to methods and strategies to ensure group cohesion and solidarity
3. the motivation to:
   • maintain health
   • sustain sound economic policies
   • prevent social disharmony
   • promote consensus on a variety of social issues affecting people's lives.

The psychology of human behaviour in relation to social policy comprises, hence, the following properties:

1. Focusing one's faculties on the analysis of situations and on making decisions. For instance, when a society faces socio-economic breakdown, re-evaluation of policies have to be done; e.g. escalation of crime and disorder can stimulate policy makers to respond. In psychological terms there is a *stimulus-response* behaviour (Fig. 7.4). Society's leaders therefore must have recourse to policy-making, to evaluate the integrity of the legal framework and to implement any required changes.

2. Human action can also generate strong emotions. In countries where social policies have failed its citizens, community aggression and violence can become the norm. On a less dramatic scale, for example, in early October 1998, the Bank of England monetary policy committee was under pressure to reduce interest rates. Strong emotions were being expressed by industrialists and business corporations concerning job losses and enterprise closures.

3. Government and its policy makers are prone to being influenced by the action of others. An American study (Monardi & Glantz 1998) aimed at testing the hypothesis that 'tobacco industry campaign contributions influence state legislators' behaviour' showed that a government's negative attitude to tobacco can be swayed, when companies increase their financial contributions to support political campaigns. In Britain, critics have found that the Government is reluctant to ban cigarette production, as it

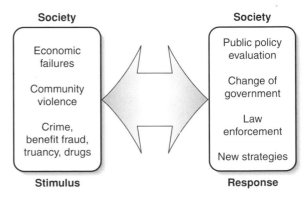

Fig. 7.4 Psychological theory to explain stimulus-response principles as applied to social behaviour in society and policy-making.

provides revenues to the treasury through taxation.

The above are some examples that illustrate the connection between social policy and psychology. Students of social policy may wish to explore other examples:

- personality types and nature of policy-making
- the effects of past learning/experience on present government policies
- compliance and conformity in relation to pressure group influences
- policy makers' perception and social realities.

Activity 7.2

1. Prepare a list of social issues. In small groups discuss their relevance to sociology, social economics, psychology and health care.
2. Draw a diagram to illustrate the many dimensions of social policy.
3. Discuss with your mentor/assessor in health care settings their views on social policy and the nursing role. Write down your findings. Now do a literature search to compare your findings with research material on the subject.

??? Question 7.3

1. Do you agree that social policy is multidimensional in nature?
2. How should nurses and other allied professionals consider their work in relation to social policy?
3. If social policy concerns health care professionals, what in your view has prevented them from participating in policy-making?

SUMMARY

Social policy is concerned with social issues as they affect individuals in any society. As an academic discipline, social policy is also related to other social sciences, namely sociology, social economics, health policy and psychology. For health care workers, social policy becomes an important subject, as their practice is influenced by the wider conceptual framework of policy-making. Further, there are elements of socio-political aspects that impinge on their practice. For students of social policy, the interdisciplinary nature of social policy provides the instrument to explore its complexities, how they relate to everyday life and their effects on individuals in a variety of settings.

GLOSSARY

Bureaucratic formal administration and organization of work, often seen as inflexible and oppressive
Consensus collective agreement by the people
Eclectic using many dimensions and ideas from other disciplines
Fabianism refers to the characteristics of an organization that believes in socialism
Health policy measures taken to ensure the provision of health care and social services; for example, the role of the Department of Health in managing health and personal social services
Motivation in psychology, the factors which stimulate and direct human and animal behaviour
Political sociology the application of sociological principles in studying the political framework of society

Poor Law a time during which the English political system attempted to combat poverty, by implementing the Poor Relief Act 1601
Recession when socio-economic activities decline
Social exclusion refers to the disadvantaged groups in society who cannot always access services provided, e.g. the person with mental illness, learning disabilities and the homeless
Socialist pertains to individuals who believe in an egalitarian (equal and fair) society
Stimulus-response in psychology, the observation that environmental stimuli elicit responses that can either be rewarded or punished

REFERENCES

Ackers L, Fordham J 1995 Contemporary social policy. Churchill Livingstone, New York
Alcock P 1996 Social policy in Britain. MacMillan, Basingstoke

Allsop J 1995 Health Policy and the NHS: Towards 2000, 2nd edn. Longman, London
Atkin K 1996 Social policy in a multiracial Britain. In: Lunt N, Coyle D (eds) Welfare and policy research agendas

and issues. Taylor & Francis, London, p 141–158

Beuret C 1991 Women and transport. In: Maclean M, Groves D (eds) Women's issues in social policy. Routledge, London, p 61–75

Bilton T, Bennett K, Jones P et al 1996 Introductory sociology, 3rd edn. MacMillan, Basingstoke, p 294

Boettcher R E 1997 Revitalizing families: a communitarian agenda for social work. Journal of Community Practice 4(3): 47–58

Boggan S, Popham P 1998 The arrangement. The Independent 21 July p 1

Bradley G 1997 Translating research into practice. Social Work and Social Sciences Review 7(1): 3–12

Burgess R 1996 For debate: Drugs prevention: watershed or threshold? Health Education Journal 55(3): 345–351

Burtless G 1995 The case for randomized field trials in economic and policy research. Journal of Economic Perspectives 9(2): 63–84

Callender C 1992 Redundancy, unemployment and poverty. In: Millar J, Glendinning C (eds) Women and poverty in Britain the 1990s. Harvester Wheatsheaf, New York, p 129–148

Chapin R K 1995 Social policy development: the strengths perspective. Social Work: Journal of the Association of Social Workers 40(4): 506–514

Cohen B J, Austin M J 1997 Transforming human services organizations through empowerment of staff. Journal of Community Practice 4(2): 35–50

Colton M, Drakeford S, Roberts E et al 1997 Social workers, parents and stigma. Child and Family Social Work 2(4): 247–257

Community Care 1998a White Paper aims to introduce tougher monitoring of services. Community Care 1234: 7

Community Care 1998b New Labour Big Deal? Community Care 1235: 16–18

Corrigan D, Bishop K K 1997 Creating family-centered integrated service systems and interprofessional programs to implement them. Social Work in Education 19(3): 149–163

David M, Groves D 1995 Editorial. Journal of Social Policy 24(1): 1–3

Deakin N 1993 Privatisation and partnership in urban policy: some comparative issues. In: Jones C (ed) New perspectives on the welfare state in Europe. Routledge, London, p 84–107

Digaudio K M 1993 Nurses' participation in policy-making initiatives. State University of New York, Buffalo

Dyson S 1999 Genetic screening and ethnic minorities. Critical Social Policy 19(2): 195–216

Dziegielewski S E 1998 Psychopharmacology and social work practice: introduction. Research on Social Work Practice 8(4): 371

Fletcher K 1998 Give them the evidence. Community Care 1233: 22

Freeman E M 1996 Welfare reforms and services for children and families: setting a new practice, research, and policy agenda. Social Work: Journal of the Association of Social Workers 41(5): 521–532

Glendinning C, Millar J 1991 Poverty: the forgotten Englishman—reconstructing research and policy on poverty. In: Maclean M, Groves D (eds) Women's issues in social policy. Routledge, London, p 20–37

Haralambos M, Holborn M 1995 Sociology themes and

perspectives, 4th edn. Collins Educational, London, p 378–379

Hill M 1997 Understanding social policy. Blackwell, Oxford

Holman B 1998 Why hopes have been dashed. Community Care 1235: 18

Hunter M 1998 No place like home. Community Care 1234: 16–18

Kingman S 1998 Editorial: New contract for health. Health Education 98(3): 83–84

Klein R 1995 The new politics of the NHS, 3rd edn. Longman, London, p 48

Latting J K, Blanchard A 1997 Empowering staff in a 'poverty agency': an organization development intervention. Journal of Community Practice 4(3): 59–75

Lawler S 1996 Motherhood and identity. In: Cosslett T, Easton A, Summerfield P (eds) Women, power and resistance. Open University Press, Buckingham, p 153–164

Levin P 1997 Making social policy: the mechanisms of government and politics, and how to investigate them. Open University Press, Buckingham

Linton M 1998 What research means to me: the use of research by political policy-makers. Social Sciences 39: 4

McCain R A 1984 Social economy and community. International Journal of Social Economics 11(1–2): 89–99

McKee A 1984 Social economy and the theory of consumer behaviour. International Journal of Social Economics 11(1–2): 45–61

Madeira M J 1998 Social action in Portugal. European Journal of Social Work 1(2): 227–230

Maslin-Prothero S, Masterson A 1998 Continuing care: developing a policy analysis for nursing. Journal of Advanced Nursing 28(3): 548–553

Mayston D 1996 Healthcare reforms: a study in imperfect information. In: Lunt N, Coyle D (eds) Welfare and policy research agendas and issues. Taylor & Francis, London, p 3–20

Meerabeau L 1996 Managing policy research in nursing. Journal of Advanced Nursing 24(3): 633–639

Millar J, Glendinning C 1992 'It all really starts in the family': gender divisions and poverty. In: Glendinning C, Millar J (eds) Women and poverty in Britain in the 1990s. Harvester Wheatsheaf, New York, p 3–10

Monardi F, Glantz S A 1998 Are tobacco industry campaigns' contributions influencing State Legislative behaviour? American Journal of Public Health 88(6): 918–923

Moore S 1993 Social welfare alive! Stanley Thornes, Cheltenham

Noble M, Cheung S Y, Smith G 1998 Origins and destinations: social security claimant dynamics. Journal of Social Policy 27(3): 351–369

Peillon M 1998 Bourdieu's and the sociology of welfare. Journal of Social Policy 27(2): 213–229

Pollitt C, Harrison S, Hunters D J, Marnoch G 1990 No hiding place: on the discomforts of researching the contemporary policy process. Journal of Social Policy 19(2): 169–190

Quilgars D 1998 Going it alone. Community Care 1240: 24–25

Rickford F 1998 On the brink of change. Community Care 1234: 18

Rowden R 1998 Storm warning. Nursing Times 94(40): 32

Royal College of Nursing 1998 EuroForum: European social policy in action. RCN, London

Sayce L 1998 Stigma, discrimination and social exclusion: what's in a word? Journal of Mental Health 7(4): 331–343

Stanley N, Manthorpe J 1997 Risk assessment: developing training for professionals in mental health work. Social Work and Social Sciences Review 7(1): 26–38

Steele L 1998 A brave face is not enough. Community Care 1240: 8–9

Stepney P, Lynch R, Jordan B 1999 Poverty, exclusion and New Labour. Critical Social Policy 19(1): 88–109

Taylor D 1998 Social identity and social policy: engagements with postmodern theory. Journal of Social Policy 27(3): 329–350

Twigg J, Atkin K 1995 Carers and services: factors mediating service provision. Journal of Social Policy 24(1): 5–30

Vostanis P, Grattan E, Cumella S 1998 Mental health problems of homeless children and families: longitudinal study. British Medical Journal 316 (7135): 899–902

Walker A 1998 The Amsterdam declaration on the social quality of Europe. European Journal of Social Work 1(1): 109–111

Ware R 1998 What research means to me: Parliament and the social sciences. Social Sciences 39: 4

Weaver H N 1998 Indigenous people in a multicultural society: unique issues for human resources. Social Work 43(3): 203–211

Wellard S 1998 Out of the rough. Community Care 1234: 20–21

White C 1998 Including the excluded. Nursing Times 94(37): 32

Wistow G, Knapp M, Hardy B et al 1996 Social care markets: progress and prospects. Open University Press, Buckingham, p 18

Zimmermann K F 1995 Tackling the European migration problem. Journal of Economic Perspectives 9(2): 45–62

FURTHER READING

Balwin S, Oxlad M 1996 Ect and minors: social sciences solutions will reform the psychiatric abuse of infants, children and adolescents. Social Sciences in Health: International Journal of Research and Practice 2(3): 174–188

Cantillon S, Nolan B 1998 Are married women more deprived than their husbands? Journal of Social Policy 27(2): 151–171

Mowbray C T, Bybee D 1998 The importance of context in understanding homelessness and mental illness: lessons learned from a research demonstration project. Research on Social Work Practice 8(2): 172–199

Randall V 1996 Feminism and child care. Journal of Social Policy 25(4): 485–505

Wyre R 1998 Register of hope? Community Care 1237: p 16–22

Yasseen T 1998 Playing the power game ... nurse executives should unite to influence policy-making. Nursing Management (London): the Nursing Standard Journal for Nurse Leaders 4(8): 6

Policy-making

Society's functioning is reliant on sound public policies. In democratic societies there are devised systems of policy-making founded on the representations of people's views and needs. Such systems are complex in nature, and there are many agents who participate in their shaping and implementation. The aims of this chapter are to:

- introduce some socio-political processes as they affect policy-making in Britain
- highlight the structures that influence policy-making
- discuss the role and functions of internal (within the government) agencies and external factors in policy-making and implementation.

THE STRUCTURE OF GOVERNMENT

THE CORE EXECUTIVE

The making of policy does not occur in a vacuum. Most people are aware that government is concerned with policy-making. What is not always made clear is the complex process that is involved in formulating policies, which will eventually be *felt* by their target populations.

One issue frequently made allusion to by both the lay person and academics is the secrecy that surrounds the activities of government machinery. Not surprisingly, when under close scrutiny from media and pressure groups, Ministers have developed communication strategies to fence probing questions from journalists and political correspondents. One attempt to demystify government functions and parliamentary activities was to introduce television cameras into the House of Commons and the House of Lords. While some contend that media intrusion gives an inkling of what goes on at Westminster, others feel that Parliament has become a stage on which astute politicians will show their adversarial skills, arguing their case in government policy-making to tackle social problems as speedily as possible.

While the electorate rely on the government to be faithful to their election manifestos, they remain in the dark as far as the intricacies of policy-making are concerned. In an ideal democratic society, the whole nation would participate in policy-making decisions. However, this is not possible, so Members of Parliament (MPs) have the function of representing their constituencies.

The majority of people are therefore not recognizant of central government policy-making processes and the constraints imposed on Ministers and their departments. An introduction to the structure of the 'core executive' is needed, and the role of internal and external agencies pertaining to government policy-making.

The 'core executive' (Fig. 8.1) is sometimes referred to as 'central governance' or 'central administration' since it is at the nucleus of government; it is considered to be the hub of political decision-making activities. The Prime Minister is deemed the highest representative of government (Hogwood 1997b) elected by the people. The Monarch represents the State, and oversees that any newly elected government is transferred into office according to set, formal procedures (Hogwood 1997b). In Britain, the role of the Queen is seen to exert formal constitutional powers by:

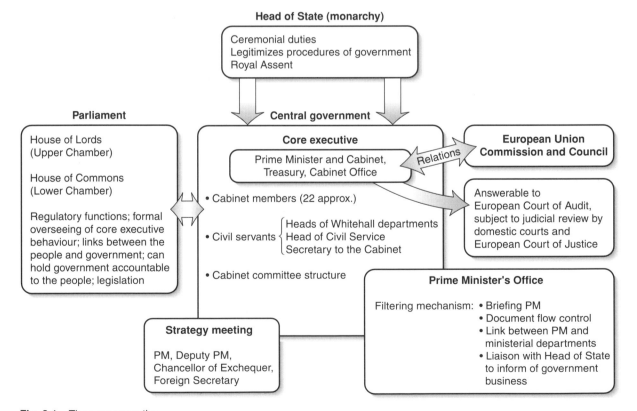

Fig. 8.1 The core executive.

1. appointing Government Ministers
2. dissoluting Parliament
3. formalizing Bills passed by Parliament and giving them 'Royal Assent'.

Parliament is an important and traditional British government institution. It is made up of the House of Lords (the upper chamber) and the House of Commons (the lower chamber); at the time of writing, the former is being reviewed by the Labour Government. The British House of Commons, together with the House of Lords have the important functions of scrutinizing discussion documents and various proposals made by Cabinet Ministers. They are hence recognized for their influential role in influencing public policy (Norton 1997).

Government Ministers, Hogwood (1997b) points out, are responsible to Parliament. The House of Commons is adversarial in nature, and is the forum for the opposition and members of the party in power to exchange views on policy matters that have implications for the nation (Peele 1995). It is now common practice for both the House of Lords and the House of Commons to be televised. Media exposure means that the Prime Minister and his Cabinet have to present impeccable arguments, in the most professional way, to make maximum use of the power of television broadcasting. It can be said that, to a small extent, the core executive political activities are made transparent in the House through broadcasting. The membership of the House of Commons (Peele 1995) has become a full-time political activity, for many MPs, with less preoccupation with developing a career outside the House of Commons. The varied experiences and education of MPs mean that they provide a wealth of information to the House for debates. Further, their close contact with constituents ensures that issues debated in the House mirror social realities. For the core executive, the diversity of MPs' contributions and counter arguments (sometimes supported by research obtained from pressure/interest groups) can be taxing. The core executive is composed of the Prime Minister and Cabinet, the Treasury Cabinet Office, Foreign and Commonwealth Office, and Security and Intelligence Services (Fig. 8.1). Within the core executive there are approximately 22 members, top civil servants who manage Whitehall departments, and the Civil Service, including the Secretary to the Cabinet. The Cabinet Committee structure also forms part of the core executive.

THE ROLE OF THE PRIME MINISTER

The Prime Minister is the role model who promotes and encourages an ethos of 'collegiality' and 'collective responsibility'. Collective responsibility has, however, been criticized for being a 'silly doctrine' (Marr 1995). It is argued that, in reality, Cabinet Ministers are not always in agreement with each other and the Prime Minister. The media have, on numerous occasions, exposed argumentative and differing viewpoints in disharmony with 'collective responsibility'. Marr explained that the rapidity with which news is communicated signifies that some Ministers may be ill-prepared to give a 'collective answer'. Journalists who have well researched their material can challenge a Cabinet Minister who is unaware of the 'detailed work and decisions of others' (Marr 1995).

The terms 'collegiality' and 'collective responsibility' are synonymous and commonly used in political literature. They refer to Cabinet members' and departmental ministers' responsibility to work in partnership; to maintain confidentiality as required; to be 'ultimately responsible to the elected representatives of the people' (Hogwood 1997b); and to be prepared to defend an agreed policy decision in public or resign.

The Prime Minister, compared to his Cabinet Ministers, has a higher degree of power and patronage (Peele 1995). The Prime Minister's style of leadership is a key factor in ensuring that his Cabinet committees run smoothly. Effective communication with colleagues (treasury officials, Chancellor of the Exchequer, Deputy Prime Minister and Private Secretaries) is needed to promote social policy goals unambiguously. Further, the Prime Minister has a duty to both departmental Ministers in the Party and the electorate, to exemplify his determination to implement the pre-election manifesto. The manifesto is naturally constantly alluded to by the mass media as the Prime Minister's strategies are scrutinized. The media provide a channel to the Prime Minister and his Ministers to publicly argue their achievements in office. It is therefore not surprising that the Prime Minister will, throughout an office term, arrange for political broadcasts on television and radio.

The aims of the Prime Minister on these occasions are to:

1. affirm the government position with regard to policy-making issues
2. reassure the electorate that the new government strategies are sound
3. expose the weaknesses of the opposition Party
4. update the nation on recent developments and achievements
5. inform the electorate of future plans (emergent policies) or intentions
6. make evident to the people that the Prime Minister and the Party keep in touch with the nation through their communication networks.

Communicating with Party members at conferences (which are televised), is another opportunity for the Prime Minister and colleagues to consolidate party partnerships, exhibit party unity, boost morale and to expose again to public view the vision and philosophy of the Prime Minister concerning social policies. This approach of media utilization has been described as 'political marketing' and is now accepted as an imperative function of a Prime Minister.

The power of the Prime Minister resides in the ability to make use of their patronage by managing and coordinating the Cabinet, to ensure smooth running of a political system that can otherwise become unwieldy. It is suggested that the Prime Minister 'shapes the structure of government' (Kingdom 1991). The Prime Minister may, for example, hold unofficial meetings known as 'strategy meetings' with the Deputy Prime Minister, Chancellor of the Exchequer and Foreign Secretary. These strategy meetings – separate from Cabinet meetings – serve the pur-

pose of specifying key policy issues for discussion, which demand specialist knowledge and keep debates focused. Policy decisions made at strategy meetings must, nevertheless, be presented to the Cabinet for debate and commentary. This approach serves to prevent alienation of the Party. Thus, conflict prevention and Party stability are two key roles for a Prime Minister. A failure to obtain Cabinet Ministers' approval on policies could result in a breakdown of Party unity, and subsequent division. Party disharmony and division supply the opposition leader with the ammunition to expose weaknesses in the fabric of government and to criticize the Prime Minister's leadership in securing collective acceptance on policy issues. Not surprisingly, the Prime Minister has to strive to keep the government well managed and integrated.

Peele (1995) and Oliver (1991) explained that the core executive is flexible and adaptable; it is nonetheless dependent on the Prime Minister's style, judgement and ability to recognize the constraints impinging on Ministers' and their departments' operations. The forging of unity by allowing Ministers, Whitehall officials (civil servants) and political supporters to function in a democratically driven political system shows the extent of flexibility that can be experienced.

The Prime Minister has power to review and evaluate the Cabinet. Cabinet reshuffles and new ministerial appointments are the Prime Minister's prerogative. Furthermore, power can be exercised by directing Ministers to consider 'policy commitments', and to expect their views on relevant matters. It should be noted, nevertheless, according to Levin (1997), that the Prime Minister does not possess 'unfettered' power.

How the Prime Minister uses the Cabinet committees is, again, conditional on leadership and personality style. Peele (1995) pointed out, for example, that Margaret Thatcher relied more on consultations with small groups of advisers outside the Cabinet for policy-making decisions. While a Prime Minister's channel of communication is expansive within the Government, there is the likelihood that sound policy ideas and initiatives communicated to the Prime Minister by Ministers and their departments' officials will be utilized. Civil Service officials have a close professional partnership with their Ministers, which is not only important, but is an 'essential feature of British government' (Nairne 1997).

An astute Prime Minister will no doubt make use of the vast experience of civil servants in his policy development strategies. In fact, in 1997, the new Prime Minister, Tony Blair – to ensure smooth Civil Service transition into the new Government – diplomatically praised the Civil Service for the 'good reception' they had shown to their new departmental Ministers (Theakston 1998). This approach prepares the way for future professional and cooperative relationships in policy-making debates. Additionally, it gives evidence that the Government value the work of Civil Service employees in policy-making.

The principal decision-making focus of the government, however, remains with the Cabinet (King 1993). A decision made by the Prime Minister alone, without Cabinet colleagues' involvement, is construed as a non-governmental decision. The British system of government organization is founded on the democratic principle. The Prime Minister is conscious of it, and will use this ideology to rally the Party and promote free expressions on policy issues, while maintaining authority, safeguarding ministerial autonomy and respecting Whitehall officials' contribution to policy-making processes. King (1993) described this standpoint as 'ensuring a highly collegial' political manoeuvre to maintain cabinet cohesion and government stability.

A Prime Minister is motivated to prove to his Party, Parliament and the nation that his vision is based on reality principles, the desire to manage social challenge and produce public policies that exemplify societal developments.

In policy-making circles, a Prime Minister who shows determination to propel their Party in dealing with society's problems, constitutes a Party's 'revolution'. In 1998, *The Times* political correspondent, Roland Watson (1998a), reported the Labour Revolution as encompassing a middle class-dominated politics (Box 8.1).

For the Prime Minister, the task of impressing the electorate becomes both demanding and imperative. Moreover, according to Philip Gould,

Box 8.1 Labour Revolution

' "We need to have a politics which is rooted in populism, but particularly rooted in the emerging middle-class" says Philip Gould, the Prime Minister's most influential adviser. "The politics of the future are going to be middle-class politics". "Modernisation is a process that never stops. The process of change increases. The revolution is never finished. It can never finish" ' (Watson 1998a).

listening to the voice of the people 'and relating their hopes and fears to the party leadership' is a democratic principle. He argued that effective government communication can translate 'hopes and aspirations' into policies (Watson 1998b). The Prime Minister has to keep abreast with socio-political change and respond to pressures from within the Party and the real world. Old policies, values and ideologies may be discarded as consequences of past experiences, research findings, and from learning acquired from domestic and foreign government policy implementation (Case example 8.1).

Case example 8.1 Thatcher was an admirer of free-market disciple Pinochet

Augusto Pinochet, the army commander of Chile ... was one of the first leaders to put into practice the radical free-market economic policies advocated by Milton Friedman, and the Chicago School of Economists ... As Prime Minister, Mrs Thatcher kept a close watch on the success of Chile's privatization programmes. General Pinochet, in turn, was flattered to see similar policies adopted in Britain (Binyon 1998).

Some critics (Garner & Kelly 1998) have highlighted 'New Labour' political trajectory, which contrasts sharply with their post-war focus on 'ensuring full employment'; evidence that there is a dilution of their egalitarianism philosophy and an abandonment of a collectivist image, in an 'individualistic age'. The Prime Minister now shows an intention to modernize Labour with a coherent set of ideas and radical long-term intentions on economic and social policy issues, which some observers argue is a continuation of Thatcherism.

The Government now aims at controlling taxation and public spending. The integration of free-market mechanism with some State intervention is also favoured, as is the promotion of individualism by creating the right economic climate, through State management.

To attain their political ideals, Prime Ministers aim to reach the ordinary person in the constituency (Box 8.1). A philosophy of pragmatism, demonstrating to the people that policies of government reflect 'policies which best meet the nation's mood' (The Times 1998a, 1998b).

Promoting a progressive image is one of the Prime Minister's primary roles by attending to the 'contemporary experience' of working-class people. In fact, Tony Blair's chief political adviser, Philip Gould, argued in *The Times* (1998b) that the working-classes who aspire to become prosperous will feel betrayed if New Labour political ideology does not reflect 'policies which are sensible and moderate' and conform to their lived experiences. Utilizing populism as a strategy can bridge government policy-making endeavours nearer to the individual.

THE ROLE OF PARLIAMENT

Parliament has differing roles (Riddell 1998):

- the maintenance of a constitutional and political and legislative relationship with the core executive
- establishing a link with the British people by voicing their fears, aspirations and needs
- teaching and informing, by expressing the 'grievances of the governed to government'
- the creation of governments
- provision of ministers
- oversight of government expenditure and tax proposals
- the scrutiny of government social policy proposals;
- general assessment of the core executive, its departments' functions and the performance of its ministers and their civil servants.

Parliament has, however, its strengths and weaknesses (Box 8.2).

While Parliament establishes a bridge between

Box 8.2 Parliament

Strengths
- Sustainment of a government
- Translating constituents' votes into clear-cut decisions on which Party should govern
- Respecting the verdict of the nation
- Ensuring fairness and equality is maintained throughout Parliament
- The Commons have a controlling influence over the core executive
- Ministers are accountable to Parliament
- Evaluates Government expenditure and tax proposal programmes
- Its Select Committee system assesses expenditure trends by checking inaccuracies and government behaviour
- Select Committees inform public debate
- Select Committees have the special function of scrutinizing Bill drafts in detail and giving advice accordingly on how improvement can be made
- Prime Minister is pressed on issues of the day
- Grievances of constituents and external agencies can be voiced
- MPs can influence change (e.g. introducing a Bill) and act as government watchdogs
- safeguarding democratic principles
- Parliament as representative of the people.

Weaknesses
- Select Committee's reports can lack details and do not change spending behaviour
- Detailed financial role now given to the executive (role is replaced by Public Accounts Committee and the National Audit Office; these committees do not make proposals to improve process on future spending policy)
- Lack of balance due to domination by MPs from majority party
- Backbenchers not invited to participate 'lest their speeches delay progress on a Bill'
- Bills can be badly drafted and rushed through
- Detailed examination can be stifled due to Government guillotines being imposed
- Not enough Bills in draft forms
- Some Ministers may not believe in exposing controversial Bills to extensive scrutiny (e.g. past experience shows that Parliament did not show pragmatism in implementing the Poll Tax)
- Full debate does not take place on the floor of the House
- Parliament less able to call Prime Minister to account due to devolved accountability (e.g. Bank of England now responsible for monetary policy)
- Alternative centres of power have weakened Parliament (e.g. Next Step Executive Agencies; regulators for privatized utilities)
- Role of the House within European Union not clearly defined
- the House has no opposition Party identified to *oppose European Union directives* if required.

the people and government by scrutinizing the latter's policy-making behaviour and by calling Ministers to account, it is itself open to public and media scrutiny. In addition, policy studies and politicians have shown a critical view of the functions of Parliament over the years, suggesting ways on how to improve its credibility. It has been suggested, for instance (Read 1993), that while Parliament provides Ministers with opportunities to question the Prime Minister and his Cabinet on social policy matters, the 'exchanges' which take place 'are simply theatre'. Marr (1995), in his comments on the role of Parliament, remarked that debates in the House lack depth, and the occasions are not conducive to 'effective probing'. He further points out the evidence of an 'underbriefed' House. Arguments are superficial in nature with no 'significant revelations about policy or ministerial thinking'. Further, the argument goes that analysis of the executive is not effective, as it lacks hold on the activities of Cabinet Ministers.

In addition, Ministers and their departmental civil servants have been known to keep most of their actions and discussions secretive, to avoid intruding examination from outside. Although Parliament has the power to influence public policy (Norton 1997) and play a reactive role in the legislative process (Hogwood 1997b), the executive can nonetheless exercise its power to control some situations, which could implicate the 'conduct of the government' (Oliver 1991).

CIVIL SERVANTS IN WHITEHALL

Government, like other organizations in the spheres of social life, needs officials to keep the executive machinery running smoothly. Civil servants are the people engaged in this process. They work in ministerial departments in Whitehall. Additionally, civil servants can be found working in organizations that implement government policies; for example as Inspectors of Taxes, staff of benefits agencies, Customs and Excise Officers; Magistrates' Court Officials etc.

Whitehall officials frequently become the focus of academic writers, political correspondents, social policy students and, of course, politicians.

They operate under strict central government guidelines within the Official Secrets Act, in their Ministers' departments. They are the servants of Ministers and have important functions in the policy-making process, as well as in policy implementation (Hill & Bramley 1986, Hill 1997).

Whitehall officials are influential in policy-making, because their wealth of experience is utilized by Ministers to inform the practicalities of making policy. They advise on the drafting of Bills, working in close professional partnership with departmental Ministers and Permanent Secretaries. Kingdom (1991) highlighted the fact that the Civil Service is at the hub of resource allocation in society (e.g. health and social care provision, managed by civil servants in social services departments and the NHS).

Although civil servants occupy differing occupational levels in the employment framework (from the industrial to the non-industrial sectors) (Kingdom 1991), social policy studies are mainly concerned with the 1% of elite officials at the pinnacle of social administration (for example, Home Office, Treasury Department, Department of Health, Defence Ministry and others).

Some writers (Hood & James 1997) have commented that the influences of the Civil Service are weakening for a variety of reasons:

- more external appointments
- decreased civil servants meetings
- the Civil Code (a regulatory, supervisory body)
- a Parliamentary ombudsman with oversight functions
- a 25% reduction of top grade jobs since 1994.

Civil servants, nonetheless, still occupy a privileged position and have valuable contributions to make in policy-making. The fact that they share with Ministers the highest posts in their functional departments (Levin 1997) creates a context which makes Ministers reliant on their experiences.

Civil Service employees have to be adaptable and flexible to cope with the changes a new government brings. Their posts are permanent, no matter how many new governments achieve office. Civil servants exercise political neutrality and approach their tasks in an objective way. Further, they are expected to function within the domain of their Ministers' official procedures and the Government code of conduct, in addition to the Civil Service Code. Policy drafts must be read and recommended changes made, while exercising an attitude of 'neutral administration' (Peele 1995).

This does not mean, however, that civil servants cannot voice their opinions on policies. In fact, Ministers invite their officials to comment on policy matters and are prepared to listen to constructive suggestions. Equally important is the ability of civil servants to remain open to making changes in their departments' policy-making activities under the direction of a strong prime ministerial leadership (Nairne 1997). Nevertheless, Nairne explained that some Whitehall officials may be inclined to adhere to 'well tried methods of administration'; an issue not to be deplored since Ministers rely on sound past experiences to guide their views on policy-making and implementation. It can be anticipated, moreover, that where contradictions occur in regard to differing ideology a degree of 'professional friction' can result.

The Civil Service has an agenda for action (Nairne 1997), which possesses some pertinent features of importance for government and policy-making:

- continuing the professional partnership between Ministers and civil servants
- improving the policy-making processes
- developing public services management.

Ministers' and civil servants' partnership

The fabric of British government relies on the essential characteristics of collaborative partnerships between Cabinet Ministers and the Prime Minister, and between departmental Ministers and their civil servants. This is so essential that, from early 1996, it has been noted (Theakston 1998) that meetings were arranged 'between Labour Shadow ministers and the Permanent Secretaries' to obtain the latter's viewpoints on

matters concerning Whitehall organizations and management – an astute strategy for a future government aiming to establish sound professional relationships with their civil servants.

Where prime ministerial leadership is strong (Nairne 1997), with a clear sense of policy direction (Theakston 1998), the Civil Service is prone to be effective. Concerns regarding the operations of the Civil Service, and how to maintain a degree of control have been so strong, that by 1994 'effectiveness issues' became the priorities of the office of Public Service *within the Cabinet Office* (Hogwood 1997a).

The reader can easily evaluate the rationale for this strategy. Such an arrangement ensures that the Prime Minister and colleagues can link in an accessible way with the Civil Service operational managers, thus indirectly superintending operations.

To civil servants, their priority is the sustenance of central administration continuity in line with their code of conduct, which specifies neutrality in their dealings across the multidimensional nature of their work: participating in policy-making review and evaluation by co-ordinating with other colleagues to improve policy drafts. Alternative policy options may have to be considered and discussed. A strong communication network that extends interdepartmentally is important for policy-making for the following reasons:

1. A public policy can impinge on other policy areas (e.g. policies related to unemployment must be coordinated with other departments, i.e. Education and Employment, Treasury, Trade and Industry, Social Security).

2. Interdepartmental integration ensures that ideas are interchanged and developments are more closely monitored. Professional isolation is also minimized.

3. Specialist knowledge may be needed (e.g. Ministers and civil servants with experience in pressure/interest group management, social security, health service management etc. may be called upon to advise accordingly).

4. A strong constitutional position has to be developed, demanding close collaboration with

other departments so that European Union directives can be debated and opposed if necessary. Bomberg and Peterson (1998) assert that bargaining skills development is necessary to access and influence policy networks in Europe.

5. The European Union is a 'highly complex negotiation system (Neunreither 1998). It is relevant for government and Whitehall to expand coping strategies in respect of bargaining for better policy-making and implementation framework.

6. The force of globalization and its impact on policy-making demands that government must understand and be sensitive to socio-political trends in addition to economic and cultural developments (Wilding 1997) in a policy context.

7. Ministers have responsibilities in making sure that training programmes are in operation to update civil servants' skills and to give them increased responsibility (Talbot 1997).

The mechanics of policy-making (Fig. 8.2) are complex. The Whitehall community is a hive of activity. Unambiguous directives are requisite for optimal performance by Ministers and their departments, as they are accountable to Parliament for policies formulated and the actions of their civil servants (Riddell 1998).

Activity 8.1

1. Draw a labelled diagram to depict the many functions of Whitehall community. Identify their policy-making roles.
2. In small groups, discuss their relationships with departmental Ministers.
3. Prepare a list of issues that need to be considered when a new government is formed.

PRESSURE GROUPS AND INTEREST GROUPS

In societies where autocratic styles of government are in operation, pressure groups and interest groups either are non-existent or they organize a form of covert resistance against their govern-

??? Question 8.1

1. It is argued that civil servants are strategically placed to influence policy-making. What are the explanations for this argument?
2. Ministers rely on their civil servants to achieve their policy outcomes. Describe the system which allows for this happen.
3. How does a Prime Minister exert power in government?
4. What agencies oversee government action?
5. How effective is Parliament in its function of exercising control over the core executive?
6. Policy-making is complex; what are the reasons for this?
7. Do you agree with the view that 'collective responsibility' can be hard to maintain?
8. Populism is regarded as commendable. How can it be achieved?

ment policies. Their strategies could be the blocking of policy implementation, which could be detrimental to their members and the rest of society.

In democratic social systems, such as Britain and the USA, pressure groups are allowed to flourish, although they can make nuisances of themselves, e.g. by intersecting whale fishing boats, by building underground fortresses to stop developers from destroying woodlands, or by gathering outside No. 10 Downing Street. Interest groups may be defined as organizations aiming to promote the interests of their group members. Some examples of interest groups are trade unions, teachers' unions, nurses' unions such as the RCN (Royal College of Nursing), farmers' unions, the British Medical Association, Age Concern and the RSPCA (Royal Society for the Prevention of Cruelty to Animals).

Some groups are known as 'promotional groups': they promote one specific model of thought, morality or beliefs, which they feel concerns the nation as a whole. In this case they are not promoting attitudes, values and beliefs for the benefit of their members, but the aim is to cause attitude change in the wider population. Some religious organizations are included in this category; another example is the NSPCC (National Society for the Prevention of Cruelty to Children). How one distinguishes the differences

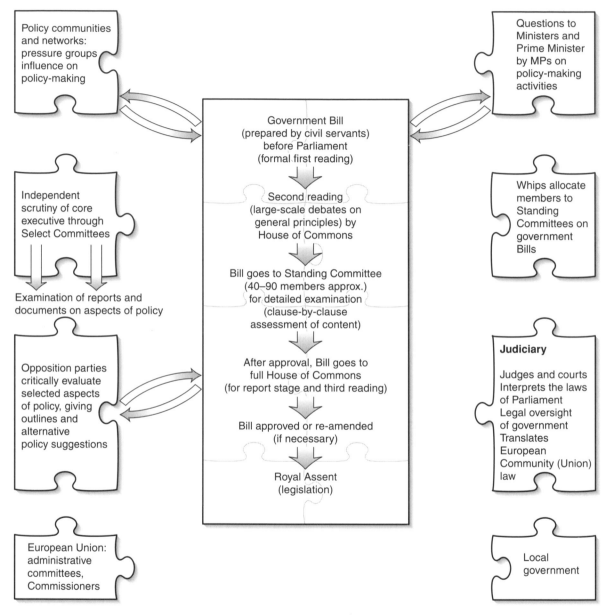

Fig. 8.2 The mechanics of policy-making.

between interest groups and promotional groups is hard to establish. Teachers' unions, for instance, promote the belief and value that society needs teachers, and the unions have an important role in the socialization of society's members. Interest groups can sometimes be described as 'associational groups'. One may, for example, make reference to the Women's Institute, the Working Men's Club, the Conservative Club, 'Wall Street' in the USA, or the 'City' in London (Britannica 1992). Associations have power too, and can exert pressure on other organizations and government.

When interest groups utilize their influence to pressure the Government into acting in certain ways, they become known as 'pressure groups'. Pressure groups represent specific sections of the community, and promote their (communities') opinions and interests (Punnett 1994). They aim to influence policy-making and implementation. With their influence they can instigate proposals for new Bills, and alter the course of public policies. In addition, pressure groups are often consulted by government officials (MPs, civil servants, Ministers), to acquire accurate data on the cause they are promoting, and to seek technical information on issues connected with their work. The Department of Health, for example, will need the expertise of the British Medical Association and the Royal College of Nursing before proposing new Bills on health care policies.

Characteristics of pressure groups

Knowledge and power

Pressure groups assimilate knowledge on specific issues over a long period. They research their subject matter and target people who are influential, e.g. MPs, councillors, community leaders, congressmen, legislators etc. to influence policy-making. They can be powerful; their exercise of power is, however, subjected to constraints by the social structures – laws, bye-laws, local and central government directives, European Union. In the USA, legislators have a controlling role in structuring the channel of communication between themselves and lobbyists who represent interest groups (Ainsworth 1997), a strategy that determines the level of interest groups' influence in the political process.

Pressure groups have, hence, to be acquainted with rules and procedures as they affect political figures. Their goal is to maximize contact with personalities likely to impact on government policies. In addition, they have to present their case in a convincing way, since there may be competing interests from other groups, as well as the policy preferences of the Ministers and their officials. Achieving credibility is therefore one key feature of pressure groups. Searching for sound scientific data is an activity preferred by committed pressure groups. It is not uncommon

for leaders to interview scientists and researchers who will supply them with the information that will buttress their cause. Specialist knowledge has the function of empowering members. On the other hand, pressure groups gain knowledge directly from legislators (Ministers and civil servants) about political activities and government intentions.

The action of the group must be compatible with 'public beliefs' and be seen to be respectable. One may find that established social issues that attract public attention and arouse constituents' feelings are more likely to increase the strength of lobbyists. Media intervention can also mobilize support from local to national level. Not surprisingly, the media has become a powerful ally for many lobbyists and interest groups.

Professional pressure groups (with many years of experience in lobbying and investigating governments and their policy-making behaviour) have structured activities. In a survey of interest group activity in the USA, Nownes and Freeman (1998) identified several roles and functions that characterize the nature of pressure groups (Box 8.3).

In addition to the tactics described in Box 8.3, militant behaviour is not an uncommon feature of pressure groups and is to be anticipated when discontent increases. Militancy confirms that the group 'means business'; it confirms that their action is founded on strong conviction and aims to precipitate change. For example, the 'nurse wave' action by Japanese nurses in 1989, organized by the Japan Federation of Medical Workers' Unions, ensured that their demands for better working conditions were met (Katsuragi 1997). One particular strategy used by the Union was to secure over 5.4 million petition signatures, and to campaign for three years, to cause health policy changes.

Money can become a powerful ally of pressure groups. Gifts and fees have been known to be exchanged for special favours. Oliver (1997) observed that, in the 1990s, many MPs were accepting differing forms of payment from lobbying organizations representing different types of pressure/interest group clients. Once payments were accepted, it was subsequently

Box 8.3 Pressure groups: their role and function in policy-making

- **Monitoring:** keeping informed of what policy makers are doing. Liaising with other groups if necessary and communicating with legislators to gain insight into departmental and governmental activities. Monitoring allows for analysis of the content of policies and gives groups a framework to decide which action to take and to agree on a common position.
- **Lobbying:** when group members approach their local representatives (MPs in Britain, Congressmen in the USA) to influence government. Contact is established with officials who can be 'alerted' to a Bill's effects on constituents. Lobbying also includes attempts to 'shape' the implementation of policy, raising new issues in line with the latest grassroots opinions and intensifying the communication networks with the media.
- **Media strategies:** talking with people from the media is useful; their daily reporting on political affairs can include a substantial and emotive issue revealed by lobbyists and interest groups.
- **Informal contact:** lobbyists can make use of informal relationships with their MPs and other officials in positions of influence. The primary target of pressure group activity is legislature and the core executive; informal contact with the right person can lead to a more formalized rapport later.
- **Finance:** wealth can help further their cause. Additionally, contributions to parties that support their cause can influence the course of legislation, with more active participation of pressure groups in the drafting of Bills (through their contact with Ministers, civil servants, Senators, Congressmen etc.).

expected of the target MPs to act in the following ways: ensuring that their clients had contact with Ministers of their choice; tabling amendments to Bills as they passed through Parliament; asking specific questions (as requested by their clients) in Parliament; and making speeches.

Hence, it is not surprising that the subject of interest group regulation is an issue that has attracted the attention of some governments. While in Britain there is a Code of Conduct designed by the Standards and Privileges Committee, which aims at regulating the behaviour of MPs (Oliver 1997) and which indirectly affects the influence of interest groups, other countries have developed other methods of establishing a degree of control/regulation.

Interest group regulation

It is understandable that any government will be interested in knowing the activities of interest groups, and if necessary to implement measures of control. It has already been argued that the presence of interest groups is a feature of democracy. Many democratic societies, however, subject interest group activity to State regulation (Yishai 1998).

In some countries (e.g. Israel and Turkey, according to Yishai), interest group activity is 'tolerated, not commended', while the Canadian and Australian governments readily 'accept and affirm' interest group activity. Various arguments are given explaining the reasons for the regulations (Box 8.4) and the differences in approaches between liberal democracies and non-liberal ones. In Britain, interest groups are tolerated and accepted as strands within the fabric of a democratic government.

Box 8.4 Reasons for regulating interest groups

Non-liberal democracies:
- Interest groups seen as threatening and viewed with suspicion and apprehension.
- State prerogative to exercise control and authoritative decision, to silence groups that may cause uprisings if seen to develop into powerful groups likely to disturb the State and its method of governing and 'its fundamental creed and institutions'.
- They are a threat to public order.
- They are accused of immoral behaviour and its promotion.
- States exploit religion to further political ambitions.
- To discourage subversive behaviour.
- To exercise centralized control if financial gains are suspected.
- Fears that subversive action might be encouraged.
- To restore order in a society where social tension can increase.
- For political reasons, e.g. if partnership with opposition parties is suspected.

Liberal democracies:
- To regulate excessive influence of lobbyists that marginalize the efforts of small pressure groups.
- Regulation ensures equity.
- Equality of access to decision-makers (e.g. civil servants, Ministers).
- To identify lobbyists formally through registration with the aim to identify the organizations they represent.
- To increase transparency of activities.
- To raise ethical standards of the State.
- To ensure political justice.

Furthermore, the Government allows that the freedom of expression and the media undoubtedly will broadcast issues that interest groups manage to bring to public attention. The media become levers in furthering the cause of the groups.

The British experience shows that government, rather than attempting to exercise regulation, aims to accommodate interest groups. In fact, Ministers attempt to *manage* the consultation process (Dudley & Richardson 1998), rather than regulating interest groups' activities. The diversity of groups' interests assures that it will be to government's advantage to create equality of opportunity among groups to voice their needs. Failure to do so could jeopardize the democratic image a government tries to further. As pointed out above, interest/pressure groups have a key role in policy-making. Not considering their contributions could undermine the foundation for sound arguments to either promote the passage of a Bill or block its progress. It is to be expected, however, that an unofficial filtering mechanism is in place, e.g. when MPs, Ministers, civil servants etc. will argue with lobbyists or pressure group leaders that a particular proposal is not worth putting on the agenda. In addition, if certain aspects of pressure/interest groups' philosophy are incongruent with a Party's political philosophy (and subversive in nature) it is expected that government officials will exercise judgement and act in a regulatory way in their dealings with such groups.

Nurses as pressure groups

The nursing profession is known for its non-political involvement in British society. Political awareness is also superficial, yet nurses have the potential to utilize their professional skills and knowledge to develop as effective pressure groups. The participation of nurses in health care policy is to be encouraged and is not a new phenomenon. As Burr (1998) argued, when the ICN (International Council of Nurses) was established in the 1890s, it was a 'campaigning organization'. Despite the example of Florence Nightingale and the writings of nursing scholars, stimulating more involvement in politics, to influence health policy, nurses only show 'tokenism' and tentative participation in the policy-making arena.

Nurses can influence policy, according to Christine Hancock, the General Secretary of the Royal College of Nursing (RCN) (News 1998). The pathway to becoming influential in health policy-making is described by Burr (1998) as encompassing the following dimensions:

1. to be professionally responsible by taking an interest in health care policy issues, and becoming participators
2. developing political 'acumen' and 'knowledge'
3. proactivity and the anticipation of broader health issues implications.

In addition to the above, nurses can apply benchmarking techniques to increase their confidence in their communications with government. Comparing their practices with other professionals in health care fields will provide them with a framework to foster purposeful action. The use of evidence-based knowledge can, moreover, accentuate their empowerment. Equally relevant is the promotion of health through sound policy. Participation in policy-making is a professional responsibility, but must be supported by good nursing research (Smith & Watson 1998).

Militant action in combination with negotiating skills is known to be the trademark of pressure groups. In late 1998, the RCM (Royal College of Midwives) showed their 'first sign of new militancy' when thousands of their members marched to 10 Downing Street, to deliver a 90 000 signature petition to the Prime Minister (Gould 1998), in connection with poor pay and a lack of career structure.

When interest groups show militant behaviour, their action soon draws media attention. Public awareness can maximize their pressure activities as the electorate can sympathize with them. A selection of tactics (Box 8.5) can be employed to sway the policy-making process.

For health care professionals, pressure group activities can be improved by accessing the ser-

---

Box 8.5 Pressure tactics

- Communicating with the Community Health Councils, to inform of any professional constraints in clinical practice.
- Lobbying: an organized process which many firms, professional groups, trade unions and charities use (Weetch 1997) to influence policy decisions. Effective lobbying, according to Weetch, must contain the following features:
  - professional approach
  - setting clear objectives which integrate realistically with the whole programme
  - group support and cohesion, with responsibilities to maintain focus
  - to aim at the right target, e.g. health authorities
  - coordination of campaign locally and nationally
  - use of the Commons Health Select Committee (Weetch 1997, Burr 1998)
  - ensure constituents support the cause at grassroots level
  - use MPs' influence
  - provide written cases to policy makers.

---

vices provided by their local Community Health Councils. These councils were set up under the 1973 National Health Service Act. They aim to represent the public interests in the health service. They can influence Health Authority decisions and have been known to delay changes in services and to be supportive to interest groups who are dissatisfied with the standards of service.

Community nurses, who are effective commissioners, are strategically placed to inform interest/pressure groups that will champion their commissioning priorities. Commissioners' monitoring role warrants that shortcomings in the system can be identified (Rowe 1998), with suitable measures executed. On the other hand, the RCN is a powerful agent of change, and will readily support health care professionals in their health policy-making contributions.

LOCAL GOVERNMENT AND POLICY-MAKING

Local government is concerned with the management of local affairs, to be distinguished from central government management, which as we have seen, relates to the core executive and its relationships with Ministers in their Whitehall departments, in the formulation of policies.

Managing 'local affairs' entails the provision of services that affect citizens living in towns, cities and villages. Such services include provisions that are taken for granted, such as the distribution of light, heat, water, gas, street cleaning, education and the management of schools, leisure facilities, fire protection services, ambulance services, health and allotment services. In fact, the term 'local government' applies to 'local politics' and 'local democracy', which have been a feature of the British political system since Anglo-Saxon times (Marr 1995).

The notion of 'local democracy' appertains to people (local government officials: councillors, mayors etc.) at local level who make decisions and participate in policy-making and implementation of public policies that impact on the daily lives of its citizens. Local government officials are therefore active participants in interpreting the directives of central government embodied in legislation, to articulate policies on:

1. the delivery of welfare services: housing, community and public health
2. the organization of libraries, town and country planning
3. protection and security: police, road safety and traffic control
4. trade and industries: transport, buildings, markets.

To supply services and meet local needs, local governments require financial support. They are not autonomous bodies (Elcock 1994, Marr 1995, Peele 1995) and have even been described as the 'creatures of Westminster legislation' (Oliver 1991). Local governments are in many ways dependent on central government to finance their services. As the costs of services increase, more reliance is placed on Westminster to help financially, and to legislate in ways that are true reflections of local needs. Local politics, however, ensure that communities pay local taxes (e.g. community tax), which aid with expenditure on service provision.

Local services can cost approximately £65 billion a year (Sykes 1998). Local authorities are aware of their limitations and can be sensitive to constant criticisms:

- that their management of local affairs lacks skills and are non-responsive to local needs (Peele 1995)
- evidence of wastefulness and incompetence (Marr 1995)
- increased expenditure, which causes increases in levy taxes (Elcock 1994)
- conflictual relationships with non-elected bodies (i.e. businesses, corporations and organizations supplying services on contract) (Painter et al 1997).

In addition, local authorities have had the inclination to adhere to traditional means of service provision, lacking innovation, at the expense of free-market, competitive mechanisms; the perpetuation of being 'providers' rather than 'enablers'.

An enabling local government is seen to be proactive and responsive in a changing competitive market. The diversity of services ensures that standards of service provision are prone to improvement, as businesses and organizations compete to provide services for local authorities. The latter will offer contracts to those corporations that can meet local demands.

RELATIONSHIP AND PARTNERSHIP BETWEEN LOCAL AND CENTRAL GOVERNMENT

Although investigators of local government's role and functions allude to states of *tension* and *conflict* between central and local government, it is nevertheless accurate to observe that without a sense of *partnership*, the policy-making efforts of the central executive will have no impact without the instrumental role of local government in translating policy-making into policy implementation. Local government must hence be recognized as one of the agencies carrying the status of *executor* in the complex equation of policy-making. Working in partnership with central government is liable to cause tension and conflict, which Elcock (1994) identified to be caused by the following factors:

1. central government has a tradition of overseeing 'local affairs'
2. legislation becomes a tool to commit local government to act in statutory ways;
3. legislation ensures compliance in expenditure control as excessive spending in one area of service provision could cause sub-standard services in other areas.

To ensure local government operates within a tight budgetary boundary, in the most reasonably efficient way, there are audit systems in place. It is common practice for all local authorities to have regular finance audits, organized both internally and externally by the Government (Chandler 1991). Furthermore, services must be of high standard. The central executive has statutory powers to investigate local authorities' services, through the deployment of 'central Government Inspectorates' (e.g. Her Majesty's Inspectors of Constabulary and Inspectors Of Schools and Colleges) (Elcock 1994).

In the late 1990s, one finds that the New Labour government, motivated by the ambition to raise local government standards, instigated a 'Best Value' philosophy: another term for value for money. Services provided must befit the high taxes taxpayers contribute. Under this scheme, the duty of councils will be to 'test the market', to guarantee that services delivered are *best* and *safe*, to remain legally unchallenged (Noble 1998). A clear statutory framework has to be devised to protect councils against legal action, a remit which officials in Whitehall's Department of Environment, Transport and Regions would undertake.

In addition to the above, the spectre of central government is reinforcing the concept of 'Beacon Status'; Local authorities that excel will be rewarded. First, they will be awarded 'Beacon Status' by Ministers – guided by an independent panel (Jones & Stewart 1998); secondly, local authorities with this award will gain 'additional powers and freedoms'.

While Councils of Excellence generate competitiveness, and act as role models to other less able authorities, it is argued (Jones & Stewart 1998) that *networks* can be effective in 'disseminating pioneering innovations of individual authorities'. Networking promoted through local government associations via conferencing, professional organizations, political parties etc., can be effective mechanisms in the dissemination of innovative practices (Jones & Stewart 1998).

It is clear from the above discussions that central government utilizes a three-pronged instrumental standpoint:

1. partnership
2. control
3. reward.

The exercise of power by virtue of legislation secures partnership. When services display competencies and distinction as per government performance criteria, a reward system ensures compliance. In this way local authorities perform under the patronage of partnership, by collaboration, control (from central executive oversight) and incentives (reward) for complying and advancing the image of local democratic government as enablers.

Additionally, there is evidence that the relationship is in a state of interdependence. Local governments are dependent on their central partners for their funding regime and for grants. It is pointed out, however (Davies 1998), that Whitehall Ministers aim to minimize the level of financial dependency by 'changing the local government finance system itself'. This necessitates raising the autonomy profile of local government by permitting councils to raise more of their own revenue; an issue which, Davies argued, is positively accepted by the local government associations, as it is compatible with the European Charter of Local Self-Government.

Increasing local authorities' financial autonomy does not signify complete freedom from central constraints. The structures and functions of local institutions are still determined by central authority (Roberts & Hogwood 1997). Local authorities will still have to be accountable to Ministers and their civil servants – who review the legislation frequently – to make sure compliance is achieved (John 1997) and service outcomes are compatible. It is possible for local government to maximize savings, e.g. by adopting some

innovative approaches used in the USA, to tackle the challenges of shrinking resources, while showing commitment to the concept of 'enabling authorities'. Florio and Raschko (1998), in the USA, described the use of the 'Gate-keeper Model' to identify the needs of an ageing population, in particular those individuals most likely to be 'resistant' to accept help or have 'the most problems in accessing help' (Box 8.6 and Case example 8.2).

Box 8.6 Gate-keeper model

This model consists of empowering ordinary citizens in the community by becoming participators in problems identification. Thus a postal worker, a milk deliverer, gas meter readers, bank clerks, shopkeepers etc. can become gate-keepers. Corporations and businesses agree to train their workforce – with the aid of health workers – to become sensitive to their consumers' health status. Their role is to alert health services in their area when they identify a community-dwelling older adult who may be in need of help. Survey has shown that gate-keepers have been able to refer at least 40% of clients, who are not found by more traditional services. Elder services provide gate-keepers training to interested businesses and community organizations at the work site. Training equips gate-keepers with the necessary information to enable them to identify at-risk older adults.

Case example 8.2 Gate-keeper model in practice

A postal worker, trained as a gate-keeper, called elder services regarding an 80-year-old widower. The carrier was concerned because the man looked 'physically run down', his clothes were dirty, he was unshaven and he sat in his chair and stared out of the front window. The carrier had spoken to him earlier and suggested that he get out of the house. The man stated he had seen everything and did not need to go out. On the initial home visit, the elder services staff found that alcohol was a part of the problem and that he was highly suicidal (Florio & Raschko 1998).

Local government is ideally placed (i.e. in their partnership with non-elected agencies in service provision) to encourage social and health services in the organization of training and education for the implementation of gate-keeping.

The prevention of mental and physical deterioration in older adults will lessen the financial burden on social and health services. Moreover, the involvement of citizens in preventative health encourages collaboration and community responsibility in local affairs.

Current trends show that services do not meet demands. Local government resources are already overstretched. One can anticipate that central government, concerned with the improvement of local standards and better expenditure management, is likely to increase its oversight functions (Box 8.7).

The prevailing ethos is now described as 'community governance': the organization of local authorities across boundaries, in partnership with non-elected agencies. Local government has, however, to uphold its responsibility in being the guardian of their citizens' interests.

Box 8.8 Agents in service provision

- Private nursing homes and residential care homes
- Opted out schools (which receive grants from central government) and are out of local authority control
- Privatized companies: water, gas, electricity
- Business Link
- Train Line
- GP fundholders
- Hospital Trusts.

Box 8.7 Other dimensions of central and local government affiliation

- **Non-passive relationships:** two-way processes where reactions and action occur due to legislation between the two parties. Councillors can express discontent and lobby in Parliament via MPs if necessary.
- **Knowledge of local affairs:** community feelings regarding services can be relayed to Parliament. This knowledge of community reactions can act as political levers to persuade Ministers to alter direction.
- **Audit Commission findings:** auditors' reports on local authorities can be utilized to substantiate the rationale for expenditure activities.
- **Relationships with voluntary groups:** it has been shown (Leach & Wilson 1998) that voluntary organizations have important functions in service provision. They have become important allies of decision-makers. Associations with voluntary groups mean that their knowledge of local affairs can be applied to policy-making and in influencing government.
- **Interdependence:** this variable bonds central government with local authorities, and conversely. Can public policies be implemented without the decision-makers at local level? Can central government policy-making gain credibility without local democracy?
- **Prescribed performance output:** one of the aims of the central administration is to maximize services' efficiency. A prescriptive stance tightens local authority performance within the boundaries of legislation. In particular, local agencies are driven to managerial accountability, and budgetary control is a major factor.
- **Local governance:** reforms of local government have weakened their structures due to loss of influence to other bodies (John 1997). The nature of local governance now consists of maintaining equilibrium in terms of 'community leadership' (Painter et al 1997) in relation to other agencies (Box 8.8), which are service deliverers.

Activity 8.2

1. Arrange a visit with your local councillors. Identify their role in policy-making.
2. Talk to your MP. Identify their role in local government affairs and democracy.
3. Select one voluntary organization. How do its members view their relationships with local authorities?
4. Arrange an interview with your Hospital Trust Executive. Find out their role in influencing health policy. Discuss their affiliation with the local authority.
5. Can you identify some pressure groups in your area? Talk to the leaders of the group. Identify the following:
   - their experience in achieving results from using specific strategies
   - their associations with local government, MPs and Whitehall
   - contribution to policy-making.

??? Question 8.2

1. What makes policy-making a complex endeavour?
2. In your view, should there be 'collective responsibility'?
3. Policy-making is dependent on many factors. Can you name them?
4. Why is the Prime Minister a key figure in making policy?
5. Central government is concerned with economic efficiency and high standards of service. What mechanisms are in use to achieve this objective?
6. Do you agree that there is tension and conflict between central and local administration?
7. How important is local government in policy-making.
8. Explain the role of Parliament in policy-making.
9. What avenues can health care professionals use to influence health policy?

SUMMARY

Policy-making is a complex process which demands the attention of politicians at all levels. It also affects the daily lives of citizens. The core executive refers to the nucleus of central government functioning. The Prime Minister and Cabinet colleagues are at the hub of decision-making. Consensus in policy-making decisions applies to the notion of 'collegial responsibility'. Policy-making and decision-making are subjected to many internal and external influences. For example, Ministers, civil servants and pressure groups can all influence public policies. In addition, Parliament has an oversight function to ensure 'fair play'; that policies are democratically formulated. The role of local government is relevant to both policy-making and implementation. Social change has meant that local authorities have had to be innovative in their approaches to provide efficient services. It is now a common trend to access the skills and expertise of private agencies by local government in delivering welfare.

GLOSSARY

Bills   a draft prepared by Ministers and their departments containing proposals for a new law
Constituencies   an area or region with voters (electorate, constituents) who have a representative in Parliament
Globalization   trends in economic, political, social and cultural developments
Liberal societies   democratic States which practise free expressions, liberty and human rights
Lobbyist   a representative of an interest/pressure group who will make necessary arrangements to present the group's case

Manifesto   a political Party's policy aims and declaration prior to election, which they declare to the nation
Populism   the political principle of attracting ordinary citizens' support
Pragmatism   a practical approach
Whip   a political Party member in Parliament who has a management role in ensuring Parliamentary discipline
Whitehall   government offices and departments in London

REFERENCES

Ainsworth S H 1997 The role of legislators in the determination of interest group influence. Legislative Studies Quarterly 22(4): 517–531

Binyon M 1998 On the privatisation pioneer who won friends in the West. The Times 19 October, p 15

Bomberg E, Peterson J 1998 European Union decision-making: the role of subnational authorities. Political Studies 46(2): 219–235

Britannica 1992 Political parties and interest groups, 15th edn. University of Chicago Press, vol 25: Chicago, p 986

Burr S 1998 Making waves. Nursing Management 5(6): 8–11

Chandler J A 1991 Local government today. Manchester University Press, Manchester

Davies R W 1998 DETR does u-turn on funding regime. Local Government Chronicle 6826: 1

Dudley G, Richardson J 1998 Arenas without rules and the policy change process: outside groups and British roads policy. Political Studies 46(4): 727–747

Elcock H 1994 Local government; policy and management in local authorities, 3rd edn. Routledge, London

Florio E R, Raschko R 1998 The gate-keeper model: implications for social policy. Journal of Aging and Social Policy 10(1): 37–55

Garner R, Kelly R 1998 British political parties today, 2nd edn. Manchester University Press, Manchester

Gould M 1998 March of the midwives. Nursing Times 94(43): 16–17

Hill M 1997 Understanding social policy, 5th edn. Blackwell, Oxford

Hill M, Bramley G 1986 Analysing social policy. Blackwell, Oxford

Hogwood B W 1997a The machinery of government 1979–1997. Political Studies 45(4): 704–715

Hogwood P 1997b Executive government. In: Roberts G K, Hogwood P (eds) European politics today. Manchester University Press, Manchester, p 158–188

Hood C, James O 1997 The central executive. In: Dunleavy P, Gamble A, Holiday I, Peele G (eds) Developments in British politics. MacMillan, Basingstoke, p 177–202

John P 1997 Local governance. In: Dunleavy P, Gamble A, Holliday I, Peele G (eds) Developments in British politics. MacMillan, Basingstoke

Jones G, Stewart J 1998 Build networks, not beacons. Local Government Chronicle 6824: 8

Katsuragi S 1997 Better working conditions won by 'nurse wave' action: Japanese nurses' experience of getting a new law by their militant action campaign. Nursing Ethics: an International Journal for Healthcare Professionals 4(4): 313–322

King A 1993 Cabinet coordination or prime ministerial dominance? A conflict of three principles of cabinet government. In: Budge I, McKay D (eds) The developing British system: the 1990s, 3rd edn. Longman, London, p 52–65

Kingdom J 1991 Government and politics in Britain. Polity Press, Cambridge

Leach S, Wilson D 1998 Voluntary groups and local authorities: rethinking the relationship. Local Government Studies 24(2): 1–18

Levin P 1997 Making social policy: the mechanisms of government and politics, and how to investigate them. Open University Press, Buckingham

Marr A 1995 Ruling Britannia. Penguin, London

Nairne P 1997 Editorial: the next government: agenda for the Civil Service. Public Policy and Administration 12(1): 1–7

Neunreither K 1998 Governance without opposition: the case of the European Union. Government and Opposition 33(4): 419–441

News 1998 Nurses can influence policy, says Hancock. Paediatric Nursing 10(8): 4

Noble L 1998 Best value shirkers face legal challenge. Local Government Chronicle 6824: 1

Norton P 1997 Parliamentary oversight. In: Dunleavy P, Gamble A, Holliday I, Peele G (eds) Developments in British politics. MacMillan, Basingstoke, p 155–176

Nownes A J, Freeman P 1998 Interest group activity in the States. Journal of Politics 60(1): 86–112

Oliver D 1991 Government in the United Kingdom. Open University Press, Milton Keynes

Oliver D 1997 Regulating the conduct of MPs. The British experience of combating corruption. Political Studies 45(3): 539–558

Painter C, Isaac-Henry K, Rouse J 1997 Local authorities and non-elected agencies: strategic responses and organizational networks. Public Administration 75: 225–245

Peele G 1995 Governing the UK. Blackwell, Oxford

Peele G 1997 Political parties. In: Dunleavy P, Gamble A, Holliday I, Peele G (eds) Developments in British politics. MacMillan, Basingstoke, p 89–109

Punnett R M 1994 British government and politics, 6th edn. Dartmouth Publishing, Aldershot, p 141–162

Read M 1993 The place of Parliament. In: Budge I, McKay D (eds) The developing British political system: the 1990s, 3rd edn. Longman, London, p 66–82

Riddell R 1998 Parliament under pressure. Victor Gollanz, London

Roberts G K, Hogwood P 1997 European politics today. Manchester University Press, Manchester

Rowe J 1998 Primary opportunity. Health Visitor 71(2): 49

Smith J P, Watson R 1998 Conference report: the leading edge. Journal of Advanced Nursing 28(3): 686–690

Sykes R 1998 Promoting local government research. Social Sciences 39: 5

Talbot C 1997 UK Civil Service personnel reform: devolution, decentralisation and delusion. Public Policy and Administration 12(4): 14–34

The Times 1998a Unfinished revolution: the need for progressives to be populist. The Times 19 October, p 21

The Times 1998b Betrayal of the working class. The Times 19 October, p 17

Theakston K 1998 New Labour, New Whitehall? Public Policy and Administration 13(1): 13–34

Watson R 1998a The Labour revolution must go on forever, says Blair guru. The Times 17 October, p 1

Watson R 1998b Sultan of spin comes out of the shadows. The Times 17 October, p 10

Weetch K 1997 Learning to lobby. Health Visitor 70(12): 446

Wilding P 1997 Globalisation, regionalism and social policy. Social Policy and Administration 31(4): 410–428

Yishai Y 1998 The guardian state: a comparative analysis of interest group regulation. Governance: an International Journal of Policy and Administration 11(2): 153–176

FURTHER READING

Beyme V K 1998 Interest groups in the German Bundestag. Government and Opposition 33(1): 38–55

Cohen P 1997 Campaigning for the future. Health Visitor 70(11): 407

Edwards J 1998 Policy-making as organised irresponsibility: the case of public conveniences. Policy and Politics 26(3): 307–319

Fenwick J, Bailey M 1998 Decentralisation and re-organisation in local government. Public Policy and Administration 13(2): 26–37

Knoepfel P, Kissling-Näf I 1998 Social learning in policy networks. Policy and Politics 26(3): 343–367

Rao N 1998 The recruitment of representatives in British local government: pathways and barriers. Policy and Politics 26(3): 291–306

Smith M J 1998 Reconceptualizing the British State: theoretical and conceptual challenges to central government. Public Administration: an International Quarterly 76(1): 45–72

Sperling L 1998 Public services, quangos and women: a concern for local government. Public Administration 76(3): 471–487

Taylor-Gooby P 1998 'Things can only get better'. Expectations and the welfare state. Policy and Politics 26(4): 472–475

Inequalities in health

9

The Green Paper 'Our Healthier Nation' (1998) has reaffirmed the Government commitment to confront major issues in connection with health inequalities. On their agenda is a list of suggested alternative approaches to narrow the health inequalities gap. The aims of this chapter are to:

- **expose the features of health inequalities**
- **identify the vulnerable groups in society**
- **discuss the factors which predispose to health inequalities**
- **emphasize the roles and responsibilities of agencies in developing effective strategies to meet needs.**

There are many disadvantaged groups in society. Very often their disadvantages are due to structural factors (i.e. the way society is organized), although some critics will argue that individual responsibility is also a factor. 'Structural factors' include the nature of organizations, their functions and loopholes in the systems which perpetuate inequalities, such as:

- the inequality of employment opportunities
- the inequality of access to good housing
- the inequality of access to welfare services
- the inequality of health care provision.

Health inequalities are caused by a combination of these determinants, which help to construct socio-economic depression in groups vulnerable to their deprived personal circumstances.

Other variables have been defined as causes of health inequalities:

- Social class
- Gender status
- Age, i.e. youth and ageing
- Family status, e.g. lower status families (unskilled, semi-skilled workers living in deprived areas) are more prone to ill-health. Their low financial status is a key to some families' deprived living conditions.
- Ethnicity and race: despite legislation which aims at ensuring racial equality, differences have been noted pertaining to access to treatment and care provision.

Shrinking resources in the health and social care fields can be expected to worsen health inequalities. Clinical staff in the British health system have for a number of years been concerned with rationing in health care, although the present Labour Health Minister, Frank Dobson, refutes the argument that there is health rationing. Funding injection is on the Government's agenda and evidence shows that expenditure on health is on the increase. Nevertheless, health care systems resources are finite (Mangan 1994), and demands for health care provision, Mangan pointed out, are infinite. Unless constructive measures are implemented, inequalities in health will continue to be perennial. Some causes of inequalities in health will now be discussed.

SOCIAL CLASS

Since the beginning of humankind, people have been classified into groups according to their social, occupational, economic and psychological status. Studies in anthropology (Béphage 1997) have shown that in the most distant non-Western countries, group affiliation is founded on kinship, traditions, cultural practices and economic status. In Britain, similar structures are evident, because of its multi-ethnic and multiracial society. While a classless society is the vision of many ambitious government officials and social leaders, the fact remains that Britain has many class systems (Box 9.1).

Box 9.1 Class systems (social grade)

A: higher managerial, administrative or professional
B: intermediate managerial, administrative or professional
C1: supervisory or clerical and junior managerial, administrative or professional
C2: skilled manual workers
D: semi- and unskilled manual
E: State pensioners or widows (no other earners), casual or lowest grade workers or long-term unemployed (Central Statistics Office 1998).

Differences in health status, based on social class, have been uncovered in many societies (Vagero 1995). For instance, the working classes are more prone to ill-health than the middle classes. The correlation between death rates and occupational status is widely recognized; there is a persistent gap in mortality rates and health differences between manual and non-manual classes (Health of the Nation 1991). Moreover, it is accepted that structural factors (poverty, unemployment, poor housing and a polluted environment) are determinants of health (Dèpartment of Health 1998). Poor manual workers are liable to develop illnesses; they are very often under-employed, and become unemployed due to poor health status. Their financial deprivation entails a predisposition to live in sub-standard housing, in deprived areas where discrimination is rife, and crime rates and the likelihood of environmental pollution are high. All these determinants empower the cycle of deprivation, which escalates the effects of health inequalities and burdens the already overtaxed resources of local authorities and health authorities. It has therefore become the mission of successive governments to promote healthy living, to improve the health of disadvantaged communities and to narrow the health gap (New NHS Modern And Dependable 1997, Our Healthier Nation 1998).

Turrell (1998) suggested that health inequalities can be attributed to socio-economic group differences in their dietary behaviours; for example, lack of purchasing power leads to consumption of sub-standard food. As indicated above, the socio-economically disadvantaged have less access to health care. This could partly explain their lack of knowledge concerning healthy eating. Further, traditional habits acquired through primary socialization can perpetuate negative health behaviours.

Families trapped in the culture of deprivation struggle to make ends meet. Community economic hardship is also connected with low birth weight (Roberts 1997): when mothers cannot afford nutritious food, this will have implications for the nutritional status of the newborn.

SOCIO-ECONOMIC STATUS

It can be deduced from the above that class status is associated with economic status. Good health can improve one's socio-economic position, as the individual is better able to participate competitively in the job market. The likelihood of increasing one's life chances is therefore greater. Social mobility can thereafter be anticipated to rise, while poor health can become an obstacle to progressive social mobility (Healy 1998).

Socio-economic status is linked with psychological status. Henderson et al (1998) reported that schizophrenia in the socio-economically deprived reduces opportunities to achieve social mobility. A negative life trajectory can precipitate the onset of schizophrenia or worsen it as the affected person becomes exposed to life stressors. Since schizophrenia fragments the personality, social isolation is often one of the features to be observed. This has the effect of increasing mental health inequalities.

Mental health services often report cases which prove that the socially excluded (the unemployed, single people, the poor and homeless with no social and psychological support) are inclined to be regular users of psychiatric resources. Poverty, which remains the scourge of social life throughout the world, remains at the base of many health inequalities.

The measurement of poverty, according to Locker et al (1996), is sometimes undertaken by assessing household income as an indicator of economic status. Thus one can compare the revenues of a semi-skilled worker with an office clerk. How they budget and prioritize the purchasing of essential commodities (food, clothing,

heating etc.) and the quality of the products acquired could provide data on the extent of poverty.

The government document 'Our Healthier Nation' emphasizes that the link between poverty and ill-health is clear. Besides, other variables that sometimes accompany poverty, such as learning disabilities, accentuate variations in health gradients. It is posited, for example, that women with learning disabilities 'are being excluded from breast and cervical screening programmes' (McMillan 1998). To be poor and female with learning disabilities increases health inequalities. It is an issue that feminist investigators have debated over the years. In the field of physical health, health trends (Box 9.2) show that the poorer classes are more likely to die of coronary heart disease. The unskilled worker in comparison with the senior executive is more predisposed to developing heart disease (Van den Bergh 1998).

Box 9.2 Class difference in coronary heart disease

The social class V, manual workers of working age, was found to have 25% higher risk of developing coronary heart disease than those among professional men (social class I) in the 1970s. The gap had widened to a 'threefold' difference in the 1990s (Van den Bergh 1998).

GENDER AND MENTAL HEALTH

It is argued that both men and women experience roughly 'equal rates' of major psychiatric conditions as currently identified in the literature (Frank et al 1998). How mental health workers perceive the differences between men and women could, however, influence objectivity. Historical attitudes toward what constitutes feminine and masculine behaviours are still partly to blame. Despite major leaps in women's position in society, which disproves the historical view that they are 'inferior' to men and that their place is 'in the home', evidence shows that traditional stereotyping and labelling prevail. Frank et al postulated that 'psychological theories of gender difference', which denote the 'masculine as norm' and the 'feminine as variant', have contributed to the process of prejudicial attitudes to women. Moreover, as discussed in Chapter 5, there are other factors (social, environmental, attitudes and beliefs) which engender differences in health among men and women. For example, women's often subordinate social role-play, their perceptions of their identity in relation to men's and their relationships with men play a part in affecting social and mental well-being.

In the 1990s one finds that the mental health professions report increasing contact with women suffering from mental illness (Hunt 1998). Arguments for this trend rest on assumptions that a Victorian psychiatric model continues to be predominant: that women may have a 'madness gene'. However, more plausible causes are given for the variations in health:

1. women compared with men are more communicative about their health problems, which has the effect of aiding health workers to define more accurately signs of mental illness
2. women are realistically exposed to tangible life stressors: rape, sexual harassment, family violence, the ill-effects of childhood abuse, which surface in adulthood.

These psychosocial factors, and women's specific responses to them, entail that their needs can be specific or unique and, as Hunt (1998) argued, 'related to their gender and position in society'. While women have traditionally been seen as being 'different' to men, one should also be conscious that gender-specific health inequalities can impact on their psychosocial well-being. Women's life experiences can be markedly different in many ways. Case example 9.1 shows how a black, lone mother's experiences of parenthood can adversely affect health. Popay and Jones (1990) pointed out that women and men who are lone parents are vulnerable groups and will continue to be at risk.

Case example 9.1 illustrates the daily experiences of many ethnic and non-ethnic mothers in the UK. However, when a person is black, female and a single parent, feminist writers have argued that their life chances are minimized. Their

Case example 9.1 Sonia

Sonia came to the UK from the island of Mauritius. She got married at the age of 29 to a British citizen. They had two children. Ten years later they got divorced. Sonia now lives in a three bedroomed accommodation with her children. Their father does not pay alimony. Sonia relies on her part-time occupation and some support from the Benefits Agency. When her children are sick she stays at home. Her manager at work complains that she is not 'pulling her weight'. When she goes home she feels depressed, isolated and hopeless. Her children try to help with the housework. At school, her children's teacher has reported that they look uninterested, sleepy and anaemic. They get bullied by other children and are victims of racist comments. Sonia has herself had to deal with racism on the estates. She feels the area is unsafe for the children and herself, yet she cannot afford to live somewhere else.

psychosocial well-being suffers too. The burden of racism, poverty, and lack of financial and emotional support for the children from fathers (Song & Edwards 1997) worsen health inequalities. Faced with socio-economic dilemmas and combining mothering responsibilities with economic roles (Randall 1996) can prove psychologically demanding. Not surprisingly, many women develop mental ill-health.

For both men and women who are in poverty, however, epidemiological studies have shown that they are predisposed to mental disorders. Beside poverty, the feelings of exploitation and powerlessness are causative factors (Albee & Ryan 1998). Living in deprived regions (where the rate of unemployment is high) with absent social and emotional support adds to the stress factor. Some researchers (Lewis & Sloggett 1998) have pointed out that unemployment could lead to alienation from the rest of society and that suicide is common among unemployed people.

A person's family environment is rarely considered in the assessment of health inequalities. In addition to material deprivation, family culture and conflicts with parent(s) have been linked to lower self-esteem, poorer psychological well-being and more biological symptoms among females (Sweeting & West 1995).

The quality of family life in adolescence can be an indicator of physical and psychological well-being in adulthood (Sweeting & West 1995). Further, women's role as caregivers in communities with shrinking resources can have a negative impact on their psychological well-being, caused by 'caregiver burden and strain' (Harrison 1998). The environmental influences on women's caring (Wuest 1997) is another dimension to be evaluated in relation to health inequalities.

Survivors of abusive relationships (e.g. homeless battered women) are distinct groups with specific needs. An investigation of health inequalities in society should encompass this vulnerable group. Studies have shown that women in abusive relationships suffer deep psychological and physical trauma (Clarke et al 1997).

Activity 9.1

Using the following headings: Social, Psychological, Physical, compile a list of problems deprived communities can experience.

AGE

CHILDREN

In spite of constant media portrayal of children as a disempowered group, and wide coverage in medical, nursing and law literature, this group remains highly vulnerable as targets of health inequalities.

In the home environment regular accidents (e.g. burns, scalds, poisoning) occur due to poor parental supervision. Outside the home, bicycle accidents are the most common cause of head injuries (Clayton 1998). At a higher level of society, it is pointed out that regardless of the fact that children represent 25% of the population, the House of Commons very rarely debate on children's issues (Burr 1998). Children's rights as human beings are persistently being violated. Abusive relationships in and outside the home, parental conflicts and family violence are some of the sources of health inequalities.

On a less dramatic scale, research findings suggest that children who belong to families where smoking is the norm are at risk of developing long-term lifestyle diseases, such as cardiovascular failure (Burke et al 1998).

A fragmented family structure (i.e. children who do not live with both parents or are parentless) causes lower self-esteem, health and educational difficulties (Baumer et al 1998). The same researchers found that children with social disadvantage and suffering from diabetes tend to have higher admission rates, which suggests frequent episodes of severe hypoglycaemia or greater reliance on health care support.

Other research findings have drawn attention to increasing rates of hospital admissions in children (Stewart et al 1998), which may be an indicator of increasing morbidity (Doughty 1998). It has been reported that children with a high deprivation score become regular users of accident and emergency facilities. While family culture can impact adversely on children's holistic well-being, Burr (1998) argued that professional help for those children is not 'always designed' to meet their health needs. However, when initial intervention takes place, follow-up services are inadequate. Studies have shown (Swanston et al 1997) that children who had been sexually abused exhibited signs of depression, were more prone to self-injury and expressed suicidal thoughts even years later, compared to their peers. Adequate preparation to identify this group is needed, with a long-term commitment to care (Brown 1998). Hunter (1998a) mooted that services can disempower children in care; i.e. structural factors such as

- reduced human resources
- care plan management failures
- deficient central recording that generates care loopholes
- failures in identifying vulnerable groups.

Under these circumstances, health inequalities can be expected to reproduce.

Children's world view can easily be manipulated by environmental images: posters on tobacco advertising and alcohol, 'soaps' programmes; marketing of goods such as 'bra top and lycra leggings which turn toddlers into mini madonnas' (Lestor 1993). Imposing sexual imagery on children at an early age can promote precocious sexual behaviour and teenage pregnancies in later years. Other issues relate to an underestimation of post-traumatic stress disorder in children (Davies & Flannery 1998); in particular, in children exposed to community violence, e.g. children of war-torn Ireland who are either victims of violence and/or witnesses of atrocities. Davies and Flannery explained that the effects of traumatic events are deep: fears, hopelessness, pessimism, flashbacks and nightmares can cause severe psychological disturbance. Inability to recognize these manifestations as after-effects of community violence widen the health inequalities gap.

Activity 9.2

1. Do a literature search on 'effects of war on children'.
2. In small groups of 10, discuss issues related to factors that maintain children's vulnerable position in society.
3. On your paediatric placements, make a list of the causes of admissions of children in your care. Can you extricate any social and/or psychological reasons for their admission in addition to biological factors?

OLDER PEOPLE

In Chapter 4, the fact that older people in a variety of social settings can be exposed to adverse circumstances was discussed. Although life expectancy is increasing, which correlates with increasing numbers of elderly, how to deal with this group is now becoming a challenging issue to policy makers and government. Newspapers, banking organizations and broadcasters on television and radio constantly remind consumers that urgent steps must be taken to organize private pension provision for retirement, because State pensions will no longer be available to future pensioners.

Many pensioners in the late twentieth century suffer health inequalities. There are numerous older adults in employment who are reaping the

harvest of an early childhood culture of deprivation: poverty, multiple pathology; abuse; discrimination; social isolation, mental health problems and lack of access to health care. It is accepted that there are many health care challenges for the next decade (Joint Committee of Professional Nursing, Midwifery and Health Visiting Associations 1997), and meeting the health needs of growing numbers of sick and frail elderly is one of them. With ageing, one can anticipate changing disease patterns and multiple pathology.

As the older person's health needs are multiple, increases in expenditure are expected. Health and social services resources are envisaged to respond to high demands. This economic dependency was predicted as far back as the late 1980s (Falkingham 1989), which has important implications for social and economic policy. It is argued (Irwin 1996) that the age structure changes are a cause of inequality. Contemporary society is changing, and the older person has higher expectations and is becoming more assertive. For instance, older people are aware of existing inequalities which concern them:

- ageism
- unfair resource distribution that predisposes to poverty
- conflict in welfare services over resource distribution between the young and the old
- the caring role of the older person: old, informal carers have unmet needs.

The burden of caring increases with age, as tasks become more complex. The old represent a vulnerable group in society who would benefit from the 'gate-keeper model' of intervention described in Chapter 8.

The multi-ethnic nature of British society means that there are now diverse ethnic groups of aged individuals whose needs are often misinterpreted and misunderstood. Consequently, the gap between specific health needs and specific interventions widens. More research is needed to acquire sensitive insight into the health behaviours of the older ethnic population.

Studies in the USA have shown that marked differences have been noted in the level of mental health between African-American and white subjects (Kim et al 1998). Differences in perception regarding health issues between the groups have also been identified. One important finding of the research suggests that the living environment of the subjects studied is correlated with mental well-being. Segregation, racism and discrimination are factors engendering tension and conflict precipitating health problems.

The personal circumstances of targeted groups (in need of support) need analysing. It has already been established that inequalities in health are nurtured by socio-economic status and personal life pathways (Blank & Diderichsen 1996).

Early life experiences – childhood culture, occupational status, exposure to adverse environmental conditions – in combination with ageing process effects, deepens the level of dependency. Inequalities in health in adulthood have been consistent, and have somehow been taken as 'unproblematic or left unexplored' (Ford et al 1994).

Once the older person adopts the new status of 'pensioner', assumptions are made that State benefits will solve their financial problems. Poverty in old age is not uncommon. Savings impairment caused by unemployment in earlier years (as applied to many older persons) and the effects of early retirement (Davey 1998) disempower the retiree. Moreover, other dimensions of poverty with psychological implications are issues which interest health workers:

• the poverty of relationships
• the social isolation that old age brings (due to loss and bereavement)
• the poverty of self-actualization. While many aged individuals resort to self-fulfilment activities – painting, writing, travels, sculpture, sports etc. – many others are disabled by physical and psychological ailments, as well as an inability to obtain the services they need.

The provision of services has become a major health issue for policy makers throughout the world. The problem of long-term care for elderly people and how to fund the services (Davey 1998) is the focus of major debates in community health care. According to the Department of Health (1996), the residential care population comprises of 500 000 residents, and approximately one million are consumers of day and domiciliary services. Further taxing of resources would be expected, with subsequent negative effects on those already facing health inequalities.

There is a growing number of homeless older people who roam the streets and live in cardboard boxes. Commonly referred to as vagrants because of their lifestyle, they often go unrecognized. In sociological terms they form the 'underclass' group of the class systems. Their needs are varied, their problems are multiple. They are liable to self-neglect and mental health problems. They may resort to drug-taking and heavy alcohol consumption. The purchasing of hard drugs is a possibility, and working for drug traffickers in the underworld is a perspective that is unexplored, underestimated and not fully recognized. Research is therefore recommended in this area, as the findings will assist policy makers to achieve objectives set by the European Union to coordinate international action against drugs (European Union in Action Against Drugs 1997).

Furthermore, older people are often victims of crime, which generates fear among the aged (Hamlyn 1998). There is a high prevalence of older people who feel prisoners in their own homes. Consequently, social isolation can compound physical and mental deterioration, with fragmentation of informal support. The quality of the environment – including housing standards – can worsen the burden of coping with life stressors.

Activity 9.3

1. Discuss with the YMCA manager issues that concern the homeless community.
2. Talk with the community psychiatric nurse, and find out the prevalence of mental health problems among the older homeless adults.
3. Ask your general practitioner to provide quantitative data on the number of old people with multiple pathology, an estimate of those who are socio-economically deprived and the number of clients with drug dependence.

??? Question 9.1

1. Why is the older person vulnerable?
2. How should social and health services view the needs of the elderly?
3. How will research help policy makers combat health inequalities among the old?

ETHNICITY

Equality of services in the NHS is being regarded as an inaccurate concept when ethnicity issues are being discussed. The way the NHS is structured prevents the promotion of health equality (Fletcher 1997). Misconceived ideas can perpetuate inequality. For example, to argue that someone's culture is responsible for the causation of illness can be inaccurate when other dimensions are ignored.

Ethnic groups are not always regular users of health and social services. This has implications for health workers' interventions. A low ethnic profile could be interpreted as 'all must be well' if it is believed that their extended families are coping with health problems in traditional ways.

As pointed out in Chapter 6, racism is a major instigator of ill-health in the equation of health inequalities among ethnic groups (Fig. 9.1). Similar to their white counterparts, many ethnic groups experience socio-economic deprivation, and often live in overcrowded conditions in tenement housing, which is not conducive to good health.

Although better awareness of ethnic groups' health needs is being developed, Fletcher (1997) pointed out that little policy implementation has occurred. Evidence shows that black people have poor access to supportive health services (Butt 1997). While there are agencies in operation to cater for ethnic groups, Butt argued that Afro-Caribbean women are not able to access those services. In the field of mental health counselling, few agencies show responsibility in this area.

Unless individuals' care needs are analysed using research data, one can argue that service provision will remain incongruent. Tokenism is

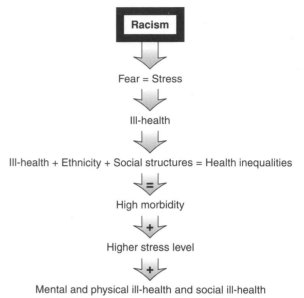

Fig. 9.1 The possible consequences of racism on the individual.

not an option that will combat the health inequalities of ethnic groups. Those who receive treatment via the mental health services can also be 'overtreated'. Butt (1997), alluding to some studies, commented that blacks compared to whites are more likely to be over tranquillized, to receive more intramuscular injections and to have more frequent electro-convulsive therapy.

A recent study (Koffman et al 1997) in a population of 3710 adult acute and 268 low-level, secure patients (Table 9.1) showed that in a 1-day survey in North and South Thames regions, a high proportion of the black community were admitted to a psychiatric unit.

Table 9.1 Ethnic origin of psychiatric inpatients in North and South Thames in a 1-day period in 1997

	Total no. of patients	
Ethnic origin	Acute psychiatric wards	Low-level psychiatric wards
White	2978 (83%)	182 (6.1%)
Black	631 (16%)	66 (10.5%)
Asian	160 (4%)	5 (3.1%)
Total	3710	268

Koffman et al also found

- an excessive use of the Mental Health Act (1983) to admit black patients compulsorily (63.5%) compared with 38.8% of Asian and 30.6% of white patients
- 10.5% of black patients were nursed in low-level, secure wards compared with 3.1% of all Asians and 6.1% of all white patients
- more black patients and Asians were diagnosed with schizophrenia.

The researchers argued that life circumstances could be ascribed to this high prevalence, such as poverty, biological causes, genetic influences and racism in psychiatry.

Further studies revealed that a high prevalence of second-generation, UK-born black Caribbean patients are dissatisfied with mental health services (Parkman et al 1997). Parkman et al concluded, from their sample of 50, that black Caribbeans may feel 'marginalized' from mainstream society. Further, the *frequency* of admission could be interpreted as a construct of victimization, bullying and discrimination, which has the aftermath of negative views of mental health services.

It should be noted, however, that in sociological parlance, statutory institutions are classified as 'agencies of social control'. When the exercise of power is targeted at vulnerable groups that are already feeling discriminated against, not surprisingly, levels of dissatisfaction are anticipated to elevate. On the other hand, as media coverage of the Steven Lawrence case in the late 1990s showed, institutional racism is a social fact. Wider social issues in relation to racism and discrimination can undermine ethnic groups' confidence in institutions designed to confront the very health problems they experience.

These constraints, which nurture psychological problems, relentlessly potentiate health inequalities. The contextual issues associated with ethnic minorities' needs have to be addressed (Gerrish 1997) in the fight against inequalities. Just as important is to widen the dimensions of ethnicity to encompass the Irish, Welsh and Scottish minorities, and other races within UK culture.

Activity 9.4

During your mental health placement, collect data on ethnic groups' rate of admissions by using case records, and by talking to the multidisciplinary team.

??? Question 9.2

1. What do you consider to be the main causes of a high prevalence of psychiatric admissions in ethnic groups?
2. In view of the findings described above, do you think that 'bad behaviour' is interpreted as 'mad behaviour'?
3. The researchers argued that blacks' behaviour is seen to be 'aggressive' and 'violent'. What could be the possible reasons for this?
4. Another finding suggests that second-generation Afro-Caribbeans are more critical of mental health services. Can you offer reasons for this?

SOCIAL SYSTEM FAILURES

In Section 1, allusion was made to society as a set of systems with specific functions. We also found that sociologists who use this perspective call themselves 'functionalists', and they believe that society functions in accordance with set rules, without 'conflict'. In reality, it is a social fact that the social system can fail many of its citizens. In the process, health inequalities are produced and reproduced.

What has been discussed so far in the previous paragraphs is a reflection of failures in the social structures that have caused numerous groups in society to be disadvantaged.

The political system is the machinery that can control or perpetuate inequalities. One finds that the Government's agenda in 1997 comprises the promotion of public health to reduce health inequalities (Munro 1997). There is also the argument that health service and social care agencies are in need of closer collaboration. The Secretary of State explained that the Department of Health mainstream functions are to tackle health inequalities (Munro 1997). The fact that health inequalities are rife proves that the present and past political systems are not achieving their objectives of guaranteeing health equality.

Financial status is another issue policy makers are concerned with. Although a national minimum wage is now established, critics argue that the health of the underprivileged will not necessarily improve. Similarly, although better occupational status is believed to improve socio-economic status, the wider dimensions (discussed above) as they affect the individual must be analysed and improved.

The role of local government in improving public health is being recognized. However, according to the Secretary of State for Health (Munro 1997) this basic responsibility has not been fully given. Moreover, a conflictual relationship between local authorities and health authorities have led to a fragmentation of their public health role. For example, integration between hospital and community services is lacking (Sims 1998). It has also been pointed out that local government, which has the potential to be a powerful player in public health, has 'lacked strategic' direction since 1974 (Reid 1997).

Since the Conservative's Community Care Act (1990), the complexity of the legislation is affecting some vulnerable groups in the community. Coombs (1998) reported how older disabled people and their carers are encountering difficulties to 'obtain well-informed support'. Inefficiency in local authorities' care plans to meet the needs of those with HIV has also been identified (Nicholson 1997).

Since many underprivileged groups rely on benefits agencies for support, it is acknowledged that the latter are failing in their responsibilities. The Commons Public Accounts Committee has discovered management failures due to £3 billion lost in fraud and errors (Community Care 1998). Additionally, the credibility of agencies is undermined by their inability to assess needs accurately, and for providing a stigmatized service.

INDIVIDUAL RESPONSIBILITY

Criticisms against social structures as causes of health inequalities can mask the potential of individuals to engender their own health inequalities by the decisions they make in managing their lives. People who choose to live in rural areas, for example, may become 'invisible' to health agencies. In a BBC Radio 4 interview on 26 November 1998, Dr Cox stated that rural poverty exists. While urban poverty receives much publicity, the poor and those in need of health intervention in the rural areas may be neglected.

It is often assumed that homelessness is caused by a society's inability to cater for those in need of housing. There are many homeless people who choose a nomadic lifestyle, sleeping rough, for personal reasons. Similarly, there are individuals who choose to remain unemployed. They may find that State benefits are sufficient, or rely on informal networks for support. Others make token applications: giving the impression that they are actively seeking employment so that they continue receiving benefits (Sheehan & Tomlinson 1998). On the other hand, Sheehan and Tomlinson pointed out, when job seekers fail to demonstrate 'motivational' behaviour and 'ability', employers are inclined to reject them. Their decisions may be founded on the applicants' duration of unemployment, which they argue indicates evidence of motivation or lack of it.

A healthy lifestyle is also dependent on one's socio-cultural beliefs and the degree of ethnocentric attitude. Strict adherence to traditional practices directs a person's choice of what constitutes acceptable health behaviours, e.g. in spite of health education information, dietary habits remain unaltered. To comply with medical instructions may be interpreted as rejecting traditional healers' recommendations. To some, attending the out patient clinics is alien. They may go instead to a Shaman, community leader, or a mosque.

Many Westerners are aware that an unhealthy diet will affect their health. A high prevalence of obesity and atherosclerosis shows that their lifestyle is not compatible with healthy living.

Some people engage in leisure and occupational activities that are dangerous to health, such as car racing, boxing and mountaineering. Others make decisions to pursue criminal careers that bring them in constant conflict with law makers.

STRATEGIES, TARGETS, RESPONSIBILITIES AND POLICIES

Research

Promoting research in health promotion to combat inequality is recommended (Millar 1998). The deep-rooted nature of health inequalities demands a multi dimensional strategy, to ensure that diverse variables are scrutinized. Research should become a major component of policy. Although many research papers have established evidence in the correlation between socio-economic disadvantage and negative lifestyle with poor health, there is a lack of research on strategies that can enable individuals to adopt a healthier lifestyle. An identification of 'disadvantaged pathways' at critical periods is suggested. Researchers, however, have to be eclectic in their methods of investigation. Quantitative methods, although useful, do not provide the richness and insight of qualitative approaches; yet it is imperative to obtain the views and reports of the life experiences of the subjects under investigation. Hence, phenomenology becomes a relevant tool in research. Comparative research is another perspective to be developed. Comparing and analysing research findings nationally and internationally allows researchers to be critical about their results, thus giving reasons to refine their research tactics.

Health focus

Regardless of advances in medical and health care philosophy, it is argued that, in the late 1990s, focus on illness is still evident (Peckham et al 1998), and most common in general practice (Case example 9.2).

The NHS is seen to apply a medical model of care at the expense of broader social dimensions. Primary care, Peckham et al (1998) pointed out, has had a 'general practice' focus, whereas the true nature of public health is within the wide framework of environmental health, and includes a community, its people and how their lives are guided by broad social policies – policies that can either constrain or liberate 'public health as a resource'. The circumstances of a

Case example 9.2 Medical focus

Mrs White, aged 80, had been coughing for the past two weeks. Her neighbour took her to the general practitioner. Her GP told her: 'It is common at this time of the year. Let me listen to your chest. Yes, just what I thought. You have got flu, and bronchitis. I will prescribe some tablets. You can go home. Tuck yourself in and keep warm. I'll ask the district nurse to keep an eye on you.'

Mrs White was living in a damp house on her own with no heating. The GP made no effort to ascertain the cause of her illness, but simply treated the symptoms.

person are key issues to consider, e.g. mode of living, dietary habits, leisure and hobbies inclinations. Peckham et al (1998) pointed out that the 'resource' aspect of public health consists of 'epidemiological' knowledge, or data that can be utilized by care managers to re-distribute resources according to needs. A public health 'action', however, applies to strategies and interventions that aim to improve health.

Local government

Local government has a central role in addressing health and well-being issues in the community (Millar 1998), and in being innovative in the allocation of staff resources (George 1995). A health strategy is recommended to create healthy communities, hinged on local authorities' initiative to stimulate collaborative work with other agencies such as health authorities, the private sector and voluntary organizations.

Although funding is a major problem, research to analyse efficiency in spending behaviours is needed. Moreover, benchmarking can be a useful tool for local government, politicians, policy makers and health workers. An awareness and knowledge of current health promotion activities in other regions can give insights into successful practices. For example, Millar (1998) explained that radio is a useful medium to communicate health issues. Local authorities, in collaboration with central government, have responsibilities to cooperate with researchers, scientists, the media and the public, in promoting critical discussions and participatory policy-making.

Some researchers, namely Arblaster et al (1996), have suggested that policy makers should target some of their health budgets on social expenditure, such as housing and employment, rather than treatment. Although local government has traditionally been a key agent in housing provision (e.g. council houses), focused strategies to improve social conditions would alleviate mental, physical and social incapacities.

As community health professionals are in a prominent position in a community model of care provision, their communication and negotiation skills can enhance professional relationships with local authority officials, and other services holding vital functions in preventative health and risk management.

A bureaucratic style of managing welfare agencies can impede a comprehensive needs assessment. However, flexible welfare organizations that are proactive and sensitive to current turbulence in welfare delivery and risk management (Alaszewski & Manthorpe 1998), are more likely to achieve successful health outcomes. For example, changes in social policy to effectively manage at-risk patients by a statutory Supervision Register, which became operative from 1 April 1995 (Goldstraw & Salib 1998), demand flexible adaptation by not only health authorities but local authorities and other welfare agencies, to achieve the local targets in the strategy for health.

Local authorities that integrate their expertise with health authorities, statutory and voluntary services to adopt 'a comprehensive approach' to reach local health targets (Millar 1997) are better empowered to tackle local health inequalities. It is, nevertheles, good practice to study the experiences of European agencies, Millar asserted. This has the advantage of offering a 'range of models of how local authorities and health authorities can work in partnerships. In addition, establishing joint projects with European countries enables agencies to evaluate each others' strategies, and to implement policy changes as required. Moreover, it is argued that European partnerships can mean access to funds to help implement new projects.

It is advantageous for local welfare agencies to foster a spirit of innovative partnership with their European counterparts. In an environment of shrinking resources, with high demands and low supply and dominated by competitiveness, local authorities and community agencies have to depend on some key principles. Elsen and Wallimann (1998) recognized these principles to be:

1. coordination of services
2. networking with other enterprises/ organizations
3. personal, professional and organizational development
4. the promotion of social, cultural and political relationships with European partners in care.

Health Action Zones

The concept of Health Action Zones (HAZs) can be defined as the combining and intensifying of health resources in a particular zone, a town or city with its community. The primary objective of HAZs, under the management of local health and social services community leaders, is to narrow the gap of health inequalities. For example, Lapthorne (1998) described the features of HAZs, and the roles of key players concerned with community health, to implement strategies that will reduce deprivation in identified areas (Box 9.3).

Box 9.3 Features of Health Action Zones

- A practical philosophy of needs assessment which is comprehensive for the area
- Rallying multi-agency support
- Community development, which is 'integrated strategy focused'
- The identification of social exclusion
- Seeking collaboration from key health promoters within the community workforce: health visitors, school nurses, pharmacists
- Community psychiatric nurses, social workers
- Extending the role of family doctor services, health visitors and pharmacists
- Developing parenting partnerships
- The assessment of public policy to evaluate effectiveness
- The development of a public health action centre
- Integration of community services, encompassing all disciplines, to target older people with multiple health problems, and the young and drug mis-users.

Health Action Zones can only succeed when a fully integrated service is in operation. Participatory responsibility cuts across all boundaries, from the individual level to statutory local management. Individuals have to be informed of their role in HAZ initiatives. Community practitioners have responsibilities to mobilize community resources (informal carers, nursing and residential home managers, schools and voluntary organizations) to raise awareness that the tackling of health inequalities through HAZs is a collective responsibility.

In regard to children services, agents of HAZs should reduce the fragmentation of services, particularly between community children's nurses, specialist out-reach nurses, practice nurses, health visitors and school nurses (Burr 1998).

Current implementation policies reflect a lack of communication between services, which culminates in either work duplication or implementation failures, because it is believed that other agencies have already intervened. It is hence useful to evaluate current models of intervention in the field of paediatric health services. HAZ managers require valid information to assist in the planning, implementation and coordination, and in the auditing of health interventions.

HAZs must have a children's home nursing action priority. This dimension entails the recognition that families need support and education to promote a healthy family unit environment.

Activity 9.5

1. Is your area a Health Action Zone? Describe the initiatives being implemented in your local community that reflect HAZ concepts.
2. Prepare a list of questions to ask health visitors on your placement.

Social capital

Social capital is not a new concept. For example, during the First and Second World Wars, communities built informal networks to help each other. Some networks were more formal in their activities, e.g. the well-known French Resistance. Their social networks were pivoted on trust, group cohesion and a code of secrecy vital for the success of their war stratagems. In addition, community participation was expected; i.e. the marshalling of available resources each member of the community was encouraged to provide. This consisted of the mustering of existing expertise from volunteering citizens. The development of a rationale for their cause to arouse a common community spirit was an additional feature. At an informal level, ordinary citizens would organize themselves into groups to talk about the War and its effects on communities. They would seek information and share practical advice on how to cope with issues as they arose, as well as showing concern about each other's well-being.

In health promotion terms, social capital has a similar meaning except that the context differs and secrecy is not a feature. Gillies (1997) explained social capital in terms of the existing resources that communities possess: 'trust, positive social norms, overlapping and diverse horizontal networks of communication and exchange of information', to enhance their abilities in developing sound health behaviours. Other characteristics of social capital comprise:

- actively participating in local community group meetings
- the development of environmental safety mechanisms to protect the vulnerable, e.g. by using surveillance systems (e.g. Neighbourhood Watch Schemes)
- establishing links with environmental health officers and the constabulary to ensure that practices are within legal boundaries.

Gillies argued that building on the strengths of the communities, by utilizing health promotion tactics, can ease access to available resources. Where communities are receptive to learning and adopting a healthy lifestyle, health promoters have to seize the opportunity to transfer skills to families with the objective of empowering them. Information-giving as a process should include diverse issues connected with determinants of health: transport, education, employment, poverty, housing.

Networks (including the latest technology, internet access etc.) and associations stimulate group cohesion and strengthen group identity. It is pointed out (Gillies 1997) that the existence of a trusting social network can help prevent disease, by promoting preventative health-related activities among disadvantaged groups. However, to assure maximum benefits from social capital, deliberate efforts must be made to raise communities' awareness that they have the potential – through social capital – to reduce their own health inequalities. For example, in 1998, the Secretary of State for Health stated during a BBC Radio 4 interview (30 November 1998) that injection of financial capital is not a guarantee that care standards will increase, whereas, very often, adopting good practice improves care. Trust, support, empathy, information- and knowledge-sharing, and integrated social networks to raise standards can be applied in practice to improve health outcomes.

One important issue for health promoters and health educationalists is to examine the meaning attached to 'social support' by diverse communities. To gain this understanding, cross-cultural studies and research are needed, and a wealth of information can be accessed from the social sciences (sociology, social anthropology).

Social capital is a key concept that needs to be considered as one of the major components in a comprehensive health model (Fig. 9.2).

Health improvement programmes

The Government's aim to build a healthier nation resides on the efficaciousness of their strategies to target disenfranchised groups. In late 1998, one finds that cave dwellers still exist in Britain: contemporary media reports indicated that in the city of Nottingham, many homeless people live in caves. This disturbing fact is a major challenge for local authorities aiming to implement Health Action Zones (HAZs).

Housing policy has been a perennial social problem. Other criticisms are connected with failure to recognize the needs of those with learning disabilities in the housing market (Holman 1998). However, some critics will argue that the

Government social exclusion unit policy aims to break the vicious circle of exclusion, by making changes in policies and intervention mechanisms.

The Green Paper, 'Our Healthier Nation', emphasizes that Health Improvement Programmes (HIPs) will target the vulnerable in various regions, with Health Authorities managing available resources. Partnerships in health delivery are emphasized. This consists of joint collaboration with local authorities and primary care groups: family doctor services, community care professionals, dentists, the public and so on. HAZ is one such initiative. HIPs are partnership-focused, stressing collaborative work between statutory and non-statutory organizations (e.g. voluntary and and business organizations).

Healthy Living Centres will aim to develop citizens' safety in the regions and within the homes, for example, by reducing the number of accidents among the very young and the aged. The role of Health-Promotion Units (Beishon 1998) in transferring their skills to develop such programmes is emphasized. Focusing on the determinants of health is important prior to the implementation of measures. In addition, local initiatives in HIPs should be compatible with the Government's public health strategy. Furthermore, consulting the European Union directives is recommended to ensure that national operations follow European standardized health policies. HIPs are of relevance to Social Exclusion Unit managers. The Social Exclusion Unit should be seen as an important force within HIPs: the coordination of services and clear-cut role identification will help prevent the fragmentation of services. A reliable communication network should be established. Moreover, to improve social inclusion Alcock (1998) and Hunter (1998b) asserted that the consequential role of social networks should be accepted. To participate in social life, access to a wide range of informal and formal social networks is required. Within the HIP, responses (interventions, strategies, community efforts) to social exclusion should be integrated. Alcock pointed out that coordinated local action within identified areas to change social relations is a priority. A combination of professional courses of action should be seen as

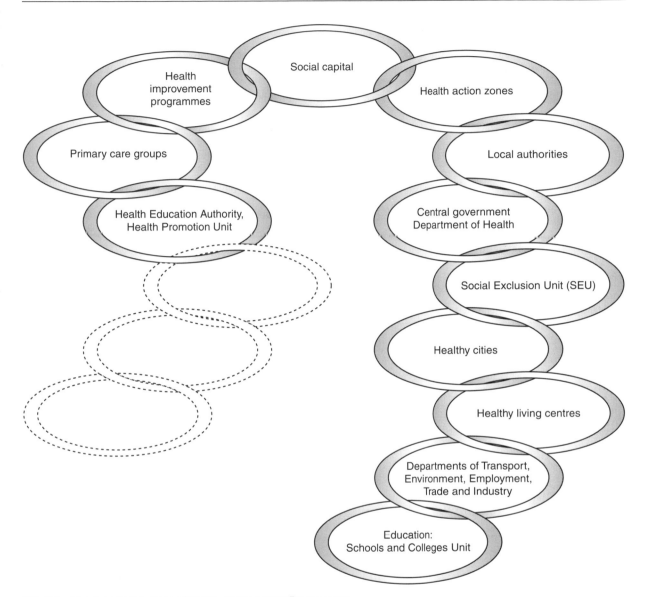

Fig. 9.2 The links in the chain of Health Improvement Programmes.

multiple links in a long chain of integrated services (Fig. 9.2) that are interdependent, thus avoiding the danger of working in isolation.

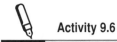

Activity 9.6

Read Case examples 9.3 and 9.4 and answer the questions.

SUMMARY

Health inequalities have been an ongoing problem in the UK for many years. Several reasons are given for this trend. These are described as the effects of being born in a particular social class. For instance, it has been pointed out that the working classes are more prone to ill-health than the middle and upper classes. Socio-economic status is another variable associated

Case example 9.3 'My ward is more deprived than yours'

Deprivation measures have become important tools in examining variations in health and are valuable to health authorities in the planning and delivery of health care.

Wards are geographical, administrative and political areas. National and local initiatives to improve circumstances of people living in poor housing and relative socio-economic deprivation often direct resources to the 'most deprived' wards in a city area.

'Most deprived' ward status can be a gateway to funding, but different agencies may use different measures of deprivation to attract and allocate funding (MacKenzie et al 1998).

Questions

1. What do you consider to be the implications of using different tools to assess deprivation?
2. In small groups, discuss issues related to the appropriateness of using 'ward boundary'/geographic areas to identify deprived communities for funding.
3. MacKenzie et al wrote that priorities for funding may be based on the ranking of ward. Can you identify any problems with this approach?

Case example 9.4 Two communities in Northern Ireland: deprivation and ill-health

Northern Ireland is one of the most deprived regions of the UK. It consistently has the highest levels of unemployment, with an even greater disparity in the rates of long-term unemployment. Average gross weekly earnings per household and per person are the lowest of any of the four countries.

The relationship between social security benefits uptake and religion probably reflects real differences between the two communities. Although the main difference between the two communities could be ascribed to different socio-economic characteristics (such as employment status), about 18% of the income gap between Catholics and Protestants is due to unequal pay for equal job qualities (O'Reilly & Stevenson 1998).

Questions

1. Make a list of opportunities for politicians and policy makers to reduce inequalities within the communities described above.
2. What do you consider to be the main priorities for the government in tackling inequalities in the two communities?

with health inequalities. Unemployment, therefore, has a detrimental effect on well-being. Whether one is male or female will have implications for health, and ethnicity has been linked to mental illness. Researchers, however, are debating whether racism and discrimination in mental health services are linked to the high prevalence of psychiatric admissions. There are health inequalities among the young and the aged. Accidents in the home as they affect children and the elderly have been reported. While individual responsibility in health maintenance is another issue, it is also argued that social systems failures are perpetuating inequalities. For the Government and policy makers, new strategies and health programmes have been suggested. The focus of policy implementation, however, is on the integration of statutory and non-statutory services, including the major roles of local authorities and health authorities in the process. Another key issue is the acknowledgement of informal social networks' role in health-promoting endeavours.

GLOSSARY

Atherosclerosis pathological changes in the structure of arteries due to formation of fatty deposits

Electro-convulsive treatment the application of an electrical pad to the temple to stimulate an artificial seizure, with the aim to alleviate some mental illness symptoms

Epidemiological knowledge knowledge related to the spread of diseases, morbidity, mortality etc.

HIV an abbreviation for human immunodeficiency virus which can damage the immune system

Multiple pathology a combination of ailments particularly noticeable among many elderly people

Qualitative related to assessing the views and feelings of subjects (i.e. people) being studied for research purposes

Quantitative to do with data collection (statistics, numbers, quantities)

Stigmatized service a service that reinforces the stigma attached to particular social problems (for example, attitude to the unemployed and benefits claimants)

Tenement housing houses where many tenants share available space

REFERENCES

Alaszewski A, Manthorpe J 1998 Welfare agencies and risk: the missing link? Health and Social Care in the Community 6(1): 4–15

Albee G W, Ryan K 1998 An overview of primary prevention. Journal of Mental Health 7(5): 441–449

Alcock P 1998 Bringing Britain together? Community Care 1250: 18–24

Arblaster L, Lambert M, Entwistle V et al 1996 A systematic review of the effectiveness of health service interventions aimed at reducing inequalities in health. Journal of Health Service Research Policy 1(2): 93–103

Baumer J H, Hunt L P, Shield J P 1998 Social disadvantage, family composition, and diabetes mellitus: prevalence and outcome. Archive of Diseases in Childhood 79(5): 427–430

Beishon M 1998 The HIP new way of working. Healthlines 54: 8–9

Béphage G 1997 Social science and healthcare: nursing applications in clinical practice. Mosby, London

Blank N, Diderichsen F 1996 Inequalities in health: the interaction between socioeconomic and personal circumstances. Public Health 110(3): 157–162

Brown K 1998 Commentary. Evidence-Based Nursing 1(3): 84

Burke V, Gracey M P, Milligan R A et al 1998 Parental smoking and risk factors for cardiovascular disease in 10- to 12-year-old children. Journal of Pediatrics 133(2): 206–213

Burr S 1998 Children: picking up the pieces. Nursing Management 5(7): 6–10

Butt J 1997 Race equality. Research Matters 3: 36–38

Central Statistics Office 1998 Social Trends 28. HMSO, London

Clarke P N, Pendry N C, Kim Y S 1997 Patterns of violence in homeless women. Western Journal of Nursing Research 19(4): 490–500

Clayton M 1998 Encouraging children to use cycle helmets. Paediatric Nursing 10(3): 14–16

Community Care 1998 MPs slam management for errors at benefits agency. Community Care 1234: 5

Coombs M 1998 Challenging the system. Community Care 1234: 22–23

Davey J A 1998 Exploring shared options in funding long-term care for older people. Health and Social Care in the Community 6(3): 151–157

Davies W H, Flannery D J 1998 Post-traumatic stress disorder in children and adolescents exposed to violence. Pediatric Clinics of North America 45(2): 341–352

Department of Health 1996 A new partnership for care in old age. HMSO, London, p 53

Department of Health 1998 Report by the Standing Nursing and Midwifery Advisory Committee. HMSO, London

Doughty I 1998 Commentary. Archive of Diseases in Childhood 79(3): 224

Elsen S, Wallimann I 1998 Social economy: community action towards social integration and the prevention of unemployment and poverty. European Journal of Social Work 1(2): 151–164

European Union in Action Against Drugs 1997 Office for official publications of the European communities, Luxemburg

Falkingham J 1989 Dependency and ageing in Britain: a re-examination of the evidence. Journal of Social Policy 18(2): 211–233

Fletcher M 1997 Equal health services for all. Journal of Community Nursing 11(7): 20–24

Ford G, Ecob R, Hunt K et al 1994 Patterns of class inequality in health through the life span: class gradients at 15, 35, and 55 years in the west of Scotland. Social Science Medicine 39(8): 1037–1050

Frank J B, Weihs K, Minerva E, Lieberman D Z 1998 Women's mental health in primary care. Medical Clinics of North America 82(2): 359–389

George M 1995 Collaborative caring. Nursing Standard 9(4): 22–23

Gerrish K 1997 Preparation of nurses to meet the needs of an ethnically diverse society: educational implications. Nurse Education 17(5): 359–365

Gillies P 1997 Social capital: recognising the value of society. Healthlines 45: 15–17

Goldstraw D, Salib E 1998 The Supervision Register: another exercise in paperwork that does not work? Psychiatric Care 5(1): 26–29

Hamlyn C 1998 Mind the gap. Healthcare Today 58: 51

Harrison G 1998 Commentary. Evidence-Based Nursing 1(2): 62

Health of the Nation 1991 HMSO, London, p 105

Healy M 1998 Inequalities in health: effects of socio-economic status. Nursing Standard 12(40): 38–40

Henderson C, Thornicroft G, Glover G 1998 Inequalities in mental health. British Journal of Psychiatry 173: 105–109

Holman A 1998 Why are people being excluded from available housing options? Community Living 12(2): 5–6

Hunt L 1998 Women's health: mental health needs. Nursing Management 5(7): 18–20

Hunter M 1998a No place like home. Community Care 1234: 16–18

Hunter M 1998b The unit in charge of social ills. Community Care 1250: 8–9

Irwin S 1996 Age-related distributive justice and claims on resources. British Journal of Sociology 47(1): 68–89

Joint Committee of Professional Nursing Midwifery and Health Visiting Associations 1997 A Celebration of Nursing Midwifery and Health Visiting. RNPFN, London

Kim J, Bramlett M H, Wright L K, Poon L W 1998 Racial differences in health status and health behaviours of older adults. Nursing Research 47(4): 243–249

Koffman J, Fulop N J, Pashley D, Coleman K 1997 Ethnicity and use of acute psychiatric beds: one-day survey in North and South Thames regions. British Journal of Psychiatry 171: 238–241

Lapthorne D 1998 Health Action Zones: taking up the challenge. Community Practitioner 71(6): 207–209

Lestor J 1993 Changing attitudes to children. Health Visitor 66(5): 162–163

Lewis G, Sloggett A 1998 Suicide deprivation and unemployment: record linkage study. British Medical Journal 317(7168): 1283–1286

Locker D, Payne B, Ford J 1996 Area variations in health behaviour. Canadian Journal of Public Health 87(2): 125–129

MacKenzie I F, Nelder R, Machonachie M, Radford G 1998

My ward is more deprived than yours. Journal of Public Health Medicine 20(2): 186–190

McMillan I 1998 Learning gap. Nursing Standard 12(49): 22–23

Mangan P 1994 Clinical reports. Nursing Times 90(34): 32

Millar B 1997 The European Union of Yorkshire. Healthlines 45: 22–23

Millar B 1998 Opening the window of opportunity. Healthlines 54: 6–7

Munro J 1997 Frank talking on health equality. Health Matters 29: 6–7

New NHS Modern Dependable 1997 HMSO, London

Nicholson J 1997 It's time to remove the inequality. Health Matters 30: 7

O'Reilly D, Stevenson M 1998 The two communities in Northern Ireland: deprivation and ill-health. Journal of Public Health Medicine 20(2): 161–168

Our Healthier Nation 1998 HMSO, London

Parkman S, Davies S, Leese M et al 1997 Ethnic differences in satisfaction with mental health services among representative people with psychosis in south London: Prism study 4. British Journal of Psychiatry 171: 260–264

Peckham S, Taylor P, Turton P 1998 An unhealthy focus on illness. Health Matters 33: 8–10

Popay J, Jones G 1990 Patterns of health and illness amongst lone parents. Journal of Social Policy 19(4): 499–534

Randall V 1996 Feminism and child daycare. Journal of Social Policy 25(4): 485–505

Reid R 1997 Securing the people's health. Health Matters 29: 8

Roberts E M 1997 Neighborhood social environments and the distribution of low birthweight in Chicago. American Journal of Public Health 87(4): 597–603

Sheehan M, Tomlinson M 1998 Government policies and employers' attitudes towards the long-term unemployed in Northern Ireland. Journal of Social Policy 27(4): 447–470

Sims J 1998 Mental health: failure to connect. Healthcare Today 58: 66–67

Song M, Edwards R 1997 Comment: raising questions about perspectives on black lone motherhood. Journal of Social Policy 26(2): 233–244

Stewart M, Werneke R, MacFaul R et al 1998 Medical and social factors associated with the admission and discharge of acutely ill children. Archive of Diseases in Childhood 79(3): 219–224

Swanston H Y, Tebbutt J S, O'Toole B I et al 1997 Sexually abused children 5 years after presentation: a case control study. Pediatrics 100(4): 600–608

Sweeting H, West P 1995 Family life and health in adolescence: a role for culture in the health inequalities debate? Social Science and Medicine 40(2): 163–175

Turrell G 1998 Socio-economic differences in food preference and their influence on healthy food purchasing choices. Journal of Human Nutrition and Dietetics 11(2): 135–149

Vagero D 1995 Health inequalities as policy issues: reflections on ethics, policy and public health. Sociology of Health and Illness 17(1): 1–19

Van den Bergh P 1998 Action on coronary heart disease. Healthcare Parliamentary Monitor 220: 7–8

Wuest J 1997 Illuminating environmental influences on women's caring. Journal of Advanced Nursing 26(1): 49–58

FURTHER READING

Balarajan R 1996 Ethnicity and variations in mortality from coronary heart disease. Health Trends 28(2): 45–51

Blackburn C 1994 Low income, inequality and health promotion. Nursing Times 28(39): 42–43

Caraher M, Dixon P, Long T, Carr-Hill R 1998 Access to healthy foods: part 1. Barriers to accessing healthy foods: differentials by gender, social class, income and mode of transport. Health Education 57(3): 191–201

Foster P 1996 Inequalities in health: what health systems can and cannot do. Journal of Health Service Research Policy 1(3): 179–182

Manor O, Matthews S, Power C 1997 Comparing measures of health inequality. Social Science and Medicine 45(5): 761–771

Smith G D 1997 Down at heart: the meaning and implications of social inequalities in cardiovascular disease. Journal of the Royal College of Physicians of London 31(4): 414–424

Webster J 1998 Time to get things rolling. Health Matters 34: 10–11

10

Mixed economy of care

A mixed economy of care is now an accepted social welfare issue. However, the participation of many agencies, both statutory and non-statutory, have increased complexity, and caused tension and conflict in many fields of health and social care. The aim of this chapter is to:

- highlight such changes
- discuss the role of government and the community in their roles as enablers of health and social care provision
- pinpoint some contemporary issues that concern the individual (users of services and professionals alike).

CONTEMPORARY ISSUES IN COMMUNITY HEALTH AND SOCIAL CARE

VALUES CONFLICT

The NHS and Community Care Act of 1990 – the outcome of a Conservative government health policy debate – has fuelled heated discussions and further controversies in regard to its integrity since implementation in 1992–1993. A plethora of literature reinforces the notion that, in some parts of the country (e.g. London) primary care, mental health, intermediate care and community services are inadequate (Porter 1998), and that there is a diffusion of responsibility, with evidence of 'appalling hospital care' (Rivett 1998), coupled with reduced patient contact with health care professionals. The issue of spending is also located at the heart of the debate. Furthermore, rationing of health care has been the focus of health care analysts. One argument is concerned with whether the NHS can provide a high quality, comprehensive and free service to its citizens (Weale 1998).

Comparing the British system of health service with that of the USA, Weale pointed out that the Americans value high tech equipment, which is costly but guarantees high quality services their clients have to afford, whereas in Britain, quality takes third rank in relation to comprehensiveness and 'free' services. Weale described this conflicting picture or dilemma as a *triad* (Fig. 10.1), because in the real world, a free service does not assure comprehensiveness and high quality simultaneously. Charges (Munro 1997a) can have a deterring effect. Munro felt that the public values free health care and an attempt to charge

for services can compel those who need help to avoid seeking out health services, thus adding to the NHS dilemma. The development of a 'new constitution' for the NHS is suggested, embodying an evaluated set of 'core values' (Munro 1997b).

Although the Labour Government advocates enthusiastic support for their dynamic strategy to improve the health of its citizens (Jowell 1998a), their Green Paper, 'Our Healthier Nation', certainly shows that their strategies can only 'narrow the health gap' and not close it. This perhaps reflects the lack of comprehensiveness described above, and the fact that public health innovation has its limitations. In addition, value conflict can be observed, e.g. in the Government's handling of tobacco manufacturing. Although successive governments have traditionally claimed they represent the best interests of the people (Jowell 1998b), their failure to achieve a total ban on tobacco production reflects the dilemma they face, i.e. tobacco manufacturing is a good source of revenue through taxation. While Jowell (1998b) explained that governments can sometimes be the only agents to act in affairs that have implications for public health, she does not make clear why tobacco manufacturing is still allowed.

Conflict in health and social care

There is a lack of harmonization between health care and social care agencies. In late-twentieth-century Britain, there are clients who have considerable health needs but receive no services (Rodrigues 1998). This may be due to inadequate coordination of services caused by interagency boundaries (Waters 1998), and a failure to recognize and accept the wider responsibilities of local authorities in social and health care.

Glasman (1997) suggested that attempts to reduce health and social boundaries in order to provide a seamless community health service could be enhanced if local authorities purchased community health services. Boundaries are erected when professionals adhere rigidly to traditional methods of intervention, e.g. an inability to exercise flexibility when faced with issues impinging on both health and social domains. The problem

• Free service inclines toward fragmentation (lacks comprehensiveness)
• Free service has to confront steep obstacles to achieve high quality
• There is linkage between high quality and comprehensiveness

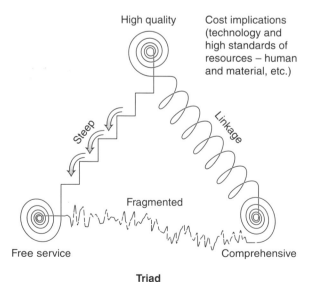

Triad

Fig. 10.1 Conflicting ideals caused by constraints. Can a service be comprehensive, free and of a high quality?

could be accentuated when agencies function in a climate that is under-resourced.

Conflict is also generated by ambiguous role descriptions. Collaboration and joint working between health authorities and social services to manage budgets (Glasman 1997) could foster better service coordination. Additionally, professional communication between health care organizations and colleagues in social care and housing organizations (Waters 1998) is recommended.

Resource constraints appear to be adversely affecting relationships between health and social services. Shrinking funds have precipitated local authorities to reassess their methods of service delivery. For example, stricter control of users' dependency levels is exercised (Edwards 1996), which has led to decreased provision of low-level home care.

The implications for the health services are:

1. Due to reduced vacancies in local authorities care homes, patients cannot be discharged, causing 'bed blocking'. On the other hand, early discharge caused by internal pressures (e.g. health managers' priorities to increase throughput) will have implications. As Henwood (1997) argued, the discharging of large numbers of 'alleged bed blockers' into the community or into care homes, prematurely, could increase re-admission rates and worsen existing problems. This causes a collision of cultures: conflicting responses between health and social care authorities. This issue confirms health and social care analysts that ineffective collaboration between agencies to set up care in the community is to be blamed (Hirst 1997).

2. Increased hospital stay means additional expenditure. Edwards (1996) observed that a hospital stay is more expensive than a residential or nursing home care.

In addition, health authorities (hospital trusts) are the recipients of higher funding, at the expense of community health services (Edwards 1996). Cutler (1998) commented that these grey areas of responsibility caused by the overlapping of health issues with social care have fuelled the conflict. Moreover, there are circumstances when health authorities are expected to exercise responsibility, such as in the care of the terminally ill. Edwards (1996) indicated that if terminally ill patients are in hospital with only four weeks to live they become the Health Authority's responsibility; for longer stays, the responsibility is no longer 'solely' the Health Authority's. This approach has been criticized for its lack of flexibility by local authorities.

Although it is argued that the public on the whole – as service users – do not care whether services provided are by health or social care providers (Leadbetter 1996, Sone 1997), the issue of accountability is nevertheless a major argument. As service users become exposed to increasing numbers of a fragmented service, Sone pointed out, confusion is created about which agency is accountable.

The integration of services is a major challenge for both government and policy implementors. Several initiatives have been suggested such as Health Action Zones, and Joint Working and Commissioning, encouraging agencies to foster a spirit of collaboration. Lack of uniformity in regard to the nature of services, resource availability and lack of funding compound the tension between agencies. Additionally, historically social services have operated more or less independently, with a different ethos. Techniques and philosophy in care delivery are hence dissimilar. For example, some social services may be charged (i.e. domiciliary care), whereas health care is considered free at the point of delivery.

CHARGING FOR SERVICES

In a review of social services behaviour connected with charging policies, Lunt (1996) identified local authorities' rationale for charging citizens for defined services:

1. Charging for domiciliary services (i.e. Meals on Wheels, domestic help) has been a traditional policy.

2. Reasonable charges are allowed within the legislative framework of the Health and Social Services and Social Security Act (1983).

3. The NHS and Community Care Act (1990), with its new challenges, has compelled local

authorities to review and adjust charges to meet new pressures and demands for Meals on Wheels, home adaptations, aids such as alarm systems etc.

4. Cost shunting by health authorities: reduced long-term beds and earlier discharge from hospital have forced local authorities to redefine services (traditionally interpreted as health) as social care. The impetus to achieve services integration with a person-centred (needs-led) approach – underpinned with equitable funding – for health and social care-related services (Whitfield 1998), is directing managers to consider how some social service functions could be carried out by health care organizations and vice versa.

5. Higher consumer expectations of a better informed, needs-led service, i.e. for community nursing, flexible and effective response to locally understood patient care need is expected, by being able to work with both health and social care agencies (DeBell 1998).

6. Central government expectations (external pressures) that local authorities should improve standards and be more accountable, while central government controls public expenditure.

To control expenditure and ensure quality of services are dilemmas faced by both health and local authorities. The redefining of both social and health needs, impelled by cost shunting, can foster professional friction between agencies. Moreover, for the recipients of care, increased charges may act as disincentives to seek health/social support, which has implications for both social and health care organizations. Lunt pointed out the possible aftermath of charges: reduced uptake of services; social exclusion; health deterioration; client–professional relationship undermined.

An ageing population will further compel the State to introduce charges. Connelly (1997) argued that social protection (social security, health and social care, compulsory occupational pensions) can be inadequate for users to buy services. For many who are on the margins of society, even small charges can be detrimental to their livelihood.

At the time of writing, MPs are seeking to implement a 'national charging strategy' (Philpot 1998) to ensure uniformity nationally. At local level, this may be criticized for being undemocratic.

Activity 10.1

List your own reasons for charges being implemented.

??? Question 10.1

Should the better off be charged more for services?

PERFORMANCE STANDARDS

We live in a consumer-driven society. While profit-making can be a powerful motivator, producers have to take clients' needs into account. From the High Street stores to the National Health and Social Services, consumers have a strong input in the way services are managed and delivered. Not surprisingly, the public now expects a high standard of service. The ethos of consumerism is integrated in the framework of health and welfare.

Performance is a key concept in service provision; in a mixed economy of care this has become more significant. Competitiveness is high on the agenda, and service providers are expected to show evidence that they are good performers. In 1998, the Secretary of State for Health emphasized that the Government would set 'new standards of performance and will publish annual reports on all councils' performance'.

The White Paper 'Modernising Social Services', issued in November 1998, recognized interprofessional conflict between health and social care services, engendered by a lack of coordination. Although the Government acknowledges evidence of 'many excellent examples of joint health and social care services' their main concern is to monitor both the NHS and social services performance frameworks (Modernising Social Services 1998).

However, good performance is also linked to being able to work as 'crucial partners' across boundaries. The Government emphasizes the role of local authorities and health services to achieve joint working. To attain this goal the Health Minister proposed three key strategies:

1. pooled budgets (joint funds pooled by health and social agencies to facilitate integrated care)
2. lead commissioning: delegating functions and allocating funds for the purchase of both health and social care
3. integrated provision: the provision of either health or social care, as needed, by an agency.

Chadda (1998) believes that efficiency savings in social services departments could be linked to performance targets, and the Secretary of State for Health asserted that improving performance is not necessarily more costly than doing things badly. Social services managers, however, point out that constraints on their fee structures by local authorities could impede their targets of upgrading standards, to meet national targets of improving protection for the vulnerable in society. The White Paper reinforces the idea that a robust system of regulation is imperative to maintain standards. This will be achieved by 'Regional Commissions for Care Standards', which will be independent structures with oversight functions for both the NHS and social care agencies. An important feature is the inclusion of representatives from both local and health authorities on health boards, as well as users' and providers' representatives. This approach paves the way for a better integrated service. In addition, as Moores (1998) stated, the involvement of both the public and patients'/clients' views, nationally and locally, takes the *quality* agenda forward. Developing and encouraging the participation of users and carers is nevertheless an important democratic process.

Performance can, however, be frustrated when the psychological well-being of staff is impaired. Halpern (1998) commented on the incidence of psychological disturbance as well as emotional exhaustion, among nurses and doctors. Scott (1998) explained that shorter hospital stays and early discharge are factors burdening staff morale. These issues have implications for care delivery. In the new health framework, provision for the maintenance of staff welfare must be included.

BEST VALUE

The concept of 'Best Value' is intertwined with the mobilization of interprofessional resources; it refers to a philosophy that promotes the skills to work across departments, disciplines and professions, and is not a clear departure from a multidisciplinary team principle. It applies to a performance framework that can be guaranteed when skills are integrated by making use of social (informal networks) and professional capital. Best Value also entails greater transparency and fairness in the contribution that people are asked to make towards social care. The Government hence aims to implement a 'Fair Access to Care' policy. Authorities will have responsibilities to ensure clear objectives are set, which will be consistent with evidence of regular reviews and risk assessments. Best Value encompasses key targets:

- the dissemination of information across professional boundaries and to users of services and the public
- preventive strategies targeting low-level support at the vulnerable in society, most likely to lose their independence; e.g. people in the community who are deprived of secure and decent homes (Cooper 1998).

The role of housing agencies in community care is underestimated, Cooper argued, as very often they are enablers too, supporting those with mental illness and disability, to stay in their own homes. The prevention of a housing crisis could also prevent health crisis, as the two are interconnected.

In a mixed economy of care, Best Value initiatives are stimulated because of competitiveness. Additionally, workforce planning is of strategic importance, a challenge to professionals engaged in meeting the health needs of local populations (Benton 1998).

Cost-effective care is dependent on sensitive management of human resources: the allocation of tasks congruent with skills, and staff deployment based on users' needs. Benton explained that workforce planning is concerned with evidence-based practice and relevant educational underpinnings, to inform service provision, leading to health strategies. It requires the integration of all these components. Moreover, a coherent policy – supported by key players in care provision – is a requisite. Best Value is best promoted when a user-focused, professionally supported and evidence-based practice is consciously practised. However, at the interface of translating theory into practice, conflict can become an issue. To maintain Best Value integrity in organizations where conflict exists, attempts to harness conflictual issues in a positive way are recommended (White 1998).

White pointed out that failure to manage conflict could constrain an organization's progress. Basic communication skills are necessary, coupled with a thorough analysis of the roots of the problems. Effective conflict management can enhance the process of building quality services. The NHS Executive (1998a) document, 'Professional activity in health promotion and care', sets clear guidelines that relate to Best Value, by stating 'quality indicators' (e.g. Kings Fund Audit, Investors in People, the Business Excellence Model) are necessary.

Social Service Commissioners have incorporated standards for care support workers in some areas, based on assessment of workers' performance. Additionally, adequate training and updating will enhance professional competence and practice (NHS Executive 1998a)

JOINT WORKING AND JOINT COMMISSIONING

It is believed that one of the ultimate steps in breaking down barriers between health and social care is best undertaken by joint working and joint commissioning. The former can be defined as collaborative caring and partnership

in the care dimensions, the latter refers to the statutory powers delegated to authorities (health, social and others) to promote measures with the main objectives of fostering high-quality care performance, by working collaboratively and in partnership. The Government aims at providing a seamless service. It is acknowledged that the Conservative administration widened the division between agencies and fragmented services; however, there is a school of thought which critically argues that the move to merge health and social services is cost-driven rather than quality-driven (Hirst 1997). Others point out that joint commissioning – although a powerful initiative (Hudson 1997) – can fail if a coherent national policy is not formulated and if agencies have unclear objectives (Case example 10.1). It has also been noted that:

Case example 10.1 A social care problem?

A research study of randomly selected sample of 90 older people (with only 48 able to take part) (Phelps & Shepperdson 1998) provides an interesting insight into variations of professionals' perceptions of 'health' and 'social' care. The researchers discovered the following:

1. acute admissions of older people were influenced by 'social' and 'domestic' situations: social isolation, dependencies, informal carers' ill-health
2. lack of social care by social services
3. only 10% of problems were attributed to failures in medical services
4. admissions to hospital may be based firstly on a 'social situation', but the 'presence of an illness' gives a good reason for admission
5. non-clinical factors are influential in increasing emergency admissions
6. a failure in social services assessment and emergency support.

- health care reform is interpreted by some to circumscribe a strategy linked with employment policy, social welfare, housing, the environment, operating in coordination (Keighley 1998)
- if there is limited agreement between members and poor understanding of other team members' roles, collaboration will be affected (Vincent 1997)

- effective joint working can be impeded by a clash of cultures (Case example 10.2) and if patterns of accountability are not coherent (Hudson 1998).

Case example 10.2 Social services versus health services

Social care managers who have no experience of medical illness and with no nursing experience will have a different outlook on the presentations of clients' needs. Functional failure (from a social care perspective) in an elderly person, for example, can be caused by latent physical pathology, which would be diagnosed by a nurse or physician; a social care managers' care plan is not likely to reflect biological conditions. On the other hand, a primary health care team may misdiagnose a *social care need* if they focus on a medical model of assessment. Further, conflicting ideology becomes an obstacle in regard to nursing and medical care being free at the point of delivery, while the social care client is likely to be means-tested, assessed for dependency level and charged for services.

It is suggested that the burdens on social and health agencies caused by re-admissions can be minimized by a smooth transition from acute hospital care to 'intermediate care' (Bowman & Black 1998). Intermediate care refers to second-stage or convalescent beds, according to Bowman and Black, but with greater focus on outcomes. The aim is to establish rapid transfer, by having intermediate care facilities near district hospitals. The prevention of health and social breakdown could be prevented by joint commissioning.

Users' views are, however, paramount in this process. Assumptions should not be made that discharge in the community is always desired by the client (Ahulu 1995). It is possible that an intermediate care programme may provide a compromise. On the other hand, measures to include new rehabilitation services to prevent unnecessary admissions to hospital (George 1998) should operate concurrently with intermediate care.

Activity 10.2

Contact your local hospital manager. How do they perceive health and social care acute admissions?

Question 10.2

How should the primary care team prevent acute admissions of clients with social care problems/needs to hospital?

Joint working has many features, according to Hudson (1998):

1. Effective communication, which can be either non-structured (informal) or structured; the latter applies to documentation and agreements on strategies needed, formally known as PASS (Practice Agreements with Social Services).

2. Coordination, which refers to organizations/agencies working across boundaries in a formal way.

3. Co-location: the location of members of different professions in other professionals' organizations, e.g. a social care worker in general practice, a general practitioner in a hospital casualty department, a health visitor in a social service agency.

4. Commissioning: a shared approach to strategies required by professionals authorized with this remit.

Joint commissioning can be described as being based on a trusting relationship (Case examples 10.3 and 10.4) and organizational interdependence, when professionals share the vision of the agencies (Hudson 1997).

Joint commissioners are anticipated to utilize their broad experience to ensure that other pertinent players are involved in the framework. For

Case example 10.3 Integrating the boundaries

One health authority and one local authority have established joint funding for their client groups. They have reviewed their management systems to help promote a more strategic focus. They aim to integrate their expertise to create a 'virtual organization', which they assert is based on the philosophy that planning is resources-led, and that joint commissioning can only be realized if resources are managed jointly.

Case example 10.4 Crucial inter-relationship

Some local health and social care agencies have identified the interdependent nature of their work in the fields of needs assessment, care management and pooling of resources. Services are coordinated, a care manager is allocated and, if necessary, a specialist is called in to participate in the assessment.

Some social services care managers are facilitating closer joint working with district nurses and other members of the primary care team. Community care agencies using this integrative approach report that clients and professionals benefit from this efficient resource allocation.

example, housing organizations, employment agencies and general practitioners can be invited to work alongside local authorities and health providers. Makin and Campbell (1997) point out that the police and education agencies are of relevance too.

The main objective is the improvement of services, to reduce fragmentation by being sensitive to the needs of communities. Transparency in the communication networks and in general management and financial planning is considered imperative.

One initiative seen to be advantageous is to have a 'generic care worker' (Poxton 1997) who is able to use a diversity of skills, without being constrained by specific job descriptions. In some parts of the country, Poxton points out, district nurses have started to take on social care management functions, and are able to access social services funds, once a comprehensive needs assessment has been done.

To ensure safe practice, central government policy is to regulate and improve staff standards (George 1998) by setting up a General Social Care Council.

USER PERSPECTIVE (PUBLIC PARTICIPATION)

A mixed economy of care with its competitive nature has led health care managers to exercise more sensitivity in regard to users' views, and to respond accordingly. Attempts to achieve custo-

mer/client/patient satisfaction can become a profitable strategy (Andaleeb 1998), but to attain this goal, users' views must be obtained. The Government White Paper, 'The New NHS Modern Dependable' (1997), recognizes this fact: 'the government will work closely with those in the NHS, users and carers, and partner organisations on implementation'. Further, the Secretary of State for Health's common objectives, stated in his White Paper 'Modernising Social Services' (1998), are: 'to actively involve users and carers in planning services and in tailoring individual packages of care …'.

We can agree that the Government's intentions to include users in the scheme of things are clear. The White Papers, however, do not specify *how* users will be involved. While (1998) postulated that the government *hopes* and *expects* that joint working with clients, individuals and families, as well as neighbourhoods, schools and employers, who are users, will help realize the vision that health is for all.

Social change and modernization of thinking have contributed in making the public more aware and critical of their rights as consumers of services. Public services are currently exposed to community scrutiny, and users have high expectations. It is therefore not surprising that efforts are being made to instigate public participation. Barnes and Evans (1998), for instance, emphasize how important it is to involve individuals and citizens in their health care.

Current political ideology welcomes user participation since the people's confidence in statutory services has declined. How user involvement can be encouraged and developed remains a challenge. Barnes and Evans (1998) make the following suggestions:

1. Direct participation: this involves respecting the users as individuals with unique experiences who can develop partnership with their clinicians, and can be counted in decision-making processes at local and national levels.
2. Informed views: as consumers the public can voice their experiences of positive and negative outcomes of service provision. Constructive dialogue between users and providers will

help gain insight into services' shortcomings or loopholes.

3. Community development: citizens to become participators in decision-making in connection with health-promoting matters.

4. Local scrutiny and accountability: to ensure transparency of managerial activities so that the public becomes aware of accountability issues, locally and nationally.

Citizens' participation is so important that mutual understanding and the user's perspective are becoming central elements in mental health courses for professionals in health and social services (Reynolds 1998). Besides, health outcomes measurements assume better validity when users and significant others give their meanings of the significance of 'becoming' and 'being ill' (Godfrey & Wistow 1997). The writers emphasize that they view this approach as an integration of users' understandings of their illness and coping strategies, with the empowering skills of the professionals in securing the best service provision. It is a clear departure from the 'oversimplistic' concept of consumerism in health, which is concerned with obtaining 'feedback' about patient satisfaction. As Barnes and Evans (1998) argued, citizens' participation is a means for achieving the objectives of the service. They become, in fact, agents of change. This becomes a possibility when clients' views are considered in decision-making.

In addition, outcomes, according to Higginson et al (1997), have to reflect the needs and expectations of service users. For example, the importance of involving users was greatly emphasized when the Department of Health consulted over 500 representatives of service users, their relatives and others in designing a framework for good practice in the field of learning disabilities (NHS Executive 1998b). Critics point out, however, that in mental health, a paternalistic stance to care has excluded the client and failed to meet users' demands effectively (Sallah 1998).

Social structures have been implicated in erecting obstacles to joint working (Hawtin 1998):

- a competitive market
- inaccessible funding
- uncoordinated directives from central government
- too many agencies without clear objectives.

Hawtin wrote that, since professionals find it difficult to implement joint working among themselves, attempts to include users in decision-making processes can prove even more challenging. He explained that there are many reasons for this:

1. staff have always assumed technical knowledge and expertise
2. users of services are not traditionally seen as 'equals'
3. power relationships (users are subservient; professionals are decision-makers)
4. users may not fully represent those they speak for.

The empowerment of users is nevertheless highly recommended. Patients can be helped to regain control, while a professionally led service adopts a more 'needs-driven' system (Benton 1995). Additionally, the benefits of social capital and networking with users (who have knowledge and experience of services), have potential to influence policy. Joint working with these aims in mind will aid strategic planning. Finally, as Hennessy (1998) explained, professionals and the community have responsibilities to utilize opportunities for policy involvement.

PRIMARY CARE GROUPS

Primary Care Groups (PCGs) will comprise general practitioners in an area, working in partnership with community nurses, having a strategic objective to commission the best services for their local communities (The New NHS Modern Dependable 1997). They will have statutory accountability to health authorities: the latter will be accountable to Regional Offices and the NHS Executive (Fig. 10.2).

PCGs will also be expected to work with NHS Trusts (which have service accountability with health authorities), agreeing on long-term service agreements, targeting specific groups as needed (e.g. children, and people living in areas where coronary heart disease is prevalent), establishing

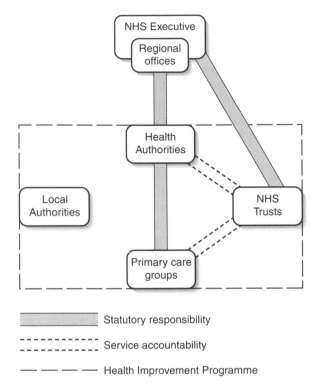

Statutory responsibility

Service accountability

Health Improvement Programme

Fig. 10.2 The new NHS. (Reproduced with the kind permission of the Controller of Her Majesty's Stationery Office from The New NHS Modern Dependable 1997, p. 21.)

specific links with National Service frameworks. This service accountability ensures that maximum input is obtained from clinicians engaged in health care planning.

Health authorities, PCGs, NHS Trusts and local authorities all work within the Health Improvement Programmes (HIPs) framework (see Fig. 10.2). It is expected that PCGs will establish joint working with social services, aiming to strengthen links. The role of local authorities is interpreted to be wider and corporate, circumscribing public health responsibilities, community safety and housing generation plans. They are the crucial partners of the new NHS (Modernising Social Services 1998), pooling budgets where appropriate.

Since the publication of the two White Papers ('The New NHS Modern Dependable' and 'Modernising Social Services') an abundance of literature has been generated by the professions. In particular, professionals at grassroot commu-

nity level have shown enthusiasm in asserting their roles and functions within the PCGs' philosophy. For the practice nurse, Swage (1998) envisaged a wide spectrum of responsibilities, which would have positive contributions to patient care (Box 10.1).

Box 10.1 Role and functions of the practice nurse in PCGs

Practice nurses have specialist knowledge invaluable to HIP development. Their experience of 'practice information systems' and networking can help identify inequalities in access to health care. Their contribution can facilitate change. They have daily responsibilities in health promotion programmes and preventative care (e.g. health advice and support to HIV/AIDS sufferers, men's and women's health, pregnant teenagers). They have a key role to play in the development of primary care, by implementing 'nurse-led clinics for asthma, diabetes and epilepsy'.

In addition, it is anticipated that the nature of PCGs will vary across the country, dependent on population size (Madden 1998) and boundaries. For example, in some areas there may be groups of only 50 000, which fall below the Government-specified target of 100 000 to form PCGs. In other areas, Madden pointed out, 'Local Health Groups' have been formed instead of PCGs. She argued that practice nurses will undertake responsibilities in commissioning services by working with general practitioners. Literature search indicates, however, that the transition from the internal, fragmented market mechanism to PCGs is proving challenging for many reasons.

1. The recruitment of nurses for PCGs is stimulating debates. It is believed that community nurses with the right calibre should be selected, and that community nurse representation is a fundamental component of PCGs, because of their expertise in community health needs and problems (Young 1998, Young & Sutton 1998). Fair representation, according to the Royal College of Nursing, can be achieved by local agreement among community and practice nurses.

2. Plans are discussed to give GPs control of PCGs, at the expense of nurses and other professionals (Lipley 1998, Smith 1998).

3. Practice nurses may be under-represented in the new structure. There is fear that 'other community' professionals may be given priorities to become major participators in the new scheme (Mayor 1998).

4. The role of the Community Health Councils (CHCs) has to be clarified if they are to be community representatives.

5. Conflicts may arise when locality groupings are identified. This may become an issue, Smith (1998) explained, because of 'pre-existing' boundaries of natural community groups, clashing with statutory arrangements of community groups 'for management strategies'.

6. The White Papers have not specified the role of midwifery services in the scheme of things. This is an issue over which critics (Gulland 1998) have expressed dissatisfaction.

The above issues indicate that, while the Government's intentions are clear, the realities at clinical level show that PCGs' implementation can prove challenging. Role conflicts, which are discussed above, are to be anticipated. However, if joint working is to be successful for PCGs, innovative ways to develop professionally integrated care must be sought. Several objectives must be made clear: how will budgets be managed; in what way will PCGs act in an advisory capacity; how can PCGs achieve independence but be accountable to health authorities at the same time, in the commissioning of care?

Commissioners and joint workers have to secure collaboration and avoid negative competition. A new role in commissioning for nurses and midwives (Payne 1997) should enhance the demise of the internal market.

PUBLIC HEALTH

Figure 10.2 depicts the major players in the Health Improvement Programmes. The broad remit of health monitors is to ensure that the public, in its widest sense, lives in a safe environment. Health improvement programmers have to exercise their powers in environmental control and health surveillance techniques as effectively as possible. Their functions are dependent upon the expertise of many, from the lay person to the core executive in government.

Inter-organizational working is now encouraged. Local government and the NHS have an important role in public protection: their professionals can develop schemes that will help promote environmental health. The focus, hence, should be on the development of healthy alliances (Clarke et al 1997). Environmental and social services functions are increasingly being recognized as the role of local government. In late 1998, for example, the Deputy Prime Minister announced that local authorities will be empowered to control environmental pollution, by minimizing town and city traffic via a system of charges for motorists. As transport control is being considered, a national transport strategy to check traffic growth is becoming a priority. As pressures magnify from the efforts of local, national and international environmentalists, local government will have to seek support and technical expertise from community health agencies. Clarke et al (1997) suggest that a review of existing local government guidelines is needed, with the possible implementation of a new model of governance. Central government agenda, however, shows clear direction that major changes are expected across statutory agencies concerned with environmental health.

Human health is reliant on environmental health. Furthermore, bio-psycho-social well-being can be undermined by adverse environmental conditions: noise, water and air pollution, unsanitary conditions, overcrowding and disease (Scally & Perkins 1998).

Healthy Cities projects are being developed to combat the causes of inequalities in health, and to identify the causes of illness. The Minister of State for Public Health has stated that Government policies are to involve agencies to review public health strategy and implement Health Action Zones (Taggart 1998). Urban and rural health are issues to be analysed by health and social care workers. Social capital and networking across population groups can be utilized to raise public health awareness and to empower the community; a means of social investment

(Stott 1998) with positive benefits for populations and in moving the Healthy Cities projects forward.

COMMUNITY MENTAL HEALTH

IMPROVING HEALTH AND SOCIAL FUNCTIONING

Services for individuals with mental health disorders are still being criticized in late-twentieth-century Britain due to inappropriate and ineffective interventions, lack of access and exclusion of some minority groups from health provision (Sallah 1998). Warner et al (1998) reported that, while evidence of good services exists, mental health service users very often do not access support tailored to their needs. They point out, for instance, that many residents are isolated from statutory mental health or social services; some were found to be without health or social services key workers. In addition, when needs change (i.e. for different types of support, housing, benefits etc.), users find themselves trapped in services no longer meeting their needs.

If maximum health and social functioning is to be attained, the views of mental health service users must be sought (Hannigan et al 1997). Social health functioning hinges on sound interpersonal relationships and support from informal networks. Users of services are aware of the importance of 'community' and 'society' in determining their mental health status. This may entail daily interactions with neighbours, friends, families and even the value of pets in companionship.

While cognitive functioning must be assessed, social functioning must equally receive a thorough examination. One emphasis should be upon public health policy (providing a healthy and supportive environment) consolidating social and personal skills (Hodgson 1996), with further emphasis on community empowerment.

Contemporary issues are in connection with community care (supervised after care) for people with severe mental illness under the Mental Health Act 1996 (Patients in Community). It has become a major public debate, since ordinary citizens and professionals have been known to be the victims of violence from psychiatric patients discharged in the community. Shacklady (1997), in a research study in one Community Trust, discovered that 50% (157 respondents) of community nurses reported their assailants were patients/clients, and 31% were clients' family members.

It is now envisaged for community psychiatric nurses to focus interventions on clients with severe and enduring mental health problems (Hannigan 1997), and to adopt the role of mental health supervisor (Slinger 1997). A supervisor is anticipated to monitor a client's health progress in the community and to initiate early treatment to prevent deterioration. A care programme approach is recommended with the involvement of the primary health care team (Schneider 1994). The care programme approach was introduced by the Conservative Government in 1991, and specifies the responsibilities of health authorities and social services departments to design care packages to meet the needs of patients requiring specialized mental health services (McDermott 1998). Brooker (1997) believed that their conditions can make them vulnerable to poor services.

Nevertheless, assumptions must not be made that community mental health services are always the best option for clients' needs, instead of long-term hospitalization. In September 1997, the Government confirmed that the mentally ill will not be moved from hospital to community care unless adequate resources are made available (Valios 1997). Care of the mentally ill is a broad concept and the primary care health team assessment tool has to be all-encompassing, targeting community groups from the very young to the very old.

Children have mental health needs too. As discussed in Chapter 3, they can have diverse negative life experiences that may impinge on their socio-psychological well-being. Professional learning in child care by hospital and community nurses can be carried out by comparing experiences, according to Perkins and Billingham (1997), who have drawn attention to an increase in mental health and behavioural problems among children. Epidemiological studies (Symington 1997) substantiate this argument, while it is pointed out that mental health services for young people are inadequate.

At the other spectrum of the human life trajectory, one finds that an ageing population is coupled with an increasing incidence of mental ill-health: cognitive dysfunction, depression, self-harm and other psychological alterations. Social and personal changes in later life (e.g. widowhood) can be a threat to personal adjustment (Thuen et al 1997). Research studies have shown that older people with depression are high users of health services (Livingston et al 1997), and that the suicide rate in the elderly is high, linked with a high mortality from completed suicide (Hepple & Quinton 1997).

The role of primary care teams in preventative health is acknowledged, and they have responsibilities to:

- detect the socially isolated older person
- investigate evidence of informal networks support
- empower users by raising awareness of early psychiatric interventions and resources
- assess factors in the older person's environment which can predispose to psychological deterioration
- establish links with GPs' services and social care workers
- develop a gate-keeper model and apply a 'patient-focused' care: the continuing evaluation of care to meet holistic needs, incorporating staff and users' perspectives (Williams et al 1997).

Activity 10.3

1. Do a search in national newspapers. How many cases of violence by psychiatric patients can you find?
2. Prepare a list of issues that should be considered in the planning of an effective care package.

??? Question 10.3

1. A person with mental illness is vulnerable. How should primary care teams protect the individual?
2. What do you consider to be the ethical issues in connection with a mental health supervisor in the community?

NEIGHBOURHOOD AND MENTAL HEALTH

The environment is a determinant of mental well-being. When tensions exist in neighbourhoods classified as unsafe (evident in many inner-city deprived areas), due to racial disharmony, unemployment, poverty and social isolation, psychological impairment is often a consequence. It has been confirmed that people who live in urban areas are prone to mental ill-health. In a longitudinal study undertaken in Oslo, Dalgard and Tambs (1997) re-interviewed 503 persons 10 years after an initial interview; their findings support the environment stress hypothesis, and they concluded that the nature of the neighbourhood is linked to the quality of mental well-being.

These findings suggest that improved environmental conditions correlate with better mental health. For care professionals in community health services, there are some clinical implications to consider (Box 10.2).

Box 10.2 Neighbourhood involvement

Local authorities have a duty to consult mental health services prior to housing regeneration so that residents' needs are discussed before decision-making, so that they have an opportunity to participate in solving environmental problems.

An integrated assessment model (bio-psycho-social) has been suggested (Jenkins et al 1998) to minimize the impact of social disability caused by neurosis and psychosis. Primary care teams have to evaluate their intervention methods: it is imperative that clients' perceptions of their environment are assessed, in an objective way, to prevent health workers' bias. Suicidal assessment techniques need to be refined. The use of benchmarking can be invaluable as it helps professionals to compare practices with those that have been successful.

THE ROLE OF THE VOLUNTARY SECTOR

Without voluntary organizations, the impact of social problems already identified in this book would be much greater. The voluntary sector has a major contribution in the mixed economy of care. As the name implies, its members are volunteers with altruistic aims. They want to help others – the poor, the homeless, the unemployed, the young and old – in fact practically any group in society whom they feel are disadvantaged and require support. Billis and Glennerster (1998) believe that the voluntary sector has a wide remit in the welfare state: it takes over where the mainstream public services have given up. Voluntary sector organizations are known for their commitment in alleviating the suffering of the stigmatized in society. In particular, Billis and Glennerster describe the characteristics of voluntary organizations as 'motivation' and 'sensitivity': the desire to act as a response to needs, when other sectors either have failed or cannot respond to societal disadvantage. They also pointed out that voluntary organizations can act as pressure groups to cause positive change in public policies.

To support those in need is not an easy matter, however. Voluntary organizations have to achieve credibility in the eye of society, and at a local level, to be accepted by their communities and local authorities. Their purpose and activities must be exposed to public and statutory scrutiny. They have duties to ensure that their welfare enterprises attain positive outcomes. Equally important, is the fact that voluntary organizations have undergone changes in their relationships with local government, due to a 'contract culture' instigated by the NHS and Community Care Act 1990. The Labour Government is currently

encouraging a 'partnership culture', desirable since voluntary organizations can benefit by working alongside government agencies, which are mainly the funders. The achievement of a partnership culture is, nevertheless, fraught with tension and conflict, as a mixed economy of care refers to the diversity of agencies, each with its own particular culture, with well established roles and functions founded on traditional procedures.

THE VOLUNTARY ORGANIZATIONS AND GOVERNMENT

Members of voluntary organizations are motivated by their personal beliefs that there are gaps in services (Case examples 10.5 and 10.6), which cause inequalities. Their altruistic/philanthropic

Case example 10.5 42nd Street

This project (Snell 1998) describes the work of a voluntary organization that aims to meet the mental health needs of young people (aged 15–25). Since set up in 1980, it strives to help young people under stress, by creating a therapeutic climate with 'youth work' as its basis. It is a non-stigmatized service, managed by 24 paid workers and a similar-sized team of volunteers. A flexible service is provided. This consists of formal and informal counselling, psychotherapy, a support group, a befriending service and helpline. The aim is early intervention. The charity's income is about £460 000 a year. Funding comes from a variety of sources (social and health services, Comic Relief, National Lottery grant).

Case example 10.6 The George House Trust

This project, established since 1985 in Manchester (Snell 1998), describes a voluntary organization aiming to improve the quality of life for people with HIV. As improvement in therapy occurred, the voluntary organization found that people needed a different kind of support, e.g. help in coping with complex drug regimen, advice, advocacy, information on treatment and benefits, as well as how to adjust to a new way of living with their illness … The Trust has a strong lobbying role and helped to set up the National HIV Alliance.

aims can instigate members to act as a pressure group. It is hence not surprising to find that lobbying is one activity the voluntary sector engages in (Leach & Wilson 1998). A local authority's predisposition to voluntary organizations is consequently shaped by a perception of their motives, and if they are likely to cause 'electoral embarrassment'. At local level, some authorities are sensitive to suggestions and ideas concerning services and a participation in decision-making by voluntary organizations. Taylor (1997) suggested that voluntary organizations 'have many dimensions' in their relationships with government. The voluntary sector has many strings to its bow, a potential that local authorities are inclined to tap into. Diverse activities by voluntary organizations are regarded as possible resources that can be utilized in the new climate of service provision. Leach and Wilson (1998) pointed out that there are three broad views demonstrating local authorities' attitude to voluntary organizations:

1. Instrumentalist/value for money: a voluntary organization may be in a better position to provide services in a more economically efficient way, for which a local authority has a statutory responsibility to provide.
2. Participative democratic ethos: a basic awareness and belief that voluntary organizations have an important role in community services, and some councils want to promote an image of participative decision-making.
3. Traditional: in this context a local authority continues to support an organization because of a long-standing partnership in service provision, rather than as an 'expression of a more explicit view of its value'.

As perceptions and attitudes vary, one can expect local government to be additionally influenced by budgetary constraints and the political system they serve. Ackers and Fordham (1995) pointed out that not many organizations receive subsidy from the Government. They may, however, claim tax relief on investments, as well as council tax relief. Others will receive grants from social services and health authority departments. Leach and Wilson documented that the level of expenditure on voluntary organizations varies from one local authority to another; for example, their research shows that Leicester City Council has spent £12 + per head, while Nottingham City Council has spent £4–12 per head, and Kettering District Council under £4 per head.

In a new partnership culture, it is envisaged that funding for projects will be further restrained, because of central government pressures on local administration to check expenditure. Thus, the voluntary sector finds itself drawn into the political structure. As resources become scarce, it pays funders to be more critical of services and to have higher expectations. The 'monitoring role' (Gann 1996) of local authorities can be a cause of tension and conflict in voluntary organizations. In addition, a culture shift, fostered by welfare pluralism, attracts bureaucratization, managerialism and interpersonal tensions between users, funders, paid employees in voluntary organizations and their volunteers (Weeks et al 1996).

A competitive climate is causing voluntary organizations to fear the loss of their autonomy as well as the true nature of their activity, which is *voluntary*-based and not seen as *work*. As government public policy on health and welfare services changes, this is propelling voluntary organizations to re-examine their activities and to manage change. Weeks et al (1996) observed that internal pressures, as in the case of voluntary organizations for HIV/AIDS and in other spheres of the voluntary sector, make it difficult to cope with new developments.

Others (e.g. Gann 1996, Taylor 1997, Harris 1998) have noted the tension and frailty of voluntary organizations as they battle to secure funding for their cause. There is insecurity due to possible loss of contract for funding or reduced funding and dependence on funders that increases vulnerability. In addition, a voluntary organization that becomes too political can lose its members and funding issues can dampen an organization's political activity: a funder may cut back funding if an organization is too critical and politically involved.

Changes are also affecting board members who find themselves entrenched in complex negotiation meetings with governmental agencies over funding. Board members can become the 'intermediaries' between local government and the organization's paid staff. The impact of government policies is described in Box 10.3.

Box 10.3 Investigating and regulating

Increased legislation means more work for voluntary organizations as they face tighter control and monitoring. For example, Thompson (1998) acknowledged that there is mismanagement and wastefulness in the voluntary sector. The role of the Charity Commission as an effective regulator is emphasized. Contracting means that funders have a right to inspect the organization's resource management. This results in committees having to review their organizations' policies and procedures. Consumerism, performance standards and Best Value initiatives, which are expected of local government, now spill over into the voluntary sector. Voluntary organizations have to conform to welfare pluralism.

In a changing welfare climate, voluntary organizations are steered by their beliefs that their functions have to be independent from any political structures. However, a dependence culture is a source of dilemma: either a voluntary organization remains unfunded, thus affording the freedom to be critical of statutory services, or the organization is politically neutral and works alongside local authorities directed by their performance standards.

Leach and Wilson (1998) felt that, in the future, a broader role is anticipated for voluntary organizations: advisory (on policy and practice), and participatory (partners in decision-making). In addition, some organizations may increase their pressure group activity. Others still may develop their services to very high standards, upon which statutory agencies may become dependent. This effect, as Leach and Wilson (1998) observed, will counteract the 'dependency imbalance'.

INFORMAL CARERS AND SOCIAL POLICY

It is estimated that there were approximately 5.7 million carers in 1995 in the UK (Office for

---

Activity 10.4

1. Prepare a list of strategies that you would consider if you were to set up a self-help group/voluntary organization.
2. Organize a debate on the following issues:
   • There are good reasons to believe that local authorities are dependent on voluntary organizations
   • Voluntary organizations can be political in their activities, but are prevented from doing so because of a contract culture.

??? Question 10.4

1. Why do public policy changes affect the relationships between funders and voluntary organizations?
2. Should the voluntary sector develop more efficient ways to fund itself? Can you suggest how?
3. What could prevent some voluntary organizations from exercising pressure group activities?

National Statistics 1998). Although they constitute the 'informal sector' of community care, the presence of carers is acknowledged in Government documents.

The role of carers in assessment and their needs are mentioned in the Conservative Government White Paper on policy guidance, 'Community Care In The Next Decade and Beyond' (1990). In the Department of Health paper from 1997, 'Voices In Partnership', the importance of involving carers in strategic planning and care programming is emphasized. The issue of empowering people at home by the provision of 'easier and faster advice and information about health, illness and the NHS, so that they are better able to care for themselves and their families' was discussed in 'The New NHS Modern Dependable' (1997), and the institution of a long-term care charter 'to empower users and carers by promoting awareness of local services' was put forward in 'Modernising Social Services' (1998). While government White Papers demonstrate an awareness of the important role of carers in the community, there are many carers that still remain invisible and have unmet needs. For instance, the White Papers do not pinpoint the increasing numbers of children who are carers. When policy documents use the term 'carers' assumptions are made that only adults are carers. The Office for National Statistics (1998) key findings (Box 10.4) do not refer to children carers. Ackers and Fordham (1995), using figures from the Carers National Association, suggested that nationwide there are 10 000 children acting as primary carers.

Box 10.4 Office for National Statistics (1998) findings

There are approximately 6 million carers in the UK, 1.9 million of whom are caring for someone in the same household. Fifty-five per cent of carers are women (3.3 million), and 45% (2.4 million) are men. This reflects the fact that there are more women in the general adult population in the UK.

Relatives and family members constitute the majority of carers (nine out of ten). Peak age for caring was 45–64. Sixty per cent of carers had dependants with physical disabilities; 15% had dependants with mental and physical disabilities; 7% had dependants with mental disabilities only. Over a third of carers reported no one else helped them look after their dependants. Over 60% of carers who devote at least 20 hours a week to caring were women, and women were more likely to be the main carers; men, however, were more 'non-main carers'.

It is possible that current legislation on the employment of children creates loopholes preventing law enforcers from reaching the private domains of family life activities. In a review and evaluation of 'family work' legislation in the UK, Bond (1996) identified the divide that exists between the public and private, in relation to social activity (family work), which is beyond the reach of the law. Loopholes in the law make children more vulnerable to exploitation. Bond (1996) confirmed that, according to section 18(2)(a) of the Children and Young Persons Act (1933) and its bye-law, children under 13 can be employed by their parents in 'light agricultural and horticultural work'. Section 18 does not, however, make reference to informal work (i.e. domestic work, caring for a frail, elderly parent etc.), which is often done without monetary rewards. Bond refers to this situation as the 'legal invisibility of housework'. Young carers, Dearden and Becker (1997) remind us, are not always known to agencies in community care, although many care for their parents, relatives and others from childhood to adulthood. Children carers can be protected, they postulated, when existing legislation is utilized, to help safeguard children's interests. For instance, the Children Act 1989 and the United Nations on the Rights of the Child can be applied to enlighten the plight of young carers.

Young carers often do not make themselves visible to professionals out of fear: they fear being reprimanded and then removed from their parents. However, if the 'welfare principle' is applied, the child carer may be more at ease knowing that the rationale for intervention is founded on the belief that their well-being is cardinal (Dearden & Becker 1997). Local authorities, under Section 17 of the Children Act, have the power to assess the health needs of a child and to make decisions regarding the implementation of statutory health provision to protect the child.

Although legislation gives guidelines and a framework for action, professionals should attempt the following:

- to promote consciously the rights of children to access information
- to empower children to make decisions about maintaining their own well-being
- to respect children's needs for privacy and dignity
- to listen to their views and to involve children in designing a self-care plan.

Helping young carers can sometimes be achieved by providing services *for the persons they are caring for*. It is suggested (Dearden & Becker 1997) that voluntary organizations can better help young carers by undertaking needs and problems assessment, instead of statutory services, which the public often associate with a 'stigmatized service'. Carers (young and old), in addition, need information on the availability of services and the costs to be expected (Millar 1998). More dependence secures service access, Millar pointed out. For other carers, however, their needs could remain unmet.

The Carers (Recognition and Services) Act 1995, implemented in 1996, makes provision for carers to be assessed at the same time as the users are assessed. The nature of the Act is to ensure that carers receive support, that their ability to cope is evaluated and that appropriate services are given to the user (e.g. attendance to a day centre, thus giving respite to the carer) (Letts 1996). The focus is on the users' needs, but the carers' views are also considered as they may feel unable to continue giving care.

It is also known for carers to be as unwell as the persons they care for. George (1995) posits that two-thirds of carers have health problems: mental health difficulties which are stress related, and physical problems related to the musculo-skeletal system. In this case, decisions have to be made to secure the best type of services for both users and carers.

Supporting carers is now a major social issue (Box 10.5) and policy makers have to recognize their invaluable contribution in community care participation. It is estimated that carers' services

---

Box 10.5 Caring for carers

Carers have a need to gain information (Case example 10.7) to help them in their caring role. They have differing needs as their personal circumstances vary. For example, Beck and Minghella (1998) recognize that many carers look after the mentally ill at home, on their own. Their needs are:

- to have greater access to services
- information on the nature of the illness and education
- access to around the clock support
- to be taught how to cope and have practical support
- guidance on entitlements (e.g. benefits, assessment of needs).

Case example 10.7 'If they'd said ...'

'If, right from the beginning, someone had sat down with us and, instead of shoving her home and saying there were no problems – when in fact she was virtually dependent – if they'd said, "she's going to need care and here are the ways we can help". If we'd been told about the financial help, the short-stay accommodation, given a wheelchair we could actually use. If someone had said, "if it gets too much, here are the options ..." ' (Hicks 1988).

---

would cost approximately £30 billion if they were paid (Wellard 1998).

Other dimensions of importance are being able to acknowledge and respond to the needs of caregivers in the fields of learning disabilities (young and old), HIV/AIDS, and the elderly infirm with multiple pathology (e.g. dementia, challenging behaviour, Alzheimer's disease etc.). The role of care professionals has to adapt to new demands from informal carers as they continue to cope with intensive home care procedures. Kirk and Glendinning (1998) asserted, for example, that nurses should complement lay care giving: there is a need to impart technical information – to assist lay carers in clinical procedures – and to educate. Further, carers' needs for psycho-social support must be understood and responded to.

Activity 10.5

1. Ask your community health service managers how many carers they have identified in your area.
2. Identify their caring role in relation to the users' care needs (i.e. mental health, learning disabilities, older infirm adults etc.).

??? Question 10.5

1. To what extent has the Carers Act raised awareness of needs?
2. What makes some carers reluctant to disclose their caring responsibilities? Can you list some possible personal reasons for this?

SUMMARY

In a mixed economy of care, multiple agencies are envisaged to participate by competing for contract. A contract culture has been responsible for causing alterations in the management of social and health services. In addition, other agencies in the independent sector have been affected. The Government has recognized that value conflict exists in social and health services and Government White Papers aim to promote a new culture of partnership in care. The ideal is to have joint commissioning and joint working, to develop best value initiatives, encourage higher performance standards, involve public participa-tion in Health Improvement Programmes and to implement Primary Care Groups, which aim at providing services tailored to users' needs.

GLOSSARY

Intermediate care   sometimes known as convalescence care. The discharge of a client to a care setting once acute care is delivered, before final discharge home

Low-level home care   care that does not require intensive clinical intervention (e.g. food preparation, house cleaning etc.)

Musculo-skeletal   refers to the muscles and bones of the body

Paternalistic   male-dominated

Primary care   care given by community professional and informal carers

Welfare pluralism   a mixed economy of care; the participation of many welfare agencies in service provision

REFERENCES

Ackers L, Fordham J 1995 Contemporary social policy. Churchill Livingstone, New York

Ahulu S 1995 Discharge to the community of older patients from hospital. Nursing Times 91(28): 29–30

Andaleeb S S 1998 Determinants of customer satisfaction with hospitals: a managerial model. International Journal of Health Care Quality Assurance 11(6): 181–187

Barnes M, Evans M 1998 Who wants a say in the NHS? Health Matters 34: 6–7

Beck R, Minghella E 1998 Home alone. Health Service Journal 108(5607): 30–31

Benton D 1995 The role of managed care in overcoming fragmentation. Nursing Times 91(29): 25–28

Benton D 1998 Workforce planning. Nursing Management 4(9): 12–13

Billis D, Glennerster H 1998 Human services and the voluntary sector: towards a theory of comparative advantage. Journal of Social Policy 27(1): 79–98

Bond A 1996 Working for the family? Child employment legislation and the public/private divide. Journal of Social Welfare and the Family Law 18(3): 291–305

Bowman C, Black D 1998 Intermediate not indeterminate care. Hospital Medicine 59(11): 877–879

Brooker D J 1997 Issues in user feedback on health services for elderly people. British Journal of Nursing 6(3): 159–162

Central Statistics Office 1998 Informal carers in 1995: Supplement A to the General Household Survey No 25. HMSO, London

Chadda D 1998 New cash tied to first ever efficiency targets. Community Care 1233: 1

Clarke M, Hunter D J, Wistow G 1997 For debate: local government and the National Health Service: the new agenda. Journal of Public Health Medicine 19(1): 3–5

Community Care In The Next Decade And Beyond 1990 Policy Guidance. HMSO, London

Connelly J 1997 The fragile welfare state: what future? Journal of Public Health Medicine 19(4): 373–374

Cooper K 1998 Report slams lack of decent homes for vulnerable people. Community Care 1223: 4

Cutler I 1998 Tributaries to the team. Nursing Times 94(2): 40–41

Dalgard O S, Tambs K 1997 Urban environment and mental health: a longitudinal study. British Journal of Psychiatry 171: 530–536

Dearden C, Becker S 1997 Protecting young carers: tensions and opportunities in Britain. Journal of Social Welfare and Family Law 19(2): 123–138

Debell D 1998 The challenge of leadership in community health care nursing. British Journal of Community Nursing 3(2): 62–63

Department of Health 1997 Voices in partnership: involving users and carers in commissioning and delivering mental health services. HMSO, London

Edwards P 1996 Community care in health and social services: divided responsibilities? Public and Social Policy 2(3): 10–12

Gann N 1996 Managing change in voluntary organisations. Open University Press, Buckingham

George M 1995 Collaborative caring. Nursing Standard 9(46): 22–23

George M 1998 Getting together. Nursing Standard 13(12): 13

Glasman D 1997 Those magical mystery zones. Healthmatters 31: 6–7

Godfrey M, Wistow G 1997 The user perspective on managing for health outcomes: the case of mental health. Health and Social Care in the Community 5(5): 325–332

Gulland A 1998 Nappy brash. Nursing Times 94(18): 10–11

Halpern S 1998 NHS staff conditions come under scrutiny. British Journal of Healthcare Management 4(4): 178–179

Hannigan B 1997 A challenge for community psychiatric nursing: is there a future in primary health care? Journal of Advanced Nursing 26(4): 751–757

Hannigan B, Bartlett H, Clilverd A 1997 Improving health and social functioning: perspectives of mental health users. Journal of Mental Health 6(6): 613–619

Harris M 1998 Instruments of government? Voluntary sector boards in a changing public policy environment. Policy and Politics 26(2): 177–187

Hawtin M 1998 User friendly. Community Care 1228: 24–25

Hennessy D 1998 The shape of things to come. Nursing Times 93(27): 6–8

Henwood M 1997 Discharging responsibilities. Community Care 1191: 7

Hepple J, Quinton C 1997 One hundred cases of attempted suicide in the elderly. British Journal of Psychiatry 171: 42–46

Hicks C 1988 Who cares? Virago, London, p 221

Higginson I J, Jefferys P M, Hodgson C S 1997 Outcome measures for routine use in dementia services: some practical considerations. Quality in Health Care 6(3): 120–124

Hirst J 1997 Health and social care: all together now. Community Care 1191: 1

Hodgson R 1996 Mental health promotion. Journal of Mental Health 5(1): 1–2

Hudson B 1997 Caring sharing. Community Care 1191: 2–3

Hudson B 1998 Prospects of partnership. Health Service Journal 108(5600): 26–27

Jenkins R, Bebbington P, Brugha T S et al 1998 British psychiatric morbidity survey. British Journal of Psychiatry 173: 4–7

Jowell T 1998a We will only improve the nation's health if everyone plays their part. Nursing Times 94(6): 3

Jowell T 1998b Lecture. Nursing Management 4(10): 14–16

Keighley T 1998 Nursing: the big picture. Nursing Management 5(7): 27–31

Kirk S, Glendinning C 1998 Trends in community care and patient participation: implications for the roles of informal carers and community nurses in the UK. Journal of Advanced Nursing 28(2): 370–381

Leach S, Wilson D 1998 Voluntary groups and local authorities: rethinking the relationship. Local Government Studies 24(2): 1–18

Leadbetter M 1996 Blair's big idea: so what's in stakeholding for social work? Professional Social Work 4: 8–9

Letts P 1996 Informal carers are at last given recognition. Community Living 9(4): 24

Lipley N 1998 Doctors get controlling role in new primary care groups. Nursing Standard 12(40): 5

Livingston G, Manela M, Katona C 1997 Cost of community care for older people. British Journal of Psychiatry 171: 56–69

Lunt N 1996 Squaring the circle: devising charging policies for domiciliary care services. Research Policy and Planning 14(1): 85–95

McDermott G 1998 The care programme approach: a patient perspective. Nursing Times Research 3(1): 47–63

Madden V 1998 Primary care groups: ready or not? Practice Nurse 16(1): 19–21

Makin K, Campbell N 1997 Breaking down barriers. Community Care 1191: 4–5

Mayor S 1998 Primary care groups: friend or foe? Practice Nurse 15(10): 578–581

Millar B 1998 Let the people come. Health Service Journal 108(5602): 16

Modernising Social Services 1998 Promoting independence, improving protection, raising standards. HMSO, London

Moores Y 1998 This government believes nurses have a crucial contribution to make. ... Nursing Management 4(10): 17–20

Munro J 1997a Public believes in free health care but fears it will be lost. Healthmatters 31: 2

Munro J 1997b NHS needs 'a new constitution'. Healthmatters 31: 2

The New NHS Modern Dependable 1997 NMSO, London

NHS Executive 1998a Professional activity in health promotion and care. Department of Health, London, p 12–13

NHS Executive 1998b Signposts for success in commissioning and providing health services for people with learning disabilities. Department of Health, London

Office for National Statistics 1998 Social Trends 28: Social Grade. HMSO, London

Payne D 1997 Primary movers. Nursing Times 93(51): 12–13

Perkins E, Billingham K 1997 Working together to care for children in the community. Nursing Times 93(43): 46–48

Phelps K, Shepperdson B 1998 Emergency admission of elderly: a social care problem? British Journal of Community Nursing 3(10): 489–495

Philpot T 1998 Let history judge. Community Care 1251: 18–20

Porter R 1998 Capital gains. Nursing Times 94(6): 18

Poxton R 1997 Brave new workers. Community Care 1191: 6

Reynolds J 1998 Directions: learning together. Mental Health Care 1(8): 276

Rivett G 1998 A return to a caring service. Nursing Standard 12(21): 18

Rodrigues L 1998 Survival tactics. Nursing Times 94(6): 38–39

Sallah D 1998 Delivering the Bevan dream: celebrating the NHS at 50 and planning for the next century. Psychiatric Care 5(5): 166–168, 170–171

Scally G, Perkins C 1998 Environment and health. Hospital Medicine 59(11): 872–876

Schneider J 1994 Care programming: mental health angle. Primary Health Care 4(7): 12–14

Scott H 1998 The NHS can seriously damage your health. British Journal of Nursing 7(7): 364

Shacklady J 1997 Violence in the community. Journal of Community Nursing 11(10): 10–15

Slinger P 1997 Supervised aftercare for clients with mental health problems. Nursing Times 93(43): 50–51

Smith J 1998 Who will deliver primary care groups? British Journal of Midwifery 6(4): 262–264

Snell J 1998 Making an impact on the community. Healthlines 57: 12–14

Sone K 1997 Joint working so near yet so far. Community Care 1195: 18–21

Stott R 1998 Rebuilding social capital. Journal of the Royal College of Physicians of London 32(6): 568

Swage T 1998 Don't miss your chance to be heard. Practice Nurse 16(2): 73–76

Symington R 1997 Mental health services for young people: 'inadequate and patchy'. Paediatric Nursing 9(7): 6–7

Taggart S C 1998 The healthy city. Journal of the Royal College of Physicians of London 32(6): 568–571

Taylor M 1997 The best of both worlds: The voluntary sector and local government. York Publishing Services, York

Thompson A 1998 Look after the pennies. Community Care 1223: 18–19

Thuen F, Reime M H, Skrautvoll K 1997 The effect of widowhood on psychological well-being and social support in the oldest groups of the elderly. Journal of Mental Health 6(3): 265–274

Valios N 1997 Grasping the nettle of mental health. Community Care 1191: 11

Vincent M 1997 Collaborative working. Journal of Community Nursing 11(7): 38–40

Warner L, Ford R, Holmshaw J, Sathyamoorthy G 1998 Homing in on need. Community Care 1233: 20–21

Waters A 1998 Breaking down boundaries. Nursing Standard 12(22): 14

Weale A 1998 Rationing health care: a logical solution to an inconsistent triad British Medical Journal 316(7129): 410

Weeks J, Aggleton P, McKevitt C et al 1996 Community and contracts: tensions and dilemmas in the voluntary sector response to HIV and AIDS. Policy Studies 17(2): 107–123

Wellard S 1998 Carers speak out. Community Care 1223: 9

While A 1998 Is health for all just around the corner? British Journal of Community Nursing 3(3): 149

White P 1998 Fighting. Nursing Management 4(8): 7

Whitfield L 1998 Paved with good intentions. Health Service Journal 108(5599): 9

Williams G, Watkins L, Laungani P 1997 Community patient-focused care: fantasy or reality? Journal of Community Nursing 11(3): 16–17

Young L 1998 Understanding primary care groups. Primary Health Care 8(3): 6–7

Young L, Sutton E 1998 Aiming high. Nursing Standard 12(47): 16

FURTHER READING

Hirst J 1998 Is labour working? Community Care 1213: 16–19

Jackson S, Zairi M, Whymark J 1998 Organisational effectiveness in the NHS: what are the measures? British Journal of Health Care Management 4(4): 180–183

Pleace N 1998 Single homelessness as social exclusion: the unique and the extreme. Social Policy and Administration 32(1): 46–59

Savage P 1998 Care in the community. Journal of Community Nursing 12(1): 4–6

Van Eenwyk J 1997 Approaches to community concerns: applied public health. Public Health 111(6): 405–410

3

The individual and health care

The contribution of psychology in developing an understanding of the individual is highlighted in this section. Some concepts of psychology are explored and their relevance in health care settings is emphasized. As the nature of human behaviour is complex, an insight into the cognitive processes, which guide behaviour, will enhance professionals' expertise.

11 Introduction to psychology

Psychology is considered essential in health care. How humans behave when sick, what they feel, the emotions they experience and their attitudes in coping are of interest to psychologists and health care workers. The study of psychology comprises an understanding of differing schools of thought and how psychologists view human behaviour. The main aims of this chapter are to:

• highlight and explain the meaning of psychology by describing some key concepts
• show their relevance to health care situations.

WHAT IS PSYCHOLOGY?

Most textbooks of psychology begin by attempting to define 'psychology' by stating that it is a scientific study of human mental life and behaviour. Although this definition is true, it does not help us to know what mental life is and how human behaviour is linked to the concept. In addition, what is human behaviour? Is it different to animal behaviour? Is mental life a form of behaviour? If it is, how can it be described? If thinking is an aspect of mental action, how can it be explained? If I say that before starting to write this chapter, I did a lot of thinking, what does this tell us about human behaviour, and what evidence can be provided that someone has *thought* so that the behaviour can be observed?

A student recently commented that the science of psychology, in contrast with biology, is an elusive subject in which answers cannot readily be pinpointed to specifics, and are inclined to be abstract in nature. This argument is true in many ways since scientists have researched mental life in order to provide definite answers in regard to its nature. So when one begins to investigate psychology, other key concepts are discovered. For example, conscious mental processes are believed to be encompassing the activities of mental life, such as thinking, feeling, imagining, recalling events, perceiving the environment, both internal (within oneself) and external (outside one's body). Any factors in our environment can trigger responses within our psyche, causing temporary reactions so that we can respond to events as they occur.

Gross (1992) pointed out that mental processes are the private domains of a person's mental life. In other words, one cannot know for certain what is going on inside a person's brain unless one is told by the person. However, one can make *inferences*. By this Gross meant that observations of individuals' external behaviour can give an inkling of the processes taking place within their psyche. For example, one can infer that a person's anxious facial expression is due to their experiencing feelings of danger, uncertainty, or impending doom. In a health care setting, observing the clients' behaviour gives the caregiver an insight into the possible course of events in the individual's mind. This does not mean, however, that the application of psychological theories makes the professional a mind-reader. In fact, psychologists have warned against adopting this stance as it is not a true reflection of psychology as a scientific discipline. Rather one should use one's knowledge of life experiences – attached to research findings from psychology – to facilitate an understanding of why a client/patient may be behaving in a particular way.

Introspection is one method used to explore one's mental processes. This approach has its limitations, however, because only human behaviour can be assessed in such a way. Human thoughts and feelings cannot be compared with animal behaviour.

Eysenck (1996) pointed out that introspection should be supplemented with the 'study of behaviour'. Behaviour, he argued, can readily be described (e.g. joy, fear, anxiety, aggression, compassion etc.), while mental processes are hidden from view. It is the latter, Eysenck postulates, which has been the focus of psychologists. They want to acquire knowledge of cause and effect: while external behaviour exhibits the effect, psychologists want to know *why* the person behaves accordingly. Put in a different way, psychologists seek to discover the complex internal brain processes that caused the behaviour.

Some psychologists will, however, argue that introspection is not easily achieved. A possible argument is that people are only partially aware of their consciousness. Deeper mental activities are not easily accessible, as it is believed that they remain in the unconscious compartment of the mind. Eysenck (1996) refers to the conscious mind as the 'tip of the iceberg'.

Other writers have attempted to elucidate the complex nature of the mind. Postle (1989) tentatively refers to the mind as a concept containing a whole range of human experience. Rosenthal (1991) alludes to 'mental phenomena' as mental states which, compared with physical and natural sciences law, remains an abstract concept and can only be described through language (i.e. the expression of thoughts and feelings).

The mind, in addition, is interpreted and understood from one's personal experience. When I say, for example, that I must focus my mind on this subject matter, to make my thoughts clear to the reader, I am in fact referring to my interpretation of internal mental processes, as I understand them.

Rosenthal argued that other people's mental states can be markedly different to one's own. This has implications for clinical practice. Individual patients in care settings may respond to their circumstances differently (Case examples 11.1 and 11.2) because of their mental states. Their views of the world are prone to differ as their personal experiences can be unique. It is hence a requisite to respect the individuality of a person's mental state experiences, and equally relevant to design care programmes that are specific to needs.

Case example 11.1 Belief in the spiritual world

Shah was admitted as an emergency to the surgical ward. He was 45 years old. He was at work when he started complaining of abdominal pain. The staff nurse who did the initial assessment was puzzled by his behaviour: although he described the pain as 'excruciating', the nurse's personal experience of pain did not match the client's behaviour as well as other patients she had encountered with similar diagnoses. Shah's relatives told the nurse that he believed in the spiritual world, and believed that a person could transcend bodily experiences by mobilizing mental resources, with support from beings in the spirit world. Shah's belief in the help he received from the spirit world helped him perceive the pain differently from the nurse.

Case example 11.2 Past experience

John, aged 89, has been an inpatient for the past 6 months. John spent time in a workhouse as a child and he now perceives the hospital as a workhouse. The nursing staff, he believes, are the attendants who want to control his behaviour. John's past experiences within a workhouse are affecting his current perceptions.

Since language is a useful tool to express one's mental state, professionals must be sensitive to clients' individual communication styles. In some circumstances, the complexity of someone's mental state can be compounded by cultural factors. The expression of thoughts, feelings and desires differs among cultural groups. Cultural and religious factors have been implicated (for example, beliefs in witchcraft, the ritual of sorcery, evil eye, in God(s) etc.). Such strong beliefs exert a powerful impact on the believer's mental state. Case example 11.1 illustrates a person whose personal beliefs have altered his mental state, so that the pain experience is controlled to some extent. In Case example 11.2 it is past experience that has influence over one's perception. Also important is the knowledge that a client's health status is linked to their mental state.

It is known that bio-chemical changes (e.g. uraemia, hypoglycaemia and bodily changes)

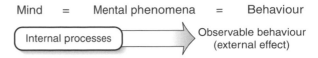

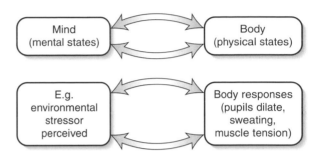

Fig. 11.1 The interconnections between the mind, mental phenomena and behaviour.

Fig. 11.2 The Mind–Body dimensions of human behaviour.

caused by electrolyte imbalance will lead to perceptual alterations, disorientation and confusion. The mind is hence argued to be equal to mental phenomena, which are equal to behaviour (Fig. 11.1). Similarly, pathological changes (biological alterations) will have an effect on mental states. The study of human behaviour has to encompass the mind–body interaction dimensions (Fig. 11.2). To explore the meanings of psychology, therefore, an analysis of consciousness and thinking has to be done by identifying its basic features (Gross 1992):

- associating human behaviour with mental processes (Atkinson et al 1993)
- focusing on what stimulates human beings to behave the way they do; in other words, 'what makes them tick' (Hayes 1984)
- general observations of people's activities (Hayes 1994).

Psychologists, however, have to study animals too, and various organisms either in natural settings or in laboratories. For example, the behaviour of the amoeba (a unicellular organism) and its response to external stimuli (heat, cold, electrical current) becomes important in research. Findings from such studies have contributed to developing our understanding of human behaviour. When psychologists study human and animal behaviour, attention is also given to the physiological–intellectual interplay processes causing the behaviour. For example, the human infant cries when parents leave the room; the baby chimpanzee clings to her mother as she moves from tree to tree; the student has sleepless nights prior to examinations. These are aspects of behaviour that can be readily observed and inferences made.

Activity 11.1

1. Describe your thought processes prior to an Interview for a job.
2. Now compare your findings with others who have been in similar situations.

??? Question 11.1

1. Can you provide some arguments to explain the complexity of psychology?
2. How would you describe the meaning of psychology?

APPROACHES TO THE STUDY OF PSYCHOLOGY

Psychology can only be studied by being aware that human behaviour occurs in a social context. Since a multitude of human dimensions is an aspect of social life, it is feasible to approach the study of psychology by raising awareness of related disciplines.

Psychology is distinct from the disciplines of psychiatry and psychoanalysis. The term 'psychiatry' applies to the study of mental ill-health, its investigation, treatment and classification (Dally 1982), and relates to the principles governing diagnosis and classification (Fulford 1994) of symptoms and clinical syndromes of mental or psychological dysfunction. There are anxiety states, for example, when individuals show the manifestations of phobias, depression and panic attacks.

Psychoanalysis, on the other hand, is considered to be a psychological method of treatment

(Hobbs 1994). Its principles lie in encouraging the patient to express attitudes, emotions, reactions that would subsequently be assessed by the psychoanalyst. Radford and Govier (1991) postulated that a psychoanalyst is essentially a therapist. Some psychoanalysts may be medically trained and are psychiatrists. A psychotherapist, moreover, is someone who provides psychological treatment and may also be a trained counsellor, using psychoanalytic techniques with clients, helping them to find solutions to their problems. An awareness of related disciplines can help psychology students in their investigation of psychological theories. Of importance too, is developing an understanding of the historical background of psychology. This particular approach, Taylor and Hayes (1990) pointed out, will indicate how psychology has differentiated itself over the years, and may clarify its definition and its specialization into so many branches.

Hence, the foundations on which present day psychology is resting may be analysed. Questions may be asked on the intricacies of the mind and its structure:

1. What methods should be used?
2. Do mental processes have functions?
3. Should human behaviour be studied from a biological perspective?
4. To what extent should the causes of psychological problems be studied by exploring the unconscious mind and its instinct?

These questions have concerned theorists in the field of psychological investigation. A multitude of ideas and theories have evolved consequently, which further explain the nature of psychology.

Another approach that may be used is to take note of social interactions. This involves using one's powers of observation. In health care settings, professionals have a duty to observe the sick person, to make notes of their behavioural responses to care and treatment. Just as important is to use the knowledge gained from such observations and to act upon them. The aim is to use a knowledge of psychology and to prevent deterioration.

Sayer (1992) wrote that it is 'communicative interactions' and the 'sharing and transmission of meaning' that will lead to an understanding of meaning. Meaningful interactions can only occur when the caregiver is enabled, through knowledge of psychology, to interact in an empathetic way.

Sometimes, knowledge of human behaviour is gained by purposeful application of theories into practice, and by observing the results of the interpersonal reactions. As pointed out above, individuals respond differently to similar situations. In some cases, a person may experience difficulties in memorizing events; the student of psychology assesses the possible variables causing the behaviour change. In addition, the links between memory and learning have to be made. Any hypotheses can be reflectively analysed, and compared with existing theoretical underpinning as suggested by researchers.

Various media are invaluable resources for the psychologist: many documentaries portray human and animal behaviour in candid settings. For example, how do people behave after a major catastrophe (e.g. a plane crash, a devastating hurricane, a bomb explosion in a city store), and how does repeated advertising influence behaviour?

Furthermore, it is important to study one's own behaviour before attempting to understand others. Williams (1993) explained that the importance of personal experiences should not be underestimated. It helps one to make sense of the world. However, it is essential to acknowledge the social context of behaviour, as existing knowledge is constantly being reshaped.

Reflection is a necessary requisite to explaining one's own and others' behaviour. As one writer pointed out, we can only begin the process of understanding by reflecting upon one's own experience (Winter 1989).

There is one further argument in connection with the study of psychology: that one should first identify the differences between psychology and other sciences (Box 11.1) and what is the nature of their interests, as this will help clarify the focus of the subject matter.

Box 11.1 Comparisons between psychology and other sciences

A **psychologist** is interested in:

- Human and animal motivation
- Personality
- Learning and memory
- Cognitive processes
- Intelligence
- The effects of stress on individuals
- Childhood development
- Compliance, conformity, aggression
- Perception

A **sociologist** is interested in:

- Social phenomena
- Group organization
- Education and its institutions
- Ethnicity and race
- Deviance in society
- Achievement and non-achievement of individuals
- The law, communities, kinship, religion
- Culture and the media
- Political systems, class systems
- The family

A **biologist** is interested in:

- The structure and functions of the human body
- Cellular structures
- The various systems of the body (animal and human): cardiovascular, respiratory, renal systems etc.

Activity 11.2

Make a list of ideas you consider to be 'psychological', e.g. reflect upon the content of a news bulletin. Ask yourself whether the topics are social, psychological or biological. Can you differentiate between these issues?

??? Question 11.2

If psychology is the study of behaviour, how would you start to explore its features?

PERSPECTIVES IN PSYCHOLOGY

A study in psychology would be incomplete without a standard discussion on its perspectives, which helps one to grasp the multi-faceted characteristics of this discipline. The complexity of human behaviour has aroused an array of differing viewpoints. The term 'behaviour', for example, not only includes external observable behaviour, but also the physiological behaviour of cells, a perspective called *physiological psychology*. Examples include:

- the biological processes occurring during learning and memorizing a task
- the production of pain, its physiological mechanisms and how they are translated into the perception of pain, accompanied by the mental anguish experienced by the person.

Biology is therefore considered to be of relevance in psychology since human behaviour is directed by many biological mechanisms.

Other psychologists will, however, use a cognitive perspective. *Cognitive psychology* propounds the notion that the human brain is similar to a computer: it processes all the information being fed into it. The term 'cognitive psychology' makes allusion to the mental processes needed to interpret the endless amount of stimuli, both internal (physiological) and external (environmental), reaching the brain. For example, when a person feels hungry the brain interprets the sensations of hunger by means of its physiological networks (i.e. hormonal, neural and cardiovascular), so that appropriate action can be taken. Or, when one looks out of a window into an open field, the brain registers the incoming data (visual, olfactory, auditory and tactile stimuli) to inform one about the external environment. In clinical settings, patients are bombarded by a multitude of stimuli, which can be unpleasant and add to their discomfort and confusion. A well-ventilated area, with the reduction of noise and odour, is conducive to rest and sleep. A calm, efficient, professional manner can further improve patients' confidence.

Developmental psychology is a specialization within psychology (Atkinson et al 1993). With this perspective, psychologists will study behavioural development from the prenatal stage to old age. Areas of interest include

- perceptual and cognitive development
- socialization
- parental influences
- language acquisition and development
- gender development

- issues related to separation and deprivation (Flanagan 1996).

In Chapter 3, the fact that children are exposed to a variety of adverse life experiences which have negative consequences on their psychosocial and physical developments was discussed. In Chapter 4, the effects of ageing on the older person, their life experiences and how adversity in late adulthood can arrest development was outlined. Recognizing the features of arrested psychological development allows professionals to initiate care as required and to communicate their observations to specialist teams.

Social factors have been known to influence behaviour. *Social psychology* is concerned with the observations of group behaviour, attitudes and responses in interpersonal relationships, and how thoughts and feelings can be influenced. Eysenck (1996) explained how in daily life one is constantly guided by 'group norms'; i.e. the rules and expectations of the group to which an individual belongs. The theory is that people are influenced by others as they interact with each other – a process known as social facilitation – and the presence of others can enhance performance. However, there are instances when a person is prone to malfunction in front of others due to nervousness, anxiety or fear.

In health care, social influences play a part in increasing compliance. The sick person complies to a nurse's request to take medications; a doctor's advice is readily accepted; the staff are influenced to perform skilfully as their activities are monitored by their peers and managers.

When a psychologist studies animal behaviour in order to obtain data that can be used to understand human behaviour, this perspective is known as *comparative psychology*. (Gross (1992) pointed out that it is also known as animal psychology.) Although animals differ from humans, many experiments (e.g. pain responses, effects of hormones on behaviour, separation and deprivation) have increased our understanding of human psychology.

Educational psychology is a specialized field and is different from the above. Educational psychologists are interested in the way individuals learn, and carry out research specific to teaching methods, to improve practice and maximize skills in order to improve learning. Educational psychologists' experience is invaluable in facilitating the learning needs of those with learning disabilities.

Clinical psychology is the application of research in psychology to solve behavioural problems. Clinical psychologists very often work with psychiatrists, who will have studied psychology and who specialize in abnormal behaviour.

Phenomenological psychology is allied to the investigation of the uniqueness of a person's perception of the world. It relates to the study of people's private experiences, their emotions, feelings and perceptions. It is subjective in nature. It is a method posited to be an approach that focuses on the lived experience (Bousfield 1997), and supplies valuable insights into the inner psychological workings of the individual. Thus personal views of events are the focus (Meldrum 1995a). For this reason this approach is also described as humanistic.

In practice, the personal world view of clients assumes great importance. Time spent to encourage the free expression of feelings and emotions allows for an accurate measurement of treatment and care effectiveness (Case example 11.3). Occasionally, due to apprehension and feelings of isolation, a person's emotional state can prevent the communication of inner feelings. A relaxed, non-threatening and friendly environment can enhance communication.

Case example 11.3 In the side-room

It is sometimes assumed that a side-room is the best option to nurse the patients. This was not the case for Tom who was in for investigation of bowel problems. Tom was an extrovert. He was told that he would find it more private and quiet in the side-room. He felt isolated, apprehensive and that he had a contagious condition. His primary nurse could not understand the change in his behaviour. He was weepy, suffered from insomnia and became withdrawn. The nurse would spend time encouraging him to talk about his feelings. He said he hated confined spaces, felt isolated from the main ward area and that he overheard another patient saying that only patients who do not have long to live are put in this side-room.

Activity 11.3

During visiting hours, spend time talking to patients/clients who are on their own. How would you describe the content of their conversations?

??? Question 11.3

Is it possible to study human behaviour by utilizing only one perspective?

CONCEPTS IN PSYCHOLOGY

When psychologists study human behaviour, they use specific technical concepts that clearly demarcate their approaches from sociological concepts. While a sociologist will focus on the organization of society into groups and systems of social functioning, psychologists are preoccupied with how individuals are mentally processing stimuli from both their internal (bodily functions) and external social environment, as well as their responses to them.

According to Chandler (1991) there is a close relationship between the two disciplines: psychology, although analysing behaviour and mental processes, is also focusing on the individual, who is the basic unit of society. Both are concerned with human beings as individuals: psychology is focused on individual human consciousness, and sociology with the individual as a member of the social system.

Motivation

When psychologists use the term 'motivation' they are referring to goal-seeking behaviour. Motivation is associated with basic needs (Burns 1980, Gross 1992, Atkinson et al 1993, Eysenck 1996), which is thought to originate from theories based on instinct and biology (Lloyd et al 1984). Since there are so many factors implicated in producing goal-seeking behaviour, psychologists have used various perspectives and theories to explain its nature:

Biogenic theories are based on the assumption that individuals are driven by needs to avoid pain and the seeking of pleasure (i.e. hedonistic impulses).

Instinct theory posits that innate and unlearned tendencies trigger specific responses spontaneously from some biological or social needs and that humans have a propensity to respond – in ways controlled by an inbred disposition – to environmental stimuli. For example, if you are hungry you search for food; if you are feeling lonely, you phone your friend for a chat. Such behaviour, however, finds its origin from a combination of factors: internal processes (physiological and cognitive) and external processes (social and cultural) which shape expressions (Wade & Travis 1993). Learning and past experience are, however, variables that are influential in triggering responses too.

Psychoanalytical theories centre on the unconscious: motives buried deep in the mind, which instinctively make people behave in ways that help maintain self-preservation.

Field theories explain motivation by including social and psychological factors: the personality of the individual and how they perceive the world at any given time, e.g. when a person hears airplanes flying low over the roof tops, they do not run for shelter; but they would if in a war zone.

Motivation is also related to stimulation levels. Many under-stimulated individuals seek situations that will keep them incited; however, a person receiving too much stimulation will attempt to reduce it to an accepted level. This theory is known as 'intrinsic motivation'.

Another theory explaining motivation follows a model designed by Maslow (1954, 1970), which is popularly quoted in psychology literature and is known as the 'hierarchy of needs' (Fig. 11.3). For example, eating and drinking are basic needs. If one is hungry, one is most likely going to seek ways to appease that hunger instead of engaging in idealistic pursuits, such as writing a book or climbing Mount Everest.

In clinical settings one finds many examples of patients whose basic needs must be met. The need to combat pain is imperative. Unless pain is

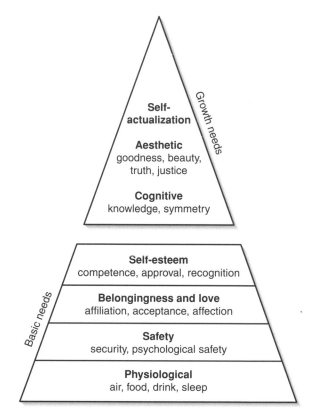

Fig. 11.3   Maslow's hierarchy of needs.

controlled, communication and cooperation are less likely to be achieved. Further, the pain factor has deep psychological implications. If pain is not alleviated, recovery is impaired, fear and anxiety states are compounded, and some patients attempt to end their own lives. Other issues related to basic needs are the prevention of constipation, to have a nourishing diet, to feel psychologically and physically safe, and to sleep and rest.

Emotion

Psychologists and social psychologists have studied the concept of emotion and established its links with physiological factors. It is believed that emotional reactions are the products of central nervous system stimulation, combined with autonomic nervous system activation (Hayes 1984) and hormone release (adrenaline and noradrenaline) from the endocrine system.

The types of physiological arousal, such as heart acceleration and muscular tension (Hall 1982, Powell & Enright 1990), created by these hormones have been described as 'instinctual survival mechanisms' (McConnell & Philipchalk 1992). Emotion, however, is also a product of the complex events that take place when social–environmental factors are perceived and interpreted by the central nervous system; e.g. bank clerks are likely to be emotionally aroused when a customer suddenly points a gun at them and threatens to shoot if they do not do what the customer says.

Biological theorists faithfully quote William James's (1884) theory of emotion. James put forward that a situation perceived as threatening (stimulus) causes physiological changes. Such changes, which precede the recognition of a threat, *cause* the emotions (fear, anxiety etc.). For example, when students on examination day say that they are experiencing a heavy, churning, 'butterfly' feeling in the stomach, they also express anxiety reactions and feelings. Using James's theory the process can be summarized as follows:

Stimulus (taking an exam) appraisal = physiological arousal (bodily changes) = emotional states (fear, anxiety, anger etc.).

Hence, it is argued that bodily changes, stimulated by hormonal factors, are what makes a person 'emotional', not the examination. McGregor (1994) explained the subjective experience of emotion, as the individual assesses the circumstances (cognitive appraisal). Opposing emotions are likely but dependent on how the person interprets incoming messages from the environment.

Emotion is hence a multidimensional concept, possessing some key features (Malim et al 1992), which have implications for clinical practice (Box 11.2). These features are:

1. it is a response to external stimuli
2. it invariably affects the autonomic system, which stimulates physical (physiological) reactions
3. it is a subjective experience
4. it has cognitive mechanisms (involving thought processes)

Box 11.2 Psychoemotional needs in clinical practice

It is acknowledged that care settings have a major impact on the sick person's emotional states. A clinical environment arouses tension, apprehension, disturbing thoughts and conflicting feelings associated with the fear of dying and death, unbearable pain, loss of loved ones, isolation and being incapacitated.

The provision of information, using a client and family-centred strategy, coupled with specialist counselling skills, can prevent psychological deterioration (Wesson 1997).

Emotional care also entails recognizing one's own feelings (Burnard 1988), and relates to the exploration of one's emotions, to enhance sensitivity to others' expressions of distress (Case example 11.4). If professionals adopt a distant, 'stiff upper lip' attitude, clients are less prone to release emotional tensions. Research findings indicate that a caring behaviour makes patients feel safe. On the other hand, impersonal behaviour on the part of nurses accentuates distress and impairs the recovery rate (Holland et al 1997).

Emotional distress is triggered by uncomfortable experiences which demand intense focus on the client's emotional needs (Giedosh 1997):

- physical discomfort caused by pain
- insomnia
- respiratory impairment
- procedures
- fear of the unknown (not being told what is happening)
- acute life-threatening illness or trauma.

Additionally, the complex interplay of physiological, psychological and situational factors (Lenz et al 1997) deepen the symptoms of the illness precipitating the emotional reactions.

Clients can, however, be empowered by the strategic use of imagery (Stephens 1993). Imagery is an effective cognitive tool to help alleviate the effects of pain and stress. Stephens asserts that its application allows the individual to exert better control on the mechanisms that link perception, emotion and bodily change. Theory of imagery states that positive thinking can impact on physiological processes, mental state, performance and behaviour, helps to reduce the effects of stress, and induces relaxation (Box 11.3).

5. expressive behaviour can be observed, such as facial alterations (Argyle 1983) and other deportment variations.

Attention

The concept of attention can be defined as the ability to focus one's mental energy on some specific sensory (e.g. auditory, visual, olfactory,

Case example 11.4 Continuing presence

'One of my allocated patients was a young woman with recently diagnosed, inoperable breast cancer. I knew no more about her than this. A consultant ward round was in progress, during which she was to learn her diagnosis/prognosis ... Was it my job to attend to this patient's emotional need in what must surely be the most devastating crisis of her life? ... I sat beside her on her bed. She said "they've just told me everything" ... I found myself saying a feeble sounding: "I am very sorry" ... She cried and raged in the following hour. We talked about her life, her husband, her hopes and fears. How could she bear to leave her children?

'I didn't bother to fight back my tears ... I wanted to thank her – for enabling me to empathize and truly share feelings; to be emotional without being unprofessional; to meet someone's needs on a level that transcended nurse/patient roles' (Allen 1992).

Box 11.3 The benefits of imagery

Imagery is a psychological concept. It requires the use of imagination. However, imagination on its own is not sufficient. Mental effort is needed. This entails applying one's cognitive skills to either recall past events with positive and relaxing effects, or to invent images one believes to be personally meaningful and beneficial. For example, you may remember the positive sensations of a holiday on a distant island; or being in the company of friends who helped in making a success of your business; or you could simply fantasize about situations you feel will help induce relaxation.

The benefits of imagery (Stephens 1993) in patient care are numerous:

- reduce anxiety
- instill a feeling of control
- a problem-solving tool: an old problem is looked at in a completely different way
- new ideas can be generated
- a link is made between imagery and healing: clients (with advanced cancer) who used imagery in combination with medical intervention have been found to increase their life span by 8–19 months.

Activity 11.4

Try to use imagery prior to writing your assignment. Now write down your thoughts and feelings. Can you make a comparison between what you felt before doing the activity and afterwards?

??? Question 11.4

1. Can you analyse what emotions you experienced when you had to give your first injection?
2. Is it possible to see emotions on people's faces?
3. How would you describe a facial expression that denotes pain, anger, joy, aggression?

tactile, gustatory) stimuli that have to be cognitively processed. For example, a writer concentrates on the visual display of a word processor while writing; cooks purposefully focus their attention on the quality of food being tasted. Attention is hence integrated with perception (Eysenck 1996). In addition, people's attention is constantly competing with a vast number of stimuli, which bombard the senses. It is for this reason that only selected stimuli are attended to. Gross (1992) explained that the brain is limited in its capacity to process all available stimuli. Further, he argued, life would be chaotic if the most important stimulation was not selected, leaving the least essential ones.

There are three main categories of attention (Meldrum 1995b):

1. Sustained attention, which is associated with powers of concentration; i.e. the ability to focus on a particular task for a defined duration, without being distracted.

2. Selective attention: this applies to the purposeful act of selecting a specific stimulus. For example, a person decides to answer the phone rather than the knock on the door, or decides to watch the television rather than read the newspapers. Selective attention is also known as 'focused attention' (Slack 1990).

3. Divided attention: this describes a person's response to differing stimulation, by attending to several tasks at once. For example, one may talk to someone on the phone, write notes on what is being said, glance at the TV channels and ask their daughters to turn the radio down.

There are some important features attached to the concept of attention. Whichever type of attention one refers to, the sensory organs are always connected with the process. This is of course dependent on the source of the stimulus. A noise stimulates the ears, a visual stimulus affects the eyes, and so on. Another relevant factor is that attention is interdependent with perception: we perceive through our senses, and thereafter our attention is drawn in different directions.

Therefore, one finds that perception and attention as psychological concepts are dependent on cognitive processes. People perceive through the senses, but the information has to be processed and 'filtered' before a particular category of attention is in operation. While psychological and biological factors are associated with this process, assumptions must not be made that they are the only variables, at the expense of cultural factors. A tourist driving across the Australian desert may be indifferent to the barren region. To the Aborigines, however, the tracks left by some ants on the sand could lead to a valuable food source. When communicating, a person's attention is drawn to the facial expressions and features of the other person. However, in some cultures people are socialized to avoid eye contact and to keep their faces covered.

Attention is likely to be impaired when a person is hungry, tired and ill. Perhaps this reminds us of Maslow's needs hierarchy. A visual display of food and a bed in which to sleep is more likely to focus the attention of someone who is hungry and tired.

Pathological changes in the brain have a negative impact on attention. Neurological impairment interferes with cognitive skills. An ageing nervous system is linked to cognitive alteration, which can interfere with attention (Meldrum 1995b). An understanding of the factors interfering with attention is an issue pertinent to health care intervention (Box 11.4).

Information-giving, Gammon and Mulholland (1996) hypothesized, increases psychological well-being and improves coping ability. One can infer that patients who are motivated to get better and to exert control over their illness, are more inclined to benefit from information that will help them to achieve their goal. In addition, as Gammon and Mulholland found out, patients whose knowledge of their condition is increased, are more disposed to be compliant with their

---

Box 11.4 Communication to increase attention levels

Research undertaken by Hart and Wells (1997) to examine the correlation between the utilization of complex language and agitated behaviour among 15 residents with dementia, showed that cognitive skills impairment (a common manifestation of dementia) depreciated their attention skills. In addition, caregivers' use of complex language increased their agitation.

Although the researchers were concerned with the degree of agitation caused by language complexity, their findings are relevant to issues concerned with attention. For example, they suggest that the client's degree of comprehension needs to be assessed to ensure that environmental stimulation must be 'in balance' with their competence. Too many stimuli can overburden them.

To encourage better attention, communication must be simplified and kept concise. Less agitation ensures the client is more relaxed to listen to the caregivers' instructions and respond accordingly.

---

care and treatment. For these individuals, it can be argued that their motivation will make them more attentive to nursing and medical instructions. As they feel that their coping ability is going to be enhanced, their attention level is correspondingly sharpened.

However, the giving of information that is meaningful to patients will not guarantee increased attention, unless the caregiver exhibits empathy, warmth and genuineness. Moreover, as stated in Box 11.4, environmental factors have to be in balance with the person's level of coping. Equally relevant is the person's bio-psychosocial status. If physical and psychological discomfort are evident, attention will be distracted. If there is evidence that social reasons (e.g. bereavement, family conflict, work pressures) are impinging on mental well-being, the propensity to focus on communication is disturbed.

Activity 11.5

1. Attempt to do a set of tasks all at once. Write down your experience.
2. Watch a TV programme. Can you focus on *everything* that appears on the screen and what is being said?
3. Can you recall a situation when you felt sad? How was your attention level at that time?

? **?** **?** Question 11.5

1. You may have read this page now. Did you notice the *size* of the printed words? If not why not?
2. As you sit reading the newspaper, you can *hear* your neighbours talking outside the window. Would you be able to describe *accurately* what they are saying? What about recalling precisely the content of what you have been reading as well?

SUMMARY

Psychology is a science that centres on human and animal behaviour. Psychologists are mainly concerned with the mental processes that accompany human behaviour. Hence, behaviour is seen as complex in nature. In an attempt to explore what makes people tick, psychologists have utilized a number of perspectives. The biological perspective looks at the physiology of cellular activity and how it stimulates behaviour. Cognitive psychology relates to the processing of environmental stimuli: messages that reach the brain and are interpreted. Cognitive theory also takes into account the internal stimuli (i.e. the biological stimulation) that people feel, and how they are interpreted.

The study of development traces the psychological stages of human progress from prenatal to old age, and how the mental framework is shaped as people grow older. The field of social psychology explores the effects of social influences on behaviour. The theory of social influence indicates that people are sensitive to group norms, that they are guided by unwritten rules, which make them conform to what they believe others expect of them.

To study human behaviour, psychologists have recourse to the study of animals, which will yield useful data that can be applied (in some cases) to the human context. This approach is known as comparative psychology. Other perspectives are linked to education strategy developed from a study of how people can learn in the most efficient way. This is commonly termed as educational psychology.

A humanistic approach to the study of human behaviour is commonly known as phenomenology. It takes into account the lived experience of the person: how someone feels, the narratives of the personal experience (i.e. emotional experiences, cognitive dimensions, their world view etc.). There are some key concepts identified in psychology. These are motivation, emotion and attention. They are all relevant to clinical practice as care professionals have to respond to their patients'/clients' needs in these areas as they arise.

Clinical psychologists and psychiatrists often work together in the treatment of behavioural problems. There are many methods of studying psychology: it can be studied alongside psychiatry; its links to social situations can be explored; on the other hand, a historical look at its development is another avenue. Comparisons can also be made between psychology, biology and sociology. Students of psychology can access pertinent information both from observing human interactions in daily life and from the media.

GLOSSARY

Autonomic nervous system systems of nerves that control physiological mechanisms, such as the heart, blood vessels, gastro-intestinal functioning etc.
Central nervous system the brain and spinal cord
Clinical syndromes a collection of symptoms that are of clinical relevance
Endocrine system systems of glands that control the release of hormones in the blood stream
Hedonistic centred on increasing one's pleasure

Hypoglycaemia reduced (lower than normal) blood glucose level
Introspection analysing one's own thoughts and feelings
Masochism propensity to derive pleasure from self-inflicted pain
Phobias extreme fears (e.g. objects, animals)
Uraemia disordered function of the urinary system causing increase in the level of urea in the blood

REFERENCES

Allen S 1992 Show some emotions. Nursing Times 88(27): 39

Argyle M 1983 The psychology of interpersonal behaviour, 4th edn. Penguin, London

Atkinson R, Atkinson R, Smith E et al 1993 Introduction to psychology, 11th edn. Harcourt Brace Jovanovich, Fort Worth, p 13, p 23

Bousfield C 1997 A phenomenological investigation into the role of the clinical nurse specialist. Journal of Advanced Nursing 25(2): 245–256

Burnard P 1988 No need to hide. Nursing Times 84(24): 36–38

Burns R 1980 Essential psychology. MTP Press, Lancaster

Chandler J 1991 Tabbner's nursing care: theory and practice. Churchill Livingstone, Edinburgh

Dally P 1982 Psychology and psychiatry. Hodder & Stoughton, London

Eysenck M 1996 Simply psychology. Psychology Press, Hove

Flanagan C 1996 Applying psychology to early child development. Hodder & Stoughton, London

Fulford K 1994 Diagnosis, classification and phenomenology of mental illness. In: Rose N (ed) Essential Psychiatry, 2nd edn. Blackwell Scientific, Oxford, p 3–16

Gammon J, Mulholland C W 1996 Effect of preparatory information prior to elective total hip replacement on psychological coping outcomes. Journal of Advanced Nursing 24(2): 303–308

Giedosh D 1997 Emotional support and the ED patient: one nurse's perspective. Journal of Emergency Nursing 23(2): 96–97

Gross R D 1992 Psychology: the science of mind and behaviour, 2nd edn. Hodder & Stoughton, London

Hall J 1982 Psychology for nurses and health visitors. MacMillan, Basingstoke

Hart B D, Wells D L 1997 The effects of language used by caregivers on agitation in residents with dementia. Clinical Nurse Specialist 11(1): 20–23

Hayes N 1984 A first course in psychology, 3rd edn. Thomas Nelson & Sons, Walton-on-Thames

Hayes N 1994 Foundations of psychology: an introductory text. Routledge, London

Hobbs M 1994 The psychological treatments. In: Rose N (ed) Essential psychiatry, 2nd edn. Blackwell Scientific, Oxford, p 225–240

Holland C, Cason C L, Prater L R 1997 Patients' recollections of critical care. Dimensions of Critical Care Nursing 16(3): 132–141

James W 1884 What is an emotion? Mind 9: 188–205

Lenz E R, Pugh L C, Milligan R E et al 1997 The middle-range theory of unpleasant symptoms: an update. Advance in Nursing Science 19(3): 14–27

Lloyd P, Mayes A, Manstead A et al 1984 Introduction to psychology: an integrated approach. Fontana, London

McConnell J, Philipchalk R 1992 Understanding human behaviour, 7th edn. Harcourt Brace Jovanovich, Fort Worth

McGregor A 1994 Catharsis: an investigation of its meaning and nature. Journal of Advanced Nursing 20(2): 368–376

Malim T, Birch A, Wadeley A 1992 Perspectives in psychology. MacMillan, Basingstoke

Maslow A 1954 Motivation and personality. Harper & Row, New York

Maslow A 1970 Motivation and personality, 2nd edn. Harper & Row, New York

Meldrum C 1995a Introduction. In: Messer D, Meldrum C (eds) Psychology for nurses and healthcare professionals. Prentice Hall, London, p 3

Meldrum C 1995b Cognitive changes in normal ageing. In: Messer D, Meldrum C (eds) Psychology for nurses and healthcare professionals. Prentice Hall, London, p 249

Postle D 1989 The mind gymnasium: a new age guide to personal growth. MacMillan, London

Powell T, Enright S 1990 Anxiety and stress management. Routledge, London

Radford J, Govier E 1991 A textbook of psychology. Routledge, London, p 640

Rosenthal D M 1991 The nature of mind. Oxford University Press, New York

Sayer A 1992 Method in social science: a realist approach, 2nd edn. Routledge, London

Slack J 1990 Attention. In: Roth I (ed) Introduction to psychology. Open University Press, Milton Keynes, vol 2

Stephens R 1993 Imagery: a strategic intervention to empower clients. Part 1 – review of research literature. Clinical Nurse Specialist 7(4): 170–174

Taylor I, Hayes N 1990 Investigating psychology. Longman, Harlow

Wade C, Travis C 1993 Psychology, 3rd edn. Harper Collins, New York

Wesson J S 1997 Meeting the informational, psychosocial and emotional needs of each ICU patient and family. Intensive and Critical Care Nursing 13(2): 111–118

Williams F 1993 Thinking, exploring the 'I' in ideas. In: Shakespeare P, Atkinson D, French S (eds) Reflecting on research practice. Open University Press, Buckingham

Winter R 1989 Learning from experience principles and practice in action-research. Falmer Press, London

FURTHER READING

Armstrong C 1991 Emotional changes following brain injury: psychological and neurological components of depression, denial and anxiety. Journal of Rehabilitation 57(2): 15–22

Morris C 1996 Understanding psychology, 3rd edn. Prentice Hall, Upper Saddle River, p 2–12

Millenson J 1995 Mind matters: psychological medicine in holistic practice. Eastland Press, Seattle, p 29–50

Personality

An understanding of individual differences is paramount in health care practice. Since there are varied personality types, it is expected that care providers will encounter individuals manifesting differing behavioural changes due to ill-health. The aims of this chapter are to:

- explicate some personality theories
- explore the many dimensions of personality disorders
- explain how relevant is the study of personality theories to health care.

WHAT IS PERSONALITY?

A person possesses many characteristics. If asked to describe someone after meeting them for the first time, most people will comment on the qualities of the person: attitude, behaviour patterns, content of conversation, the mood, the physical features of the individual and general impressions of their social background.

In describing the person, the narrator will probably utilize such terms as 'she is jovial, with a good sense of humour'; 'rather forward I think' or 'he is a loner really'. Other comments could be: 'he was so aggressive and "pushy" ' or she is 'motherly but shy'; 'he is an eccentric'; 'they are great party-goers, hate staying in and revel in the high life!'.

Upon hearing these impressions, a psychologist will classify them in technical terms, by using traits terminology, e.g. some individuals are introverts or extroverts; the woman shows expressive behaviour and is nurturing; her joviality shows her affective states; his aggression could be due to a sociopathic trait. Psychologists will hence apply specific terminology based on psychological concepts to describe the individuals' characteristics or attributes. These clusters of traits (Box 12.1) form the 'personality'.

Box 12.1 Personality traits

- Anxiety, anger, hostility
- Extraversion (preference for social activity and interactions)
- Neuroticism (proneness to unpleasant emotional experience)
- Subclinical depression
- Intraversion
- Emotional stability
- Self-confidence
- Self-control
- Agreeableness
- Conscientiousness
- Emotion regulation tendencies
- Dominant behaviour
- Defensiveness
- Locus of control
- Need for control
- Psychoticism.

Gross (1992) understood personality to comprise other dimensions: first, that personality emanates *from* the behaviour, and inferences are subsequently made from the latter. Second, that personality cannot be directly observed, but the behaviour of the person can be. Third, personality is a meaningful concept and influential in interpersonal behaviour. For example, our perception of others (how we interpret or expect their character to be) will accordingly impinge on our interactions with them. Fourth, the development of the self-image occurs in the context of interpersonal behaviour. In other words, we acquire our personality development while engaged in interactions with others, responding to others and comparing behaviours. Fifth, that personality is concerned mainly with *how* people relate to each other and 'deal with the world'. Put in a different way, our attributes determine how we cope with life experiences.

The idea that others' personalities affect our

behaviour towards them is another perspective suggested by Eysenck (1996). His arguments relate to 'cognitive processes' – how impressions and information (whether accurate or not) have been cognitively processed and stored in memory. We hence have 'concepts and schemas' of other people, and our social perception is influenced by them. The impressions one has collected of others' personalities in some ways will determine the quality of the perception and the interactions. This has implications for practice.

Knight (1995) found in his research that care professionals' behaviour is influenced by their clients' level of attractiveness: they are inclined to be less critical of attractive clients and to perceive them to want to get better quicker. Conversely, clients' perception of their caregivers' personality has influence over their behaviour: a warm, caring, empathetic approach is most likely to instil confidence and increase cooperation. The processes of forming impressions (perception) of aspects of people's personalities have interested psychologists and social psychologists. The term they apply to this theory of making inferences by using our knowledge of the presence of others (Sabini 1992) is 'implicit personality'.

This theory can be explained as follows. When we encounter someone, our impressions are generated from the store of concepts (e.g. intelligent, warm, determined, practical, cautious etc.) we have acquired and would select accordingly. For instance, we may decide that the person is 'intelligent'; this further leads us to make other assumptions that this person would be 'studious', 'intense', 'practical', 'understanding' and may be 'observant'. Sabini (1992) argued that we use language (which consists of concepts) to make explicit our organized and structured impressions of people. The theory is said to be 'implicit' because we only need to be given one trait of a person (e.g. intelligent) and we start making inferences of other traits, thus providing our own theory of how 'personalities hang together' (Sabini 1992).

One important feature of personality, however, with which we are familiar is identity. Identity makes the person. We not only recognize someone's identity from evidence of their psycho-

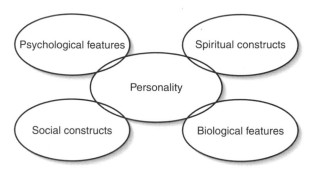

Fig. 12.1 The bio-psychosocial and spiritual dimensions of personality.

logical make-up (traits: intelligence, mood, attitude etc.) but in association with their biological, spiritual and social features. The combination of bio-psycho-social-spiritual characteristics makes the conceptual framework of personality (Fig. 12.1), which identifies a person's uniqueness. To be a person, therefore (Open Learning 1998a), applies to the integration of genetic inheritance with psychological experiences (learning, memory, perception etc.), their social constructs (the social and cultural experiences, internalized over a period of time) and their spirituality (their world view, lifeways, understanding of abstract forces, meaning of religion etc.).

In health care, recognizing the uniqueness of an individual is emphasized, which entails being sensitive to their identity and personality framework. Besides, an awareness that the client's personality may be disturbed through ill-health (thus not being a true representation of the usual stable features of their identity) assumes great importance. For instance, it is established that psychopathology is correlated with aggressive behaviour, hostility, anger and antisocial activities (Berman et al 1998).

The task of caregivers is to exercise tact and patience during interactions, aiming to deal with the source of the problems, in a non-judgemental way. In addition, how a person responds to ill-health and health is determinant upon their personality (Oliver 1993). Since personality is developed as a result of bio-psycho-social influences, any adverse life exposures can impinge on a person's attitude formation. Very often

uncooperative and resistive behaviour shown in health care settings is the outcome of such past experiences.

Activity 12.1

1. Describe the traits you consider make you an individual.
2. Using a dictionary, identify words you think help to explain the meaning of personality.

??? Question 12.1

1. If personality is behaviour and vice versa, how would you explain the expression of emotion among individuals?
2. How would you describe the personality of your friends and/or family members?

THEORIES OF PERSONALITY

The study of personality is a complex task for psychologists. There are so many dimensions attached to its concept that, not surprisingly, a multitude of theories have contributed to the debate. An eclectic approach to the understanding of personality is nevertheless recommended, as each theory complements the other to form the whole.

In this section some main theories shall be considered, namely:

- phenomenology
- social–environmental
- trait
- psychoanalytic theories.

These theories highlight the essence of human behaviour: we behave the way we do because of our constitution, which is contingent on our genes and environment (social and psychological). Additionally, the theories show similarities and differences between individuals. For instance, we all have subjective experiences and possess mental and affective states, but we differ in the way we respond and/or interpret the same circumstances.

Phenomenology

Phenomenologists believe that human experience is best understood by listening to the uniqueness of individual lived experience. In fact, the self becomes the core of the exploration. It analyses a person's world views: how they relate and understand their social environments; their methods of survival; the relevance they attach to their physical, psychological/emotional and spiritual dimensions. Phenomenologists will, therefore, argue that if we want to learn the psychology of the individual, the best propositions are to capture their personal (subjective) experiences.

This approach ignores the observation of observable behaviour (behaviourism) from which inferences have to be made. Furthermore, phenomenologists are not concerned with cognitive processes, but only with the account given. The features of phenomenology, described by Atkinson et al (1993), consist of the following:

1. It is a humanistic way of studying human behaviour, because it focuses on individuals' perception (and their version of events) in the context of people's social interactions.
2. What individuals do to achieve their 'potentials and capabilities', by exploring their personal attitudes and beliefs.
3. Individuals' inclination toward growth (potential for self-actualization and progress).
4. Maturity (to develop a stable personality compatible with their lived experience).
5. The drive to do better; how to cope with adversity, and become agents of change.
6. To evaluate experience in relation to the self-concept; e.g. after the loss of a loved one, a person analyses the feelings endured and assesses how congruent these are with the self-concept.

Emotional disturbance and anxiety (Atkinson et al 1993) can be aroused if feelings are not congruous with the self-concept. Moreover, Staden (1998) argued that for some individuals, life experiences have helped them in emotion management. Subjective experiences, hence, widen the the dimension of personality theory.

A knowledge of humanist personality theory bridges the gap in our understanding of clients' behaviour in health care settings. A client whose self-image is fractured by ill-health can verbalize hostility and anger to the nurse. If the nurse misunderstands the deep psychological reasons for the behaviour, and responds inappropriately, worsening of behaviour is a possibility.

Smith's (1998) research into problem drinking, from a phenomenological research method, shows the depth of bio-psycho-social-spiritual distress among problem drinkers. The guilt and shame felt destabilizes the personality, and heightens their dependence.

Although an undermined personality cannot be immediately recovered, a professional has the responsibility to gradually enhance the sufferer's self-image, to regain lost self-esteem and to stabilize the frail personality. Just as important is to investigate the client's personal reasons for using alcohol as a coping mechanism. Only by providing the sufferer with the freedom to expose, at their own pace, the distressing lived experiences, can positive therapeutic outcomes be attained. Psychological safety can facilitate the uncovering of motivating forces that have caused the personality dysfunction.

Social–environmental

Social–environmental theorists believe that personality develops from the interactive processes occurring between the individual and environment. It is through social interactions that one learns what constitutes acceptable and unacceptable behaviour, which is an argument sociologists will readily accept, as it applies to the socialization mechanisms that concern society as a whole. Psychologists, however, refer to the two-way processes – between the person and his environment – and how each is shaped and influenced accordingly. They are therefore interested in the 'characteristics' of both person and environment.

The core of the social–environmental theory stipulates learning, reward and reinforcement. A person aims to be accepted by others; subsequently their behaviour has to be compatible with social expectations. Personal experiences inform the individual that some actions will be approved (rewarded, praised) and others will be unacceptable (and not reinforced).

While personal experience helps to acquire certain characteristics, observing the behaviour of others (vicarious learning), and learning the context that encourages approval and disapproval, helps to shape personality. For example, a teenager watches his brother being scolded for leaving his dirty clothing on the kitchen floor, and decides to pick up his own clothes. Observing the environment, appraising it (evaluating whether social approval is likely or not) and applying one's past experiences, will direct the person to behave in set ways.

Social learning theory also informs us that we gain our individuality (personality differences) from the varying life experiences we have internalized as we grow up. The main features of this personality theory can be summarized as follows:

1. environmental factors determine how personality will develop
2. humans are shaped by their environment, and they can also cause changes in their environment
3. biological analysis and psychoanalysis concepts do not form the theory
4. behaviour that is constantly reinforced in many settings will be repeated in others: a process called generalization
5. traditional social learning focuses on process (human–environment–human interactions) and not on individual types or differences (i.e. classifying personality types and traits)
6. the theory applies operant and classical conditioning to support arguments.

Operant conditioning refers to the shaping of human behaviour, making it adaptable to the environment (using reward and punishment). **Classical conditioning** applies to conditioned responses learned after either a positive or negative experience. In Chapter 3, for example, children who have been abused and conditioned to a life of misery were discussed, and in Chapter 5, women conditioned to home violence, with fragmented personalities, living in fear were described.

Trait

Trait theory relates to a person's temperament. Professionals who use this theory postulate that personality is made up of a collection of characteristics, which make the whole person. When one says someone is introverted (Box 12.1), it means that one anticipates this person to show features of aloneness, a degree of isolation (preferring to avoid groups and the company of others) interpreted as asocial, an inclination towards self-centredness, preoccupation with one's own thoughts, distant, reflective, moody and intense. Introversion, although seemingly an undesirable trait, can be a useful personality tool. The ability to exclude external influences means that one is better able to focus mental energy on specific tasks.

While trait theory describes the attributes of a person, it lacks the dynamic processes of lived experiences which have shaped personality. Trait theory does not inform us of the 'what and the how': **what** caused an individual to adopt introverted behaviour and **how** this was achieved.

Psychoanalytic (psychodynamic)

Psychodynamic theory explains personality in terms of psychic mechanisms, as they occur in the early years of childhood development. It makes explicit the notion that people are driven by instinctual impulses (innate drives stored in the unconscious) and that they experience mental conflict and tension, but manage their consciousness by using morality to help them cope with the process of living.

Psychoanalytic theory originates from the studies of Sigmund Freud (1865–1939; e.g. Freud 1972, 1993). Freud believed that personality evolves from biological instincts, in combination with the idea that the human psyche has capacity to process information (cognitive skills, memory, perception) and is mapped at three levels: unconscious, conscious and preconscious.

The **unconscious** is the deepest level of the mind, in which resides emotions of fear, anxiety, ambition and belief, as well as varying impulses. Although these desires and fears are repressed,

Freud believed that the unconscious is dynamic in nature; it constantly relates to the preconscious and conscious mind and stores the basic instincts, e.g aggression and sex drive.

The **conscious** mind filters the content of incoming information from the environment, which is subsequently stored in the unconscious. Also known as the **Ego**, the conscious is said to contain all the moral values: an awareness of what constitutes ethical and moral behaviour, which Freud claimed to be under the control of the **Superego**, also part of the conscious (Fig. 12.2).

The **preconscious** (sub-conscious) relates to our awareness of the self and the environment at a secondary level. Unless we focus our mental energy on being aware of *how* we are breathing and what our pulse rate is, most of the time we do not pay attention to these physiological mechanisms, unless something goes wrong. Some basic primitive desires can be processed by the sub-conscious which, however, remains under conscious (Ego) control.

The psychodynamic structure of personality can be summarized as follows:

1. Personality develops in the early years of childhood (first 5 years).

2. Biological drives (e.g. eating, drinking etc.), which are innate and present at birth, represent the Id (basic primitive personality structure).

3. The Id seeks immediate gratification by unleashing all instinctual impulses.

4. The conscious mind (Ego and Superego), however, controls basic impulses since it is reality oriented: conscious of what is morally acceptable behaviour.

5. Socialization (parental control, rewards, punishment) processes develop the Superego. Thereafter, as the individual reaches maturity, the Superego directs behaviour according to internalized moral codes, independent of family control.

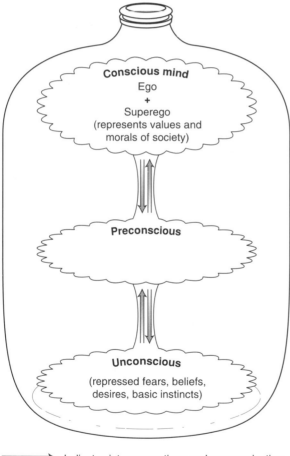

Indicates interconnections and communication networks, and the dynamic nature of the psyche according to psychoanalytic theory

Fig. 12.2 The psyche (psychoanalytic-psychodynamic process) – relationships between the conscious, preconscious and unconscious.

Activity 12.2

Observe 3- to 4-year-old infants at play. Explain their behaviour from the theory outlined above.

??? **Question 12.2**

1. How would you use the theory to explain antisocial behaviour?
2. If the Id is to do with basic impulses, what mechanisms help to prevent loss of control?

THE RELEVANCE OF PERSONALITY TO HEALTH CARE

We have an innate potential for survival. The basic forces that influence behaviour (Open Learning 1998b) motivate individuals to satisfy their basic needs. As pointed out in Chapter 11, individuals have a hierarchy of needs (see Fig. 11.3, p. 240): the drive to realize one's potential and to strive towards personal growth. Ill-health, however, becomes a major obstacle for both the ambitious and non-ambitious personality. Nevertheless, sickness and disease mean that one has to relinquish some control over how to meet one's basic needs to care professionals. When in the grip of pain, for example, we rely on quick nursing and medical intervention. Further, our inherent tendencies prevent us from active listening and information-taking, when we are apprehensive and feel psychologically unsafe.

PERSONALITY AND SUBJECTIVE WELL-BEING

A person's well-being is not only dependent upon biosocial factors but on personality variables as well. This has implications for care professionals in practice. Gosling (1995) explained how a patient's and nurse's personal characteristics can significantly affect health outcomes, e.g. an anxious personality can worsen psychological well-being. In addition, professional sensitivity can buffer the impact of anxiety-provoking situations (e.g. surgery, chemotherapy, emergency procedures etc.).

Researchers (DeNeve & Cooper 1998) have attempted to identify personality traits that are connected with subjective well-being. When one is feeling subjectively well, DeNeve and Cooper (1998) wrote, better work satisfaction is expected, positive physical health can be experienced and there is a better standard of living.

Subjective well-being nevertheless, according to Orley et al (1998), differs from quality of life (QOL). The former, they explain, entails the presence of positive and affective states. QOL, although affect-laden, is a representation of a subjective evaluation of oneself and one's social and material world.

In clinical practice, the clinicians potentiate a client's inner resources to maximize their well-being. It is through interactions that personality traits are revealed. Subjective well-being levels (Deneve & Cooper 1998) are subjected to change according to the nature of life events. Arguably, positive events increase well-being, while adverse factors reduce well-being. A stressful care environment, caused by interpersonal and professional conflict, can affect well-being. DeNeve and Cooper (1998) point out, however, that personality traits – extraversion, neuroticism, for example – are correlated with how well-being will be supported. Other researchers have explained that introverted individuals are more prone to anxiety than extroverts (Gershuny & Sher 1998). Additionally, Gershuny and Sher pointed out that introversion and neuroticism are linked to increased sensitivity and vulnerability to anxiety-provoking circumstances. Being sensitive to patients' individual responses to their environment is essential for good practice. Observational skills are important, since facial expressions and other non-verbal cues can transmit distress signals. Moreover, an attempt to assess the degree of discomfort and its causes should be done using phenomenology. As discussed earlier, an account of the subjective lived experience should be obtained. Expressions of hopelessness and powerlessness, for example, are common features in the critically ill. Strategies to support their locus of control should be developed.

In relation to health and subjective well-being, DeNeve and Cooper concluded that, although health and wealth are necessary, they are not sufficient conditions for subjective well-being. *How* individuals feel at a given stage in time (i.e. not feeling healthy) will affect their well-being.

Many behavioural problems (e.g. uncooperativeness, aggression, hostility, suspiciousness etc.) in health care are due to how the patients feel. A failure to investigate patients' feelings is conducive to inappropriate care intervention. While a focus on personality variables is desirable, other impinging factors should be assessed; e.g. sensitivity to the effects of institutional routine on the client is a requisite, and ineffective social activities management can affect clients' participation. Assumptions that professional decision is congruent with patients' needs – without prior assessment of needs – can affect mood and well-being status.

Mood states in relation to personality have been the subject of research. How people process emotional stimuli is associated with personality traits. Rusting (1998) theorized that there are individual differences in emotional processing. Some people, she posited, are inclined to process information according to their psychological make-up. People who score high on positive emotional traits (happy, affectionate, warm, jovial) are believed to perceive events in a positive way, whereas those who are emotionally negative (angry, anxious, depressed, hostile) are prone to see their world negatively and to remember unpleasant experiences.

Individual differences in information-processing based on personality traits and mood states have implications for practice. Clients who feel positive about themselves are more likely to assimilate information and take positive self-care initiatives; their subjective well-being is more pronounced and the nurse can detect in their behaviour, attentiveness, confidence and cooperation. The introverts may show more self-preoccupation and self-doubt. An understanding of the processes causing altered behaviour can enhance the therapeutic aims. Rusting (1998) pointed out that ability differs among people in the habitual use of strategies to directly change, maintain or eliminate emotional states. People, she argued, are continually evaluating their mood states and subjective well-being. However, one can expect that during ill-health, the capacity to continue avoiding unpleasant memories and maintaining subjective well-being is impaired.

Very often a client's present behaviour is a reflection of his past experience. Rusting made reference to 'emotional self-schemas' (constructed from past knowledge and experience). In child abuse cases and home violence stories, for example, the acquisition of 'dysfunctional self-schemas' (through negative childhood experiences), exposes the person to depressive feelings when current negative life events, which match past painful memories, impact on their well-being.

PERSONALITY DISORDERS

Psychological dysfunctions effect personality alterations. There are various causes attributed to such changes:

- psychopathology (mental illness)
- lifestyle instability factors (socio-environmental: criminality, substance abuse, poor living arrangement).

Being able to describe a person's personality is important for mental health workers (Deary et al 1998). The rationale for this is because personality changes very often are the causes of psychiatric problems; one or more personality disorders can be manifested. Mental health workers should, therefore, exercise caution in their personality traits assessment, because mental illness syndromes overlap with the pre-morbid personality (Deary et al 1998). In addition, assumptions and beliefs exist that individuals with personality disorders are prone to aggressive behaviour. Although research in this area has provided mixed results (Berman et al 1998), it has been put forward that other variables should be considered apart from psychopathology. For example, socio-economic status, institutionalization and legal problems can contribute to violent behaviour. Furthermore, aggression may not be due to personality psychopathology, but by the presence of some major mental disorders.

Research undertaken in the USA (Berman et al 1998) indicates that personality disorders constitute a heterogeneous group in connection with the manifestation of aggressive and antisocial behaviours. Individuals with a paranoid personality are sensitive to perceived environmental threats, and prone to be aggressive. People with depressive disorders may have recourse to psychoactive substance use, which increases their susceptibility to violence. Lower levels of aggression have been observed among schizoid individuals, due to their asocial (as they have limited social interactions) and indifferent behaviour.

Other researchers have attempted to establish a correlation between mental disorder and criminal behaviour (Bonta et al 1998). Their American findings suggest that a broader view should be taken in the assessment of the individual, in addition to clinical indicators (e.g. psychiatric ill-health, psychoticism). Social variables, economic factors and psychological reasons should be sought to explain antisocial personality.

While psychopathology is seen as important in the management of mentally disordered offenders, the findings also highlight that *non-disordered* individuals experience family dysfunction, and show features of antisocial personality.

In Britain, a special (high security) hospital study to examine the association between mental disorder and violence (Taylor et al 1998) concluded that

1. psychiatric illness leads to violent behaviour, but is precipitated by delusions
2. alcohol and other substance mis-use is a common feature among people with a mental disorder
3. psychotic personality traits and personality disorder traits can both manifest themselves in one individual.

Implications for clinical practice are numerous. Antisocial personalities are known to be high-rate offenders. An important goal for mental health workers is to initiate early effective preventative and treatment programmes. Risk assessment should include the role and functions of family members and how supportive the networks are. Psychopathic offenders often come from broken homes and are relatively resistant to rehabilitation (Lynam 1998). Lynam proposed the early identification (from childhood onwards) of behavioural problems, which are possible precursors of adult antisocial personality. For example, hyperactivity, which applies to impulsive behaviour, in association with restlessness and inattention, as well as conduct disorder evident in overt antisocial actions. Lynam classified these manifestations as HIA (hyperactivity-impulsivity-attention) and conduct problems.

Intervention should be intensive and ongoing and a comprehensive assessment of family needs is recommended. Family members may need support to undertake their caring role. On the other hand, mental health workers must be sensitive to the fact that family characteristics have influence on the course of major psychiatric disorders (Simoneau et al 1998). Family members who are continually hostile, negative, critical or emotionally overinvolved with a kin who is mentally ill, have a damaging impact on recovery. Families exhibiting these facets are said to be high in expressed emotion. To reduce and prevent relapse, it is suggested that a psycho-educational family treatment programme is implemented.

Restabilizing family relationships becomes a long-term challenge. The main objective is to reduce stressful events in the psychiatric patient's life. The positive effects of interpersonal relationships should not be underestimated; as Erickson et al (1998) argued, a patient finds 'arm's length' supportive relationship beneficial.

Meeting the needs of people with personality disorders is recognized as a clinical and social issue. Educational programmes are not conducive to the clinical demands of staff and patients (Storey et al 1997). Many clients with personality disorders are in security hospitals, because they are classified as serious offenders for criminal acts committed. Personnel need specialized training to recognize and treat personality-disordered clients. Similarly, as clients' needs for treatment and care are specialized, provision has to be tailored accordingly.

SCHIZOPHRENIA AND PERSONALITY

Schizophrenia is a serious mental illness (Repper et al 1995) that can develop slowly or suddenly (Atkinson et al 1993). As the illness progresses, significant others in the sufferer's immediate environment notice uncharacteristic behaviour alterations (Case example 12.1).

Subjectively, the schizophrenic is experiencing the world through altered perceptions and hallucinatory symptoms. Major psychological alterations impact on personality, e.g. a shy, introverted person, preferring isolation most of the

Case example 12.1 Changes in personality

Sam was well known in his neighbourhood for his quiet, self-preoccupied behaviour. Although aloof, he was considerate and polite. He had the occasional friend. He lived with his parents. He was keen on sport: swimming and jogging. He enjoyed reading and drawing.

His parents began noticing that his personal hygiene began to suffer: he looked unkempt, he did not change his clothes regularly and stopped going to the barber. He stayed much longer in his room than he used to, staring out of the window. His conversation became parsimonious and he became more indifferent to his parents' presence in the house. The nature of his drawings was changing too, as they looked less defined, more complex and distorted.

Case example 12.2 R's history

The following is an account of schizophrenic manifestations described by Kendler (1999): 'At this time, R also became preoccupied with religious themes, spending hours reading the Bible, sometimes becoming convinced that he was a great religious leader. Immediately before his second hospitalization, he stood in one posture in the backyard of his parents' house for a long time believing he was communicating with others by telepathy. In discussing these symptoms years later, R noted that they occurred with great veracity and at the time "it was impossible for me to believe that these experiences were not true" … R developed staring episodes, withdrawn behaviour, inattention to work-related tasks and irritability. He made repeated inappropriate advances to women in the administrative programme, persisting despite discouragement. He had agitation, emotional withdrawal, blunted affect, unusual behaviour, cognitive disorganization, and auditory and visual hallucinations'.

time could, with schizophrenic symptoms, reject the presence of others all together. Problems with the processing and memorizing of information are common; concentration and attention become impaired. Subjective phenomena such as perceptual disorders, thought and feeling impairment (Brennan 1997) augment the personality fragmentation. False beliefs are common and those not in keeping with the client's social–cultural background and education. Hallucinatory experiences are mainly auditory in character, although visual hallucinations can be expected. Olfactory, tactile and gustatory senses are rarely implicated in hallucinatory phenomena, but are additionally detrimental to well-being when they occur.

These subjective phenomena disrupt the personality (Case example 12.2). Onlookers may see the changes as a metamorphosis. Previous personality traits are heightened; e.g. introversion is followed by complete social withdrawal: communication breakdown associated with thought block and poverty of content. On the other hand, new personality features, characterized by the belief that thoughts are being controlled and broadcast (passivity phenomena), or are being 'taken out of their mind', are observed. Feelings are blunted and incongruent with the context, e.g. there is a burst of laughter when sorrow should be expressed.

All these features add to negative social func-

tioning. The illness impacts on families and their coping skills, as they lack understanding of the sufferer's subjective world. Attempts to engage conversations can arouse suspicions and hostility, and delusional beliefs can precipitate violent behaviour.

Practice implications are:

1. A clearer understanding of what living with a mental illness is, as opposed to having a chronic mental illness (Hayne & Young 1997).
2. Meaningful care that focuses on the person and their daily experiences of symptoms; how they describe their subjective world is important as caregivers should not impose their world view.
3. Hayne and Young suggest recognizing the client's need to grieve: the personhood of the past has been replaced by a new self, which requires adaptation and empathetic caregiving to allow 'personal meaning' to be made of the illness experience.
4. Education, self-help, follow-up and support programmes can maximize health.
5. Community nurses are ideally placed to identify 'trigger' events, which could cause relapse and enhance clients' coping strategies.

6. The prevention of a stigmatized service is recommended. Behaviour stereotyping negates health outcomes by demoralizing the client. Research shows that nurses are prone to having negative thoughts of schizophrenia (Box 12.2).

Box 12.2 The mentally ill and stereotyping of behaviour

According to Rogers and Kashima (1998), therapeutic relationships in health care can be impaired if clinicians cannot 'inhibit stereotypical representations of people with schizophrenia'. They explain the mechanisms of stereotyping as comprising stored images of stereo-typed groups (e.g. schizophrenia, learning disabilities, physical disabilities, delinquents, paedophiles etc.) in memory; each group possessing some key 'attributes', which are negative in properties. Once in the presence of a member of the group, these 'stereotypical attributes are activated'. Nurses, Rogers and Kashima argue, are not free from this process. Rogers and Kashima's study discovered that professionals' perceptions of schizophrenia 'were not less negative' than lay people's perceptions; that overt behavioural responses were more positive than their thinking and feeling. General and psychiatric nurses were more negative in their thoughts, while their feelings matched their positive personal beliefs.

7. Repper et al (1995) advised that a humanistic approach to care is essential to ascertain that clients' basic needs are met. Valuing the client, recognizing their potential and supporting their motivation for independence are the objectives.
8. Packages of care must be monitored, by key workers who liaise with community mental health teams (Brennan 1997).

THE DRAMATIC PERSONALITY DISORDERS

In a literature review, Peterson (1996) identified other dimensions of personality disorders clustered as the antisocial personality, borderline personality disorder and the histrionic personality disorder.

The antisocial personality

Persons with an antisocial personality show a lack of remorse towards their fellow humans. They lead a fragmented social life with a history of being unable to hold a job for very long, and interpersonal relationships tend to be brief, superficial and cold. Their activities can lead to conflict with law enforcers. Peterson believed that criminal activity is not synonymous with this disorder, as the rationale for illegal activities may not be related to being antisocial.

Antisocial personalities are sometimes wrongly described in media reports as 'charismatic', or 'charming', because of so-called manipulative behaviour. They are prone to lie and can create good impressions of themselves, which can sway people who are unaware.

Borderline personality disorder

Peterson applies this classification to individuals who are constantly in need of attention from others. They can show impulsivity and quick mood changes. There is evidence of instability in relationships. The person seeks reassurance from others, demanding closeness and support due to feelings of being deserted by others. In addition, the person may feel dissatisfied with their social life and work, and show fluctuating moods. Reactions to small incidents may be explosive; engaging in petty thieving, as well as experimenting with drugs have been known. They often become victims to their feelings. It is argued that the diagnosis is made more often among women than men (Peterson 1996).

Histrionic (hysterical) personality disorder

Hysterical personalities are considered to be dramatic in their behaviour. They are inclined to be self-centred and shallow in their emotions. Hysterical personality disorder is most commonly diagnosed in women. Peterson explains that hysterical features are only applied to such individuals when they have persistently and regularly exhibited such characteristics over a period of time.

They seek attention, reassurance, and have high expectations. There is over concern with physical appearance and they are in constant need of praise from others. Hysterical personalities can easily feel 'let down' and will respond to ordinary situations (e.g. meeting a regular acquaintance) in the most dramatic way. Frustrations are often expressed in an exaggerated fashion over matters that others would consider trivial, such as being unable to put the key in a keyhole.

The dimensions of personality disorders outlined above make it clear that there is a wide range of differing needs that professionals in practice have to be aware of. Each personality has to be assessed and sensitively understood on its own merit.

As pointed out already, the lived experience of a person is as different as one fingerprint is to another. Care and treatment have to be adjusted and changed as required to suit needs.

The psychological background must be assessed, and is ongoing and intensive. Mental health workers and practitioners in general nursing and medicine have to apply the many personality theories and human development research findings to gain insight into the behaviour of their clients.

Activity 12.3

1. Arrange a visit with the community mental health worker. Discuss the incidence of borderline personality disorder in the area.
2. Design an assessment tool to measure personality disorders.

??? Question 12.3

How would you differentiate the eccentric personality from the dramatic personality?

PERSONALITY AND AGEING

As one gets older, the accumulation of past experience consolidates the personality. It is argued that people are more self-centred in old age (Stuart-Hamilton 1994). They become more preoccupied with their cognitive and affective states (Coleman 1993) and bodily functions. A common observation is that with ageing some 'not so nice personality traits' can become a source of behaviour problems (Chiu 1991), or that the personality may become more entrenched, causing recalcitrant behaviour (Windmill 1990) when change is suggested.

Although the process of ageing is given as an argument, socio-cultural factors are also implicated. How societies view their older citizens reinforces the notion that old age means withdrawal from active participation in social activities. Individuals with a previously outgoing personality may resort to staying indoors and to caring for the grandchildren, due to role change and social expectations. Coleman (1993) pointed out, however, that old age does not make an extrovert into an introvert. Behaviour patterns in personality theories are responsive to life events; one expects the older person to have acquired values and beliefs that have shaped their personality, hence their present behaviour patterns. Past experiences and conflicts are re-evaluated on the basis of current life issues and more mature understandings (Huyck 1994). Keefover (1998) refers to the accumulation of knowledge base as 'crystallised intelligence', which a person continually accesses and expands throughout the lifespan. 'Fluid intelligence', on the other hand, is described as the ability to respond to changing and novel situations in a flexible way. Many older adults find it hard to change their attitude. In addition, they rely on crystallized intelligence to cope with new situations, which may not always be appropriate.

Wilkinson (1996) wrote that there is no personality type typical of elderly people as they do not represent a homogeneous group. As people age, they become carriers of 'unique life span experiences': the characteristics they possess remain unchanged, except when situations arise instigating them to behave differently (Wilkinson 1996). For example, an emergency hospitalization can overwhelm the aged person used to being cared for at home by relatives. On admission, they may be suspicious, aggressive and hostile.

Personality consistency varies according to memory status in ageing. When memory fails, the ability to retrieve memories is reduced. Information processing (cognitive speed) is sluggish, and the person may fabricate answers to camouflage memory loss.

The impact of biological changes on personality is also relevant. Sensory impairment (i.e. visual and hearing skills deterioration) is likely to distort perceptions, affecting behaviour when environmental signals are misinterpreted. Subsequently, the individual's responses may not meet social approval (Case example 12.3).

Case example 12.3 The effects of misperception on personality

George's hearing has been deteriorating insidiously. Although his carer would raise her voice when communicating with him, he always shouted out some expletives, which was uncharacteristic of him. His hearing impairment distorted the message he received. He believed his carer was being rude to him.

Further, myths exist that sexual impairment is a norm among the older generation. Showing interest in sexual matters has traditionally been concealed among the old for fear of being regarded as 'promiscuous' or being labelled as a 'dirty old man'. The media reinforces the image that sex concerns young people only (Stuart-Hamilton 1994).

Sexuality is one of the attributes that makes a whole person. Ageing, according to research findings, does not impair sexual interest and sexuality. A postal survey of 534 men and 758 women over the age of 60 in Washington DC, USA, found that 37% of respondents were satisfied with the amount of sex they were having. A similar proportion said they would have liked to increase their sexual activities. The sexually active respondents (43%) described their sex life as good as or even better than in their younger days (Elderly Care 1998/9).

PERSONALITY AND CULTURE

Culture is an integral dimension in the shaping of personality. There are stories of children who have been abandoned to live among animals in

Activity 12.4

Examine the content of women's and men's magazines. How many articles can be identified that relate to older people's sexuality?

??? Question 12.4

How can older persons be helped to express feelings concerning their sexuality?

the wild and how they grow to integrate the cultural lifestyle of the beasts that adopted them. Such children, Hogg and Vaughn (1998) state, are referred to as feral children, since they demonstrate characteristics of those reared in the wild by animals: they learn how to growl and bare their teeth; how to search for food and communicate according to the language of their foster animal parents. Children reared in more civilized, human surroundings are also shaped by their cultures. In cultures where passive behaviours are taught, either through religious rituals or the practice of ancestral traditions, one can anticipate the individual to assimilate such values. Personality moulding occurs when beliefs, values and attitudes are inculcated upon and internalized.

Nemeroff and Rozin (1994), in their analysis of the 'magical law of contagion' in American adults, agree that to study magical contagion is broadly applicable to the study of personality and the self. The law of contagion refers to the cultural belief that once a person has touched an object or someone else, they thereafter influence each other 'through the transfer of some or all of their properties'. The influence continues even after the contact has ended.

It is a social construct, with a spiritual dimension that, nevertheless, holds the person's attention and directs behaviour. As it is an internalized belief, it belongs to the personality framework, which it continues to influence.

In other cultures, strong beliefs in the supernatural (witchcraft and demonic forces) impact on personality (Pfeifer 1994). We find hence that psychological function and dysfunction are often explained in terms of abstract factors.

Cultural beliefs, health and the self-concept are interrelated. An understanding of the meaning of symptoms is a nursing practice requisite (Fry & Nguyen 1996). Additionally, the study of psychosocial variables and health status is considered uniquely appropriate for health care practice (Johnson-Saylor 1991).

Fry and Nguyen point out how our world views develop from our appraisals – founded on norms, expectations and culturally determined values. They compare, for example, a Western view of the self-concept based on the 'individual' – using a self-centred model of being, with the Eastern concept of the self. The latter view the self in relation to their communities: their attachments to family values and social networks (Fry & Nguyen 1996). These links are inseparable. Harmony among relations is invaluable and must be preserved. Vietnamese people see their identities as 'not their own', but as connected to a 'web of human relationships'.

Such views are important as they determine personality characteristics and supply explanations of their behaviour, their thinking and the emotions felt, as well as how they relate to social contexts, in particular the rapport between the self and others (Fry & Nguyen 1996). In contrast to the Vietnamese, the researchers found that Australians strive for independence, focusing on the self and projecting their individuality, personal identities and 'inner attributes'.

An understanding of the complex nature of the self-concept across cultures is necessary, as individual differences in the perception of health and illness exist, with implications for practice. The quality of health care is contingent upon care providers' accurate perceptions of patients' physical and psychological states (Molzahn & Northcott 1989). Fry and Nguyen's study shows clearly the contrast between the Western and Eastern perception of depression (Box 12.3).

Personality differences and cultural diversity mean that care providers should exercise caution in their assessment of clients' behaviour. Avoiding preconceptions and stereotypes is essential. A client's perception is contextual: analyse the

> **Box 12.3 Cultural differences in the perception of depression (From Fry & Nguyen 1996)**
>
> In comparison with Vietnamese, Australians recognize symptoms of depression more significantly. Western psychiatry is said to influence Westerners' perceptions. As Westerners are more individual-centred they are able to link their cultural norms to an understanding of emotions affecting the self. Vietnamese participants generally did not 'perceive or recognize' depressive features in others. Although they were able to identify emotions such as unhappiness, sadness and feelings of loneliness in the scenario described to them they considered these affective states to be aspects of normal life experiences (i.e. part of the maturation and human development process).

source (e.g. social, religious, ritualized practices etc.) of their rationale, and better understanding of why they feel and behave the way they do will be reached. As perception is a subjective and individual process, one should anticipate numerous and contrasting experiences.

Further, group membership could have major significance, and this factor will exercise influence on perception. Moreover, it is suggested that personality style affects the way a person seeks help and accesses services (Rosowsky et al 1997). In old age, for instance, changes in context (e.g. new culture environment with new people etc.) can adversely affect the personality. Rosowsky et al argued that personality styles are prone to suffer when systems of care 'endorse traits' that are not in keeping with those of the client's (Case example 12.4).

Case example 12.4 Residential home culture

Now aged 85, Fred has become a residential home client. Prior to this new experience, he enjoyed his own company and the occasional visits from his daughter and grandchildren. He loves classical music, has a great interest in gardening and enjoys long walks on the promenade.

The home, however, has strict regulations. It is recommended that group outings should be staff supervised. Residents do not do the gardening, and walking alone on the beach is discouraged for safety reasons.

Participation in recreational activities is encouraged: bingo, dominoes and ballroom dancing, none of which Fred is interested in.

Activity 12.5

Evaluate the literature on ethnicity and race. Can you identify issues connected with personality traits and culture?

??? Question 12.5

How should care providers prepare themselves to deliver care pertinent to personality differences?

SUMMARY

Personality is a concept that has been extensively studied by psychologists. It refers to the collection of attributes that make up a person's individuality and identity. There are many theories of personality, including:

- phenomenological
- social–environmental
- trait
- psychodynamic.

Each theory explains one particular dimension, exposing differing influences, and showing that one cannot study personality without using a bio-psychosocial approach.

The study of personality is relevant to health care. An awareness of individual differences means that care providers are able to tailor care according to needs and behaviour patterns. In addition, a knowledge of personality theories helps professionals to anticipate future behaviour in specific circumstances (e.g. hospitalization). Further, knowing that a person's unique life experiences have shaped their personality, allows professionals to gain some insight into their subjective world.

Changes in personality structure are expected when mental ill-health occurs. For example, in schizophrenia, previous personality traits such as introversion, aloofness and suspiciousness, become more pronounced as the disease progresses.

There are different types of personality disorders: antisocial personality, borderline personality and the hysterical personality, which have been categorized as dramatic disorders because of their presentations. Cultural influences have been attributed to shaping the personality. Biological changes in old age and role alterations can affect behavioural patterns.

GLOSSARY

Affective states   mood; emotional states
Emotion-regulation tendencies   inclination to control one's emotional states
Locus of control   empowering ability of a person
Neuroticism   anxiety traits with rather unstable emotions
Paranoid personality   personality characterized by suspiciousness and mistrust, with feelings of being persecuted
Psychoactive substance   drugs or chemicals affecting the mind or behaviour (e.g. LSD, cocaine, Ecstasy)
Psychoeducational   programmes aiming to improve psychological coping mechanisms, and to raise awareness of psychological issues

Psychopathology   mental disorders caused by pathology
Psychoticism   emotionally cold and antisocial features
Schizoid   traits depicting introversion, social withdrawal, aloofness and shyness
Sociopathic trait   pertaining to antisocial personality. Individuals who never learn from past experience and are prone to manipulative and remorseless behaviour
Sub-clinical depression   without clinical manifestations; in the early stages when the signs and symptoms of depression are not apparent to the observer

---

REFERENCES

Atkinson R L, Atkinson R C, Smith E et al 1993 Introduction to psychology, 11th edn. Harcourt Brace Jovanovich, Fort Worth
Berman M E, Fallon A E, Coccaro E F 1998 The relationship between personality, psychopathology and aggressive behaviour in research volunteers. Journal of Abnormal Psychology 107(4): 651–658
Bonta J, Hanson K, Law M 1998 The prediction of criminal

and violent recidivism among mentally disordered offenders: a meta-analysis. Psychological Bulletin 123(2): 123–142

Brennan G 1997 Schizophrenia. Primary Health Care 7(4): 17–24

Chiu E 1991 Psychiatric disorders in later life. In: Shaw M W (ed) The challenge of ageing, 2nd edn. Churchill Livingstone, Melbourne, p 116

Coleman C 1993 Psychological ageing. In: Bond J, Coleman P, Peace S (eds) Ageing in society, 2nd edn. Sage, London

Deary I J, Peter A, Austin E, Gibson G 1998 Personality traits and personality disorders. British Journal of Psychology 89(4): 647–661

DeNeve K M, Cooper H 1998 The happy personality: a meta-analysis of 137 personality traits and subjective wellbeing. Psychological Bulletin 124(2): 197–229

Elderly Care 1998/9 Ageing in the USA. Elderly Care 10(6): 10–11

Erickson D H, Iacono W G, Beiser M 1998 Social support predicts 5-year outcome in first episode schizophrenia. Journal of Abnormal Psychology 107(4): 681–685

Eysenck M 1996 Simple psychology. Psychology Press, Hove

Freud S 1972 A general introduction to psychoanalysis. Pocket Books, New York

Freud S 1993 New introductory lectures in psychoanalysis. Norten, New York

Fry A G, Nguyen T 1996 Culture and the self: implications for the perception of depression by Australian and Vietnamese nursing students. Journal of Advanced Nursing 23(6): 1147–1154

Gershuny B S, Sher K J 1998 The relation between personality and anxiety: findings from a 3-year prospective study. Journal of Abnormal Psychology 107(2): 252–262

Gosling J 1995 Personality. In: Messer D, Meldrum C (eds): Psychology for nurses and healthcare professionals. Prentice Hall, London, p 135

Gross R D 1992 Psychology the science of mind and behaviour, 2nd edn. Hodder & Stoughton, London

Hayne Y, Yonge O 1997 The life world of the chronically mentally ill: analysis of 40 written personal accounts. Archives of Psychiatric Nursing 11(6): 314–324

Hogg M A, Vaughn G M 1998 Social psychology, 2nd edn. Prentice Hall Europe, Hemel Hempstead, p 445

Huyck M H 1994 The relevance of psychodynamic theories for understanding gender among older women. In: Turner B F, Troll L E (eds) Women growing older. Sage, Thousands Oaks, p 202–238

Johnson-Saylor M T 1991 Psychosocial predictors of healthy behaviours in women. Journal of Advanced Nursing 6(10): 1164–1171

Keefover R W 1998 Aging and cognition. Neurologic Clinics 16(3): 635–648

Kendler K S 1999 Long-term care of an individual with schizophrenia: pharmacologic, psychological and social factors. American Journal of Psychiatry 156(1): 124–128

Knight D 1995 Interacting with patients/clients:impressions, attributions, and adhering to medical advice. In: Messer D, Meldrum C (eds) Psychology for nurses and healthcare professionals. Prentice Hall, London, p 32

Lynam D R 1998 Early identification of the fledgling psychopath: locating the psychopathic child in the current nomenclature. Journal of Abnormal Psychology 107(4): 566–575

Molzahn A E, Northcott H C 1989 The social bases of discrepancies in health/illness perceptions. Journal of Advanced Nursing 14(2): 132–140

Nemeroff C, Rozin P 1994 The contagion concept in adult thinking in the United States: transmissions of germs and of interpersonal influence. Ethos 22(2): 158–186

Oliver R W 1993 Psychology and healthcare. Baillière Tindall, London, p 21

Open Learning 1998a What it means to be a person. Learning Curve: Your Essential Guide to Professional Development 1(11): 9–13

Open Learning 1998b Personality and forces that influence behaviour. Learning Curve: Your Essential Guide to Professional Development 2(7): 9–13

Orley J, Saxena S, Herrman H 1998 Quality of life and mental illness. British Journal of Psychiatry 172: 291–293

Peterson C 1996 The psychology of abnormality. Harcourt Brace Jovanovich, Fort Worth, p 389–394

Pfeifer S 1994 Beliefs in demons and exorcism in psychiatric patients in Switzerland. British Journal of Medical Psychology 67(3): 247–258

Repper J, Brooker C, Repper D 1995 Serious mental health problems: policy changes. Nursing Times 91(25): 29–31

Rogers T S, Kashima Y 1998 Nurses' responses to people with schizophrenia. Journal of Advanced Nursing 27(1): 195–203

Rosowsky E, Dougherty L M, Johnson C J, Gurian B 1997 Personality as an indicator of 'goodness of fit' between the elderly individual and the health service system. Clinical Gerontologist 17(3): 41–53

Rusting C L 1998 Personality, mood, cognitive processing of emotional information: three conceptual frameworks. Psychological Bulletin 124(2): 165–196

Sabini J 1992 Social psychology. W W Norton, New York, p 177

Simoneau T L, Mikklowitz D J, Saleem R 1998 Expressed emotion and interactional patterns in the families of bipolar patients. Journal of Abnormal Psychology 107(3): 497–507

Smith B A 1998 The problem drinkers lived experience of suffering: an exploration using hermeneutic phenomenology. Journal of Advanced Nursing 27(1): 213–222

Staden H 1998 Alertness to the needs of others: a study of the emotional labour of caring. Journal of Advanced Nursing 27(1): 147–156

Storey L, Dale C, Martin E 1997 Social therapy: a developing model of care for people with personality disorders. Nursing Times Research 2(3): 210–218

Stuart-Hamilton I 1994 The psychology of ageing, 2nd edn. Jessica Kingsley, London

Taylor P J, Leese M, Williams M 1998 Mental disorder and violence. British Journal of Psychiatry 172: 218–226

Wilkinson J A 1996 Psychology 5: implications of the ageing process for nursing practice. British Journal of Nursing 5(18): 1109–1113

Windmill V 1990 Ageing today. Edward Arnold, London, p 2

FURTHER READING

Callahan P, Young-Cureton G, Zalar M et al 1997 Relationship between tolerance/intolerance of ambiguity and perceived environmental uncertainty in hospitals (Research into personality variations among psychiatric nurses and their coping strategies in a climate of change and uncertainty). Journal of Psychosocial Nursing 35(11): 39–44

Eurelings-Bontekoe E H, Brouwers E, Verschuur M et al 1998 DSM-111-R and ICD-10 personality disorder features among women experiencing two types of self-reported homesickness: an exploratory study. British Journal of Psychology 89(3): 405–416

Flack W F, Laird J D, Cavallaro L A 1999 Emotional expression and feeling in schizophrenia: effects of specific expressive behaviours on emotional experiences. Journal of Clinical Psychology 55(1): 1–20

Stewart A J, Ostrove J M 1998 Women's personality in middle age, gender, history and midcourse corrections. American Psychologist 53(11): 1185–1193

Perception

In this chapter the aims are to:

- explore the concept of perception from a bio-psychosocial perspective
- introduce some pertinent issues related to the perceptual systems and their influences on a person's behaviour
- describe how an understanding of perception can facilitate health care interventions
- suggest ways to identify clients' needs and problems in specific clinical situations.

WHAT IS PERCEPTION?

THE NATURE OF PERCEPTION

Perceiving is an active process whereby stimulation (e.g. stimulation of sensory organs: eyes, nose, ears, skin, mouth) is converted into organized experience. The resulting experience follows a systematic information-processing pattern by the organism. Not all stimulation reaching the senses is perceived, however (Govier 1980), because the perceiver always discriminates between incoming stimuli.

If humans were non-discriminatory in their ability to perceive events, their perceptual capacity would be overloaded, causing confusion. It is for this reason that 'focusing' perception (Hayes 1994) becomes a necessity. Hence people selectively pay attention (called selective attention) to what is going on in their environment. Some researchers (Smith et al 1998) have shown, however, that humans have innate capacity to process visual and auditory stimulation spontaneously. They point out that 'seeing and hearing' are inextricably linked in the control of visual attention. For example, when we hear a sound, our visual attention is shifted toward its source. It is also possible to be aware of tactile stimulation. For instance, as a person attends to both sound and visual stimulation, a small spider lands on his sleeveless arm; one anticipates the person will be conscious of it.

Bertenthal (1996) provides some insightful information on perception in relation to processes (information-processing) connected with object recognition.

1. People recognize objects in their environment, by linking present experience (perceiving the objects) with contact with past information. In other words, perception of current events depends upon past experiences stored in memory. It is a view shared by psychologists researching face perception and recognition (p. 269).

Successful recognition relies on the arrangement of the 'visual scene' and on 'how' similar past experiences are representationally stored in memory (Bertenthal 1996). This argument is evidence that perception is connected with the learning process, and that perceptual experiences (interpretation of external and internal (bodily) events) are meaningfully organized.

2. Some objects are not consciously processed, hence are *not* perceived, and not stored in memory. This perhaps explains the selective attention theory: people only perceive what is of interest to themselves. Recognizing involves directing attention toward selected objects.

Perception, therefore, is of importance to humans and animals. It is a survival mechanism. In interactions with the physical world, humans are dependent on both sensory organs and perceptual skill: how environmental conditions are interpreted and processed.

Nasar and Jones (1997) studied the fear of crimes as perceived by 26 college females in an urban area in the USA. Their research is of relevance to an understanding of perception for several reasons:

1. it shows how environmental factors impinge on perception
2. conversely, it shows that perceptions can be psychologically *projected* into the assumed external world (Gregory 1996)
3. that perceived environmental stressors (Box 13.1) help communities to improve safety standards
4. some specific groups (e.g. the poor, the elderly and females) perceive environmental threats more readily and are prone to higher levels of fear.

Box 13.1 Perception of environmental stressors

Nasar and Jones (1997) found that the female students being studied perceived some specific features in their environment at nightfall to be associated with increasing fears. For example, poor lighting conditions, dark pathways, being unaccompanied, and the character of some identified sections of the area which can be assumed to harbour some unknown threats.

Holaday et al (1997) showed in their US studies that perceived safety is correlated with race (i.e. white children are expected to be perceived as safer in their neighbourhood than non-white); that occupational status is also related (higher income groups are perceived to be safer in their environment); vulnerable children (e.g. with neuromuscular disorders) are seen as less safe. A perceived lack of safety caused by fear of crimes has health implications.

Activity 13.1

On your way home from work/college this evening, identify your perception of the environment you think can be unsafe. List your feelings and compare your perception with that of your friends/peers.

A perception of environmental threats is a common feature among patients in care settings. Unfamiliar environmental conditions – the formality of clinical procedures accompanied by a strict professional code of conduct – the anticipated perceived fear of pain and death, impinge on the patients' coping skills.

The perception of pain and the experience of pain are, however, two different dimensions. The pain sensation is associated with biological mechanisms: physiological processes and anatomical nervous structures. Perceiving is psychological in origin, but occurs within a brain chemistry framework. For example, a patient sees the nurse approaching the bedside with a syringe and needle. Perception consists of the patient's evaluation (information-processing, using cognitive skills) of anticipated event: the giving of the injection. However, the patient experiences the pain sensation during and after the injection. Sensations are therefore biological in origin. Perception is concerned with the understanding and the integration of learned experience. As Colwell (1998) reported, an object or a situation is interpreted by using knowledge and past experiences associated with the object or situations.

PERCEPTION AND BIOLOGY

The process of perceiving is linked with neurochemical activities within the brain. The inherent capacity of the brain in organizing and integrating incoming signals from one's environment should not be underestimated. In fact, when one is studying perception, it is difficult not to include neurochemistry in the process.

Some researchers in their studies of face perception for example, assert there is a connection between perception and brain activity (Lusher & Martin 1998). They report the findings obtained in the UK, by using magnetic resonance imaging in the examination of brain activation during the perception of facial expressions such as strong fear or disgust. Their results showed increased activation in the anterior insular cortex for perception of mild and strong facial expression of disgust, and amygdala activation during perception of the fear faces.

Other experiments reported by Lusher and Martin, using positron emission tomography, showed that subjects exposed to complete (undegraded) pictures of objects and faces before and after they were exposed to fragmented versions of the same pictures, demonstrate the neural mechanism associated with perceptual learning. The temporal cortex and parietal cortex of the brain were activated during identification of the degraded images. The perception according to these findings was particularly linked with 'medial cortex activity'. In addition, the researchers observed that face recognition areas in the brain did not operate in isolation; there is an interconnected neural system with areas (the parietal cortex) responsible for spatial attention during perceptual learning (Lusher & Martin 1998).

Rakover and Teucher (1997) in their studies on face perception acknowledged the complexity of the human brain in perceptual processes. For instance, they agree that several complex cognitive mechanisms are in operation prior to and during face perception. As discussed in Chapter 14, cognitive processes are the products of healthy neural mechanism, an important foundation in perceptual organization.

How the brain works, its organization and its role in perception is of interest to psychologists (Colwell 1998). According to the psychologist Richard Gregory (Colwell 1998), the brain is made up of modules, each with specific functions. Brain imaging is a useful assessment tool to discover what types of activities take place, in particular the role of cells in perceptual learning. While imaging and other techniques in brain studies are useful, other methods concerned with making inferences about brain functioning are utilized. Introspective analysis is such an approach. As pointed out in Chapter 11, introspection refers to people's descriptions of their subjective experiences. Behaviourists, however, view this method as unreliable since private experiences (individual perception of events) cannot be directly observed. The behaviour shown by the perceiver can nevertheless be observed objectively, from which inferences can be made of the perceiving experiences. Thus, to gain an inkling of brain functioning, behaviourists will focus on the information-processing behaviour of the perceiver through objective observations of the behavioural patterns.

When normal brain chemistry is impaired by chemical interferences (e.g. medication, electrolyte imbalance, toxic substances), perception can be disturbed. It is not uncommon in clinical practice for health care personnel to meet patients in confusional states with gross perceptual disturbances. Cognitive impairment interferes with perceptual mechanisms. Some clients in hypoglycaemic states, for example, are unable to express the strange sensations and visual stimulation they experience. Their behaviour is uncharacteristic, and they look vague and disorientated in their perception of time, person and social surroundings. Disjointed speech patterns can be observed, as they are unable either to integrate thought processes effectively or to perceive their language disturbance. An intravenous injection of glucose restores their cognition to normal level.

In other acute states such as *delirium*, defined as a temporary mental dysfunction due to nonspecific biochemical causes (Milisen et al 1998), one finds manifestations of disturbed cognition: memory loss, disorientation, language disturbance, or the development of disturbed perception.

Confused thinking in these states is evidence that the person is struggling to process environmental stimulation. Since perceiving is an active process allied with cognition, any impairment in the latter presents the perceiver with an array of disjointed or degraded images from the surroundings. Laboratory findings normally show that physiological dysfunction is implicated (Milisen et al 1998).

The role of professionals in acute states of perceptual alterations

The prevention and reduction of negative consequences of delirium demands reliable identification by professionals (Roth-Roemer et al 1997). Since delirium is not always recognized due to being under-researched, Roth-Roemer et al suggested that frequent assessments be undertaken.

Continuing assessment and evaluation will help to increase better understanding of the patient's needs and problems. Additionally, assessing the degree of perceptual changes allows the clinician to collect data on the effectiveness of the treatment programmes, evidenced in perceptual improvement.

The accurate assessment of perceptual changes using a defined sensitive tool is recommended. Roth-Roemer et al point out the difficulties associated with finding an assessment tool that can be implemented in a standard way, to measure disorganized thinking, perceptual disturbance, delusions and psychomotor activity alterations. Other US researchers have, however, shown that a carefully designed assessment tool, such as their Memorial Delirium Assessment Scale (MDAS), is reliable in assessing delirium severity amongst the medically ill (Breitbart et al 1997).

Clinical practice implications are related to the prevention of delirious states by a thorough understanding of the client's clinical presentations. Observing and assessing information-processing performance, including the degree of attention and alertness and fluctuations in the level of consciousness, will help detect early perceptual changes.

Although psychological assessment is an important care component, it should be accompanied with comprehensive physiological investigations to determine altered biochemistry often associated with delirious states. The implementation of procedures is anxiety-provoking for the patient and can be met with uncooperation, aggression and further confused reactions. It is important to maintain care continuity, by ensuring the same caregivers attend to the person's needs. Familiar faces are more reassuring and should enhance the client's feelings of safety, which is disturbed in delirium.

A re-evaluation of drug therapy is also a requisite, since some medications (e.g. antidepressants, anti-parkinsonian drugs) are known to cause delirium. In elderly patients, in particular, who are prone to delirium (Milisen et al 1998), the ageing process slows down the excretory functions of the renal system, causing waste product accumulation, a common cause of delirium.

PERCEPTUAL ORGANIZATION

According to Gestalt theory, the basic feature of perceptual organization is founded on the principle that visual stimulation is perceived as 'whole forms' or organized configurations.

People organize what they see and hear in an organized way; e.g. a dog barking outside is perceived as a whole sound amidst other sounds. When one looks at an object, a painting for example, one sees whole forms of objects (people etc.) in the picture. In fact when one does not see whole forms one looks for them: some abstract paintings appear nebulous and one's perceptual system seeks meanings and shapes to help one's understanding.

A person may distinguish figures and objects in their environment prominently against a background, a perceptual phenomenon described as 'figure and ground' effect (Atkinson et al 1987, Hayes 1994). This feature has implications in the psychology of object identification in daily activity, working and training settings, as when the military relies on the accurate identification of enemy targets (artillery, tanks, aircraft). O'Kane et al (1997) emphasize the importance of training military personnel to develop better perceptual organization, to recognize enemy vehicles, which may appear similar to their own. It is expected that trainees will re-organize their perceptual system so that they can distinguish parts (elements) of an object, their arrangements, as well as whole configurations. One's perception can be deceived when manipulation of figure and ground is achieved by blending an object into the background through camouflage.

CONTEXT AND PERCEPTION

The context in which perceiving takes place is important. When one sees and perceives stimulation from the environment, the occurrence (the event) being observed, determines *what* is being perceived. The brightness of an object, for example, is determined in relation (context) to the brightness (or colour density) of the background: a grey patch looks dark against a white background; conversely, a grey patch looks lighter against a black background.

Memory is also linked to context and to what one perceives. Gugerty (1997) refers to the concept of 'perceptual tracking', a mechanism needed in everyday life activities, which needs the use of a working memory (see Chapter 14).

Gugerty wrote that driving a car demands the driver's attention to surrounding traffic (context). This knowledge (spatial knowledge) is essential for maintaining situation awareness in many daily tasks. Research shows (Gugerty 1997) that when an individual perceives a situation to be hazardous, their perceptual organization becomes more focused and they maintain safety demands using memory resources. Past sensory experiences are therefore significant in enhancing perceptual adaptation to new circumstances. Perceptual organization is of equal relevance in face perception, a complex psychological activity, in which humans engage.

FACE PERCEPTION

Psychologists are showing increased interest in face perception. This interest can be explained in terms of the importance attached to recognizing social signals from facial expressions, during face-to-face interactive communication. Other reasons are concerned with the development of better understanding in the field of perceptual processes.

Since perception is integrated with cognition, psychologists are keen to learn the role of face perception in the theoretical framework of cognitive psychology. Additionally, knowledge of factors impinging on the accurate perception of faces is of utmost importance in many spheres of professional life: the criminal justice system, police work, health care organizations, teaching, counselling, job interviews and so on.

There are clear individual differences in perceptual functioning. In the late Catherine Cookson's novel, *The Blind Years*, Laurence Overmeer commented on Bridget Gether's painting by saying, 'That hill looks brown to me. It is brown; why do you paint it purple and orange?'. To which Bridget replied, 'Because that's how I see it'. Similarly, we perceive people's faces differently.

Our differing perception and recognition of facial features is dependent upon our experiences and our interpretation of such experiences (Colwell 1998): attention level, people's attractiveness, our personal interest and occupation or training. Lowe (1998), for example, found that police officers make better eye witnesses. As police officers rely on accurate visual assessment to detect criminals, one assumes that their attention level and observational skills in face perception will be more comprehensive.

Studies show that face perception is an intriguing psychological concept, with many other complex domains. Murphy (1998), commenting on Professor Vicky Bruce's lecture (University of Stirling), described some findings applicable to face perception. For example, he pointed out that there are 'independent representational routes' in face perception, indicating that there are several perceptual systems. These routes are said to be specialized, each with a specific function (Murphy 1998): language and face processing occur independently of each other. Facial identities and facial expressions are processed in cognitively different ways. Perrett (1995) argued that specialized cells in the brain will respond to particular features of faces and bodies. The human brain, it is posited, has the capacity to be responsive to a specific set of facial features or aspects of a face. Perrett (1995) explained that some brain cells have a tendency to respond more to only one orientation of a face.

Face perception, on the other hand, relies on efficient brain activity in the temporal cortex interacting with the parietal cortex, which is responsible for spatial attention (Lusher & Martin 1998). Normal face perception (images of faces not deliberately distorted) depend on two systems:

1. a face-specific system that connects with image orientation
2. a feature and object-based system.

According to Lusher and Martin, the latter can be impaired in some cases of closed head injury.

The findings described above have implications for clinical practice. Any interference with brain functioning due to biochemical agents or pathology can affect clients' face perception capacity. As described previously, occasions arise in clinical practice when confusion and disorientation heighten anxiety states and aggression levels. As their perception of familiar faces around them becomes distorted, it is expected that clients will become more apprehensive and anxious. It is not unusual for some clients to perceive their carers as complete strangers in such circumstances. In addition to physiological factors affecting perceptual organization, it is important to identify the role of environmental factors in the assessment of causes.

Drake et al (1997) described a small study of 52 residents in a nursing and residential home. A correlation was made between the residents' level of confusion and the environmental light intensity. The onset of late afternoon was associated with increased confusion, a condition described as 'sundown syndrome'. When improved lighting conditions were introduced within the home, increased wakefulness and reduced confusion were observed. Research has also been undertaken to assess the effects of shade caused by the reflections of light on people's faces, which can affect our perception and recognition of faces. Bruce (1998) provides an interesting account of the difficulties encountered with face recognition when lighting differs to previous recognition circumstances. She argued that an unfamiliar face can be difficult to verify when different images (under different light reflections) of the same person are presented. Conversely, a familiar face is more readily recognized because the perceiver is able to tap into face-memory stores, which contain representations of the familiar face as seen 'across numerous views, lightings and expressions' in which the face has been seen (Bruce 1998).

The relevance of face perception in the assessment of facial expressions of emotions, and as non-verbal signals in communication is important (Young & Bruce 1998). Light has a role in influencing our perception. While line drawings of faces preserve *feature* information (Young & Bruce 1998), recognition can still be difficult if variations in light are not included in the representations. Observations show that the recognition of faces and how one responds to them will be affected according to their attractiveness (Stevenage 1997, Young & Bruce 1998), i.e. faces perceived as more attractive will be recognized more easily.

In care settings, practitioners use their observational skills as one of their repertoire of communication skills, to identify their patients' psychological needs from facial expressions. In most cases clinicians encounter unfamiliar faces, so individuality of expressions of needs can prove difficult to identify. In particular, caution must be exercised during night-duty care, as poor lighting conditions are known to mask signs of distress.

Face observations must be accompanied by eliciting information from clients, encouraging them to express their needs verbally, and listening to the intonations, pitch and volume of speech to achieve better visual and auditory perception.

Bruce (1998) observed that people were better at identifying faces from varied angles when they were lit from above rather than below. At night time bedside lamps, which mostly light from below, are frequently used. In view of Bruce's and other studies, it may help to reposition lighting sources to help professionals in their assessment strategies. Equally important is to ensure that the client has a good view of the caregiver's face during communication, so that reciprocal non-verbal expressions can be simultaneously observed by both parties.

The face provides us with a rich source of information (Stevenage 1997), for example, how people feel, their moods, attitudes and so on. An insight into processing features (Box 13.2) is of relevance to health care, as psychological understanding of face perception improves anticipation of clients' needs.

Stevenage (1997) believes that part face perception is a normal occurrence, which refutes the Gestalt understanding that we process whole images rather than the parts or elements. The region around the eyes is found to be significantly important in perception. Perceivers focus more on the eye region, Stevenage argued, because it demands the most attention.

Such findings are of relevance to health care practice for several reasons:

1. If people normally focus on salient features (i.e. top half, or lower half of the face), there is the likelihood that other significant facial expressions and saliency may be omitted during interactions with clients.

2. People can control social interactions and gain knowledge of how the speaker is feeling 'from gaze direction and other facial cues' (Young 1997).

3. It is critical that an awareness of one's perceptual behaviour is developed, so that sensitivity to the client's other facial cues is demonstrated.

Young suggests that facial cues and expressions are monitored during conversation to locate subtle changes in the person's attention, intention and emotions. This can be achieved by considering the holistic features of the face to include facial distinctiveness (Stevenage 1997).

Since visual perception is required in daily interactions concurrent with spatial negotiation and analysis (Halligan 1995), a person whose perceptual organization is bisected, due to right brain hemisphere damage, will be unable to perceive environmental stimulation from the centre left of his body. Halligan observed that patients whose right brain hemisphere is damaged suffer visuospatial disorders, including being unaware of their left arm and hand. The person's safety is jeopardized due to frequent collision with objects and furniture in the environment, situated on the left side of space. Additionally, eating and dressing are affected as the individual is unaware that they have left food on the left side of the plate or may be half dressed.

Box 13.2 Approaches to explain face processing

- **Face processing** – to achieve face recognition – according to Farah et al (1998) is holistically undertaken by the perceiver. This theory fits in with Gestalt psychology, which comprises a configural (**holistic**) approach, by considering facial features in relation to one another (Stevenage 1997) rather than just looking at isolated features (e.g. a nose, a chin etc.).
- **Piecemeal processing** (the perceptual organizing of distinct salient features, e.g. a forehead, the eyes) to make sense of the whole is another approach used.
- **Independent** perceptual systems in the brain analyse some of the differing non-verbal (facial) messages independently of each other (Young 1997).

Activity 13.2

1. Place an eye patch on the left eye. Now spend the next 15 minutes walking around the house and the garden. Write down your feelings.
2. Look out of the window for 15 seconds. Now write down what you have perceived. Can you think why your attention was drawn to specific features in the environment?
3. Ask clients you have cared for to describe their initial perception of the ward during admission. Can you describe your own perception of the patients you are caring for?

??? Question 13.1

1. Do you think that perceptual ability can be improved?
2. Can you suggest ways to improve one's perceptual skill?
3. What connection can you make between perception and memory?
4. Can you provide an argument to support the idea that perception is linked to cognition?

CULTURE AND PERCEPTION

While perception is described as a biological and psychological process, it also constitutes a socio-cultural dimension. Culture influences people's world view and how they perceive themselves in relation to their living conditions.

Cultural traditions integrate with personality, acting as a driving force, while they underpin beliefs, attitudes and expectations. Such factors are relevant to how a person perceives internal events (subjective thoughts and interpretation of body functions), plus any external events (environmental issues separate from body experiences), with implications for well-being. According to Wilkinson (1996a), the combination of person (personality), culture and experiences, as well as perceptual processes, produce and facilitate interactive processing. In fact, it is impossible to conceive human experience without due consideration being given to a holistic framework approach. Wilkinson felt that several issues must be considered when the psychology of perception is studied:

- attention
- expectations
- person perception
- attribution theory.

Other domains, such as attitudes, values and beliefs (Wilkinson 1996b), are associated ideas to investigate in order to reach an understanding of how one perceives oneself and one's environment. Of particular relevance is the development of professional awareness of the relationship between health beliefs and perception.

ATTENTION

Attention has an important function in nursing care, but is a quality that can be developed (Wilkinson 1996a). Moreover, Wilkinson posited that professionals need to recognize their own sensory deficiencies, as well as the client's perceptual problems.

A client's level of attention, according to Wilkinson, is in a constant state of fluctuation, which entails that not all information-giving will be attended to. It can also be argued that if a person's health status is impaired, one can anticipate that their perception of events may not be congruent with nurses' expectations. Consequently, the client's attention may not be focused if their needs are related to pain alleviation, rather than listening to nursing information on a different subject.

Jandt (1998) postulates that humans have the inherent inclination to *select* from the environment only stimuli relevant according to *need*. The sick person is hence most likely to attend to nursing and/or medical information, that they both need and can identify with.

Attention behaviour is reliant on one's perception of events. A person who feels vulnerable, anxious and helpless in an unfamiliar setting, which is perceived to be threatening, is less able to pay attention to what is happening and being said. Deliberate effort should be made to give reassurance first and foremost. As the process of perception is interconnected with interpretation (Jandt 1998), sensitivity is needed to understand the culture context in the processing of events, and the degree of attention that will accordingly be obtained.

Attention may not be totally achieved with some clients who have entrenched personal health beliefs. The issue is of course concerned with cultural diversity and conflicting world views that can exist between professionals and their clients. For example, health, illness and disease perceptions differ among some black Americans, who practise folk medicine (Giger et al 1992): cancer, for instance, is viewed as punishment from God and a sin. In this context, attempting to provide a Western view of disease process may be received with incredulity and a lack of attention. Conversely, a professional's attention may not be in adequate harmony with the client's narratives.

As Wilkinson (1996a) explained, a professional and a lay person experiencing the same event will interpret and understand the situations differently. It is, however, recommended practice to avoid cultural imposition and to prevent ethnocentric attitudes from distorting one's perception of a client's cultural beliefs, which possess special significance.

Since caregivers need the person's attention to achieve positive health outcomes, attending by listening to their accounts of events and experiences will ease the therapeutic relationship.

EXPECTATIONS

People have numerous expectations which over the years have been shaped and modified according to life experiences. Other factors with a bearing on expectations are education, gender and socialization (Wilkinson 1996a).

The psychologists Atkinson et al (1987) point out that conscious expectations are common and related to the context in which someone is situated; for example, an inpatient consciously expects to be well cared for during his stay and when discharged into the community. Similarly, professionals have expectations regarding their clients, founded on their perception of the professional role. Atkinson et al made reference to 'prescribed behaviours': that professionals expect their clients to be 'good' and to want to 'get

better'. Most clients are perceptually aware and sensitive to their caregivers' expectations. They know that in health care settings it pays to co-operate and to comply with treatment regimens. It is important, however, that professionals' expectations do not override the clients' personal feelings and needs for support. This can become an issue when interventions are impersonal and regimented (Chamberlin 1998) (Case example 13.1).

Case example 13.1 'Playing the game'

'I learned to hide my feelings, especially negative ones. The very first day in the State Hospital I received a valuable piece of advice. Feeling frightened, abandoned and alone, I started to cry in the day room. Another patient came out and sat beside me, leaned over and whispered, "Don't do that. *They'll* think you're depressed". So I learned to cry only at night, in my bed, under the covers, without making a sound …

I was expected to be appreciative and grateful. In fact anything less was taken as a further symptom of my illness …

A patient who refuses psychiatric drugs may have very good reasons … But professionals often assume we are expressing a symbolic rebellion of some sort when we try to give a straightforward explanation of what we want and what we do not want' (Chamberlin 1998).

Assumptions are often made that clients who religiously follow the clinicians' instructions are being cooperative and compliant. As Case example 13.1 shows, passive cooperation does not reflect the true feelings of the sick person. In fact, compliance becomes a facade, to assure some harmony that supports professional expectations of their clients. The case example also illustrates the person's covert rebellion against a system that heightens the inequality of the relationship.

Expectations co-exist with personal views on health matters. In some cultures any health deviation is attributed to abstract forces, spirits and sorcery. The expectations that sacred medicine grounded in magic, divination and alchemy can combat disease is therefore high (Hiskins 1995).

When a patient's perception of events differs to their expectations, disillusionment is felt. For example, the pain experience is interpreted at an individual level, and people will respond in ways that are compatible with their cultural norms (Wenger 1993). Now, if patients perceive that caregivers cannot grasp their interpretations of the sensations they are experiencing, it is likely that patients' expectations will be unrealized. Wenger explains that if a search for the cultural meanings of symptoms (in addition to bio-psychological factors) is omitted, clients will be denied their right to receive culturally sensitive care.

PERSON PERCEPTION

How one perceives others is grounded in past experiences, which are representations stored in memory. If one is told, for example, that a group of psychologists are doing some experiments in the laboratory, one's expectations should match the images stored in memory of what experimental psychologists are.

Person perception, similar to object perception, is a common experience. Most of the time people are unaware of the thoughts, meanings, fleeting views that cross their minds when perceiving other people. Yet, what a person experiences is a daily ongoing perceptual behaviour. The study of experience using an eclectic psychological approach (Henry et al 1997), encompasses the need to consider the meanings people attach to their world experience, to include person perception.

One's social perception is continually changing as one encounters diverse groups of people and the context in which they exist. Hayes (1994) points out that person perception is concerned with many features:

- how someone's personality traits influence others' perception
- the impressions one has of others, based on stereotypic behaviour
- one's own personal social representations (known as social constructs), to do with theories of others' behaviour

- a self-fulfilling prophecy component, which in addition to being a psychological concept is also social in character.

Sociologists have studied pupils in deprived inner city areas and perceived them to be low achievers. Consequently, some teachers in their interactions with such pupils unwittingly feel that facilitating their learning can be fruitless. In nursing and medical practice, professionals' perception of their clients' social and personality traits (Wilkinson 1996a) has implications in health assessment. A patient's social background can influence professionals' perception of their health behaviour. The literature frequently refers to a culture of deprivation among the poor working classes, which has negative effects on their health lifestyles. This knowledge can impinge on practitioners' attitude during the assessment procedure if it is believed that the individual is the cause of the social and health problem.

While forming first impressions of others is human nature, it is a behaviour with significant influence on one's judgement of a person (Wilkinson 1996a). Impressions are often linked to stereotypes which if negative, according to Jandt (1998), affect our 'perceptual screen', leading to communication impairment.

In the early 1990s, some social psychologists (e.g. McConnell & Philipchalk 1992) observed how impressions can be created by significant others in the environment. They suggested that people can 'bias our perceptions' predetermining how someone is perceived by others, by giving *their* impressions of the person being encountered. It is an implicit powerful psychological force, when one's attitudes can be influenced before the actual social event: meeting a person for the first time for example. One can argue hence that the plethora of nursing literature available has the possibility of shaping and developing the professionals' impressions and perception of the sick person.

A feature of the self-fulfilling prophecy, Wilkinson (1996a) explains, is the 'halo and thorns' effect common in person perception. Halo effect applies to favourable impressions, while the thorns imply negative views. A knowledge of how person perception influences attitudes is critical in health care. Conversely, an awareness that the patient's person perception is similarly influenced by professionals' presentations must be borne in mind.

Patients may possess negative stereotypes of female nurses and their male counterparts. The media may have contributed to this process by portraying female nurses as the stereotypic, sexually motivated nymphomaniac. On the other hand, male nurses may be viewed with suspicious sexual orientations, because they are in a profession traditionally perceived as feminine.

McConnell and Philipchalk point out that 'reputation' is another attribute in person perception. In the above example, the media build the reputations of specific groups in society through communication. So, our 'internal processes' – attitudes, reputations and stereotypes – determine the quality of the interactions in the nurse–patient relationship.

Whitehead (1997) observed the negative consequences of stereotypes, which act as barriers to effective health promotion. She wrote that stereotypes are not uncommon among professionals, whose attitudes are influenced by their perception of the clients. For example, a practice nurse reports that the external appearances (self-presentations) of a client, e.g. 'looking prim and proper', will determine whether she will actively promote safe sexual practice to her client. Conversely, a midwife, according to Whitehead's findings, argued that someone with rings and tattoos and 'who looks' promiscuous, will be targeted for safe sex health promotion. One issue with implications for practice is concerned with how patients perceive 'holistic caring' (Williams 1997). This is of relevance to person perception simply because the client perceives *the person* behind the act of caring. A sensitive patient-focused care approach with the aim to alleviate anxiety and establish comfort is perceived positively.

When a patient's expectations are met, person perception is more positive. Recent research on patient expectations in clinical practice (Staniszewska & Ahmed 1998) shows the occurrence of negative person perception when clients felt their needs were unfulfilled. The researchers quoted patients as saying the nurse was 'abrasive' and nursing staff were 'abrupt in manner'. It has been known for people to have a positive attitude change when their caregivers show dedication in meeting their needs.

Activity 13.3

Identify ways which can help to prevent the stereotyping of groups.

Attribution theory

Attribution theory can best be described as a process that entails how we 'attribute', or ascribe certain characteristics to other people and explain our own behaviour, by attributing the rationale for our actions (McConnell & Philipchalk 1992, Hayes 1994) to some external factors. In other words, we are inclined to omit 'our own internal disposition' in the explanation. Our actions are hence attributed to 'situational determinants' (Gross 1992, Hayes 1994, Wilkinson 1996a).

In clinical practice, mistakes can be made when clients' behaviour is defined according to their 'dispositions': for example, assumptions are made that they do not follow health advice because they are uneducated. In reality, many people are aware of their individual responsibility for health maintenance, but their socioeconomic position (situational determinants) prevents them from achieving the desired health outcomes. Moreover, individuals rarely blame themselves or recognize their own shortcomings. Thus professionals may ignore their internal disposition and project criticisms onto others when their care interventions are inadequate. It may be perceived that patient care is undermined because of poor management from senior officials. The current Secretary of State for Health often states in public debates that good care can be given by maintaining basic professional standards; e.g. listening to patients, being supportive and sensitive to their needs despite a lack of resources.

Attitudes, values and beliefs

A person who has strong health values will accept that exercise, a healthy diet, not smoking and moderate alcohol consumption are worthwhile. Additionally, these values are linked to the beliefs that a healthy lifestyle comprises some of these key attributes. For example, if I value regular attendance at the gymnasium to keep fit, I must evidently believe in exercise as a means to good health. Consequently my attitude is related to my perceptual orientation that good health can be achieved through exercise. When I go to the gym I am indirectly (implicitly) expressing an attitude. However, this can be verified when I am asked to explain my point of view on exercise and health. Therefore an attitude can be verbally expressed.

Wilkinson (1996b) explains how beliefs, attitudes and values are interconnected and influence how a person perceives the world. These concepts are abstract in nature and cannot be assessed accurately. However, one can argue that inferences can be made about a person's attitude, beliefs and values by observing their behaviour (a behaviouristic approach).

In care settings, for example, some patients may refuse to eat pork. Cultural expectations and socialization influence their perception of pork-eating as a taboo subject. Inferences can thus be made that their beliefs are expressions of an attitude towards the value they attach to religious beliefs.

In a multicultural society, one expects to find a diversity of health perception, associated with attitudes, values and beliefs. In the USA, Flaskerud and Rush (1989) found evidence of misperception among some black American women concerning AIDS: many women believed AIDS to be caused by sinful behaviour as predicted in the Bible and that the Devil was also involved in its causation. Beliefs in religion, magic and the use of charms and herbs convince the believers that these are the only ways to combat illnesses.

Clark (1993), in his anthropological study of the Huli in Papua New Guinea, found ingrained attitudes that women are often believed to be the cause of illness among the men, due to beliefs in menstrual pollution. Cautious male behaviour was common in interactions with women in case the men contracted any infections. Such examples demonstrate varied extremes of attitudes, values and beliefs driven by socio-cultural traditions, which engender specific perception of events. When care plans are designed, it is a professional responsibility to include evidence that interventions circumscribe attention to variants in health beliefs in the client population, a necessary approach in the provision of individualized care.

Older people's perceptions of exercise in old age

At the other spectrum of life, some knowledge on how elderly citizens perceive ageing and the importance of exercise is relevant. Their personal beliefs, reflected in the values they give to exercise, have implications for health care, particularly now that an increase in the number of old people in the new millenium is expected.

Research findings reported by Stead et al (1997), in a qualitative study of nine groups of six to eight older respondents (aged 55+), show the challenging task faced by health promoters. The researchers found that the respondents held stereotypic attitudes that old age meant inactivity and disengagement. Several observations had implications for health promotion in practice. The respondents in Stead et al's study perceived themselves and exercise in the following ways:

1. A conventional way of seeing themselves as powerless against the effects of the ageing process. A higher significance was attached to being mentally alert, rather than attempting to improve physical performance as well.

2. In spite of advanced age, the respondents had a self-image of being younger than these people they considered old, which had a positive connotation. The researchers gave the example of an 80-year-old man who would not attend a local day centre 'because it was for old folk'.

3. Health professionals' attitude that a physical problem was due to old age (age stereotype) was noted.

4. Old age was associated with being cautious about avoiding overactivity and this meant, in some cases, not exercising for exercise's sake.

5. Previous lifestyle consisting of regular exercise and sport had an influence on some to continue their exercise in later life.

6. Physical ailments strengthen the attitude and perception that exercising is not beneficial and could cause more harm.

7. There was evidence amongst some respondents that rewards can be gained through exercise; improving self-worth, feeling good and socializing.

8. Some situational circumstances, such as poor access (e.g. poor public transport) and youth-oriented services, discouraged uptake of services that provide opportunities for exercise.

9. Information-giving by professionals was focused on 'smoking, alcohol and diet', showing a lack of pro-activity on other health issues, such as regular exercise and attending community services that provide access to exercise sessions.

Such findings give the foundation on which to design future health promotion strategies. An aspect not considered in Stead et al's research was identifying the respondents' definition of 'exercise'. From the answers obtained in Stead et al's survey, many older people associate 'exercise' with 'walking', 'pull the weight and pump the iron', 'biking' and 'golf'. However, identifying hobbies practised such as gardening, dancing, swimming and jogging could reinforce the notion that such activities are forms of exercise that many older people enjoy doing.

The research highlights a degree of stereotypical attitude from professionals, which implicitly conveys to the old person that ageing is the cause of their problems, when in fact it should be perceived as a period of fulfilment and enjoyment. Positive messages should be transmitted, bearing in mind individual differences in the perception of health beliefs and self-image. Personal experiences can embed some deep mind-set, i.e. smoking is not always harmful (Box 13.3) because a person is still alive and active (Mitchell 1996).

Box 13.3 Health beliefs

'They say smoking's bad for you but I was brought up in smoky atmospheres, bars, dancehalls, you name it, so why have we lived 70 … 90 years … and I'm still healthy' (an active 73-year-old smoker).

Some individuals perceive exercise as an irrelevant activity because they had not practised it in their younger days. While many respondents in the research outlined above (Stead et al 1997) recognized the social component of exercise, health promoters should adapt their strategies, encouraging positive perception of exercise as a productive activity with socio-psychological and physical benefits.

MENTAL ILLNESS AND PERCEPTION
Auditory hallucinations

Hallucinations are sensory experiences in the absence of any external stimulation. Auditory hallucinations are common in psychiatry, particularly among patients with schizophrenia. The sufferer feels plagued with voices in the head, or from external sources; in fact, auditory hallucinations commonly consist of voices, and sometimes of noises (Johnson & Smith 1994).

The person who is hallucinating believes in the experience and is psychologically distressed, especially when it is felt that the voices are threatening and persecutory in character. While mental changes can trigger different types of hallucinations (Box 13.4), it should be pointed out that

---

Box 13.4 Types of hallucinations

- **Visual hallucinations**: disturbed perception of object, people and animals. Fevers, due to typhoid and cholera, can cause these perceptual changes.
- **Gustatory hallucinations**: sense of taste disturbed; the person believes that food may be poisoned.
- **Olfactory hallucinations**: there is the conviction of an unpleasant smell (e.g. gases, fumes), possibly poisonous.
- **Tactile hallucinations**: the feeling that the skin or internal organs are invaded by insects, or being manipulated in some ways.

hallucinatory states can also be induced by drugs (e.g. LSD, cannabis etc.) and alcohol-related mental health problems, as in Korsakoff's psychosis.

The connection with cultural factors is often underestimated and misunderstood when the topic of hallucinations is discussed. Very little is understood of the nature of mental illness and its presentations among ethnic groups, an issue with implications for health care practice. Despite cross-cultural networking being established nationally and internationally, professionals still lack knowledge of the best way to tackle behavioural changes in their ethnic clients.

It is not uncommon for the ethnic client to have their values, beliefs and religious rituals misperceived. During needs assessment, the practitioner should consider varying perspectives, from biological and psychological to cultural and spiritual domains.

Traditionally, Western psychiatry has classified hallucinatory states according to set categories, with a lack of awareness of social factors pertinent to the person's present behaviour. George (1998) poses the question whether someone who hears voices or sees visions has mental health problems? The argument is founded on evidence that many groups of people have beliefs underpinned by the presence of 'spirits', with which they communicate ritually: a spiritual world peopled by deities and beings with special powers. In these circumstances, if one hears voices it is probably from a religious–spiritual source. Such beliefs can be strongly adhered to. George explained how, to many users of mental health services, keeping their religious orientations private is significant, since it is thought that their mental health care assessors are prone to misunderstand and misperceive their religion.

As far back as the early 1980s, Cochrane (1983) reported the attitudes of those concerned with identifying psychiatric problems among West Indian born patients diagnosed as schizophrenic. The issue was linked to the extent with which schizophrenia was associated with the expression of 'religious ideation'. In 1998 George pointed out that mental health workers still experience difficulties in elucidating religious expressions from mental health problems. As signs and symbols are an established method of communication among many ethnic groups, it can be argued that inadequate knowledge of these social issues will compound problems and needs identification. Moreover, as Stockman (1994) explained, in African cultures it is impossible to conceive of the African individual without simultaneously situating the person within the hub of their social environment, the family and ancestors.

A Central African, Stockman emphasized, is fully integrated with the 'super and paranatural' world, so that there is a strong bond between the spirit, soul and body. With this dimension a distinction can prove hard to establish between the physical and mental deficiencies. To the spiritual believer, it is normal practice to receive messages from one's forebears, in the forms of signs and symbols. When 'deviant' behaviour is suspected, Stockman observed that in both Central Africa and China, the family steps in to attempt to rectify the 'disordered' behaviour. In some cases, however, a person in the early stages of mental illness may acquire a special social role within family networks which is respected. Nevertheless, as the mental illness progresses the individual may be expelled from the family for a while until their behaviour is restored or stabilized.

In Britain, evidence shows that a positive move is taking place in the understanding of auditory hallucinations. There is a clear departure from traditional psychiatric interventions, which used to concentrate on the suppression of symptoms, to:

1. an understanding of the person's experience according to belief system (Allen 1997)
2. a recognition that voices may serve a compensatory function with personal meaning to the individual (Clarke 1998)
3. that 'hearing voices' does not necessarily mean mental illness (Westacott 1995)
4. assessing the coping capacity of the sufferer – in activities of daily living – is of importance since it indicates the degree of disablement caused by the hallucinations.

Hearing voices is perceived by care professionals as more prevalent among the population than originally envisaged, and many appear to be functioning in the social world adequately (Romme 1998). This evidence, Romme points out, questions conventional beliefs of psychopathology as the origin of the disorder. It appears that the coping skills adopted by those with auditory hallucinations will determine how effectively they function in society. Hearing voices is a personal and individual experience that is integral to the human experience (Pembroke 1998), and care professionals should acknowledge that many choose to live with their voices. It is good health care practice to be attentive to the client's account: obtaining an accurate description of *what* the voices say is essential, as it is important to the person concerned. As Pembroke explained, although voices can be threatening at times, they are also 'life enriching', with some positive features, such as the giving of 'precognitive insights': an intuitive function. A phenomenological approach is thus recommended, as it provides a medium to obtain insight into the nature of the experience.

Baker (1995) emphasized that adopting the attitude that consists of accepting voices as a variant of human experience (rather than an expression of a mental illness syndrome) will enhance our understanding of voice-hearers. By listening attentively to the voice-hearers'

accounts, professionals are given opportunities to 'learn' from their personal experiences, since the voice-hearers are the experts (Baker 1995). It is, however, pertinent to apply some basic strategies (Box 13.5) during interactions with clients, founded on recent debates and research on auditory experiences.

 Activity 13.4

1. Write down your views on the effects of culture on perception.
2. Explain how you would respond to symbolic messages from your client.
3. Observe the impact of perceptual changes on client's behaviour. Describe the features presented.
4. Assess the extent of dysfunctional interactions with family and others caused by altered perceptions.
5. Develop an alliance with clients and their relatives. Involve them in the care programme. Can you record their thoughts and feelings on their understanding of perceptual changes?
6. What activities can you recommend to redirect a patient's energy that is focused on listening to voices?
7. Investigate the way values and beliefs of others have shaped their perception.
8. Find out how your local community health service plans the care of those with disordered perception.

??? Question 13.2

1. How would you assess and monitor for the presence or absence of disordered perception from cultural expressions?
2. What strategies would you use to determine whether the auditory hallucinations originate from external sources or within the individual?
3. What instructions would you give to someone who is hallucinating?
4. If a person is experiencing sensory disturbances, how will a reduced-stimulation environment help?
5. Can you identify any benefits in exploring the hallucination with the client?
6. What do you consider to be the possible advantages of using a client-focused care approach to an understanding of altered perception?

Box 13.5 Client-focused approach

1. Be prepared to accept the client's version of events as the possible consequence of religious/ spiritual/paranormal belief systems.
2. Consider ways to complement the client's own strategies in coping, with other well-informed methods (e.g. thought-blocking, diversional activities), thus widening their options.
3. Boost confidence in exercising control over the voices, rather than allowing the latter to be in control, e.g. by listening to, but not doing, what is being said.
4. Encourage better awareness of the voices, so that knowledge of their occurrence can be anticipated, and prevention of intrusion attempted and blocked at its source.
5. Utilize self-help groups, so that networking and sharing of information can be established.
6. Be prepared to allow cathartic reactions and the uncovering of repressed memories.
7. Voices are real to the person: allow space and time so that free associations (a Freudian approach to promote free recall of hidden meanings) can occur.

SUMMARY

The study of perception consists of discovering how the sense organs receive stimulation from the environment, and the cognitive processes involved in integrating the experience. Perception is also linked to working memory and to biological functioning. A common theory used in explaining perception is known as Gestalt. This consists of the explanation that humans perceive whole configurations, rather than parts or elements of an object. For example, a circle made up of dotted lines is perceived as a whole; a dotted line is perceived as a straight line rather than a series of dots.

Perception is of relevance to humans as a survival mechanism since it helps one to assess one's environment. The perception of threat and danger drives individuals to take action and increase safety mechanisms. It is known for certain biochemical changes to cause altered perception, such as in toxic states and conditions of delirium. Professionals have a duty to ensure accurate assessment of clients' perceptual integrity by using effective cognitive tools.

The context of perception is of importance since it determines what is going to be perceived. The brightness of an object will be assessed in relation to its surroundings. What is perceived and understood relies on perceptual tracking, a mechanism that depends on what is stored in memory.

Psychologists agree that face perception allows individuals to detect social signals from facial expressions during interactions. Several systems have been identified in face perception, which explain the neuro-cognitive mechanisms located in the brain.

Altered perception is often found in psychotic states, such as schizophrenia, when auditory hallucinations are often present. It has been found that hearing voices is not uncommon among many people, who have managed to adapt their lifestyle to cope with their voice-hearing. It is also suggested that a patient-focused care approach be used to help clients who hear voices.

GLOSSARY

Amygdala   a mass of grey matter in the anterior portion of the temporal lobe of the brain
Anterior insular cortex   frontal and outer layer of an organ or structure
Gestalt theory   the concept that objects' configurations are perceived as whole rather than individual elements
Korsakoff's psychosis   personality characterized by disorientation, delirium, illusions and hallucinations, caused by chronic alcoholism

Medial cortex brain activity   pertaining to the middle part of the brain
Parietal cortex of the brain   outside brain layer, beneath the parietal (crown of the skull)
Positron emission tomography   a method to measure brain activity (e.g. blood flow, oxygen uptake, neurotransmitter activity etc.)
Temporal cortex of the brain   outer layer of the brain near the temples region

REFERENCES

Allen D 1997 Finding a voice. Nursing Standard 11(52): 21–23

Atkinson R L, Atkinson R C, Smith E, Hilgard E R 1987 Psychology, 9th edn. Harcourt Brace Jovanovich, Fort Worth, p 181

Baker P 1995 Accepting the inner voices. Nursing Times 91(31): 59–61

Bertenthal B I 1996 Origins and early development of perception, action and representation. Annual Review of Psychology 47: 431–459

Breitbart W, Rosenfeld B, Roth A 1997 The memorial assessment scale. Journal of Pain and Symptom Management 13(3): 128–137

Bruce V 1998 Fleeting images of shade: identifying people caught on video. The Psychologist 11(7): 331–336

Chamberlin J 1998 Confessions of a non-compliant patient. Journal of Psychosocial Nursing 36(4): 49–53

Clark J 1993 Gold, sex and pollution: male illness and myth at Mt Kare, Papua New Guinea. American Ethnologist 20(4): 742–757

Clarke L 1998 Voice-overs. Nursing Times 94(9): 28–29

Cochrane R 1983 The social creation of mental illness. Longman, London, p 98

Colwell C 1998 The sense of seeing. Psychologist 11(6): 274–275

Drake L, Drake V, Curwen J 1997 A new account of sundown syndrome. Nursing Standard 12(7): 37–40

Farah R J, Wilson K D, Drain M, Tanaka J M 1998 What is 'special' about face perception? Psychological Review 105(3): 482–498

Flaskerud J H, Rush C E 1989 AIDS and traditional health beliefs and practices of black women. Nursing Research 38(4): 210–215

George M 1998 A gulf in understanding. Nursing Standard 12(26): 24–25

Giger J N, Davidhizar R E, Turner G 1992 Black American

folk medicine health care beliefs: implications for nursing plans of care. The Association of Black Nursing Faculty Journal 3(2): 42–46

Govier H 1980 Basic perceptual processes. In: Radford J, Govier E (eds) A textbook of psychology. Sheldon Press, London, p 249

Gregory R 1996 Twenty-five years after the intelligent eye. Psychologist 9(10): 452–455

Gross R D 1992 Psychology: the science of mind and behaviour, 2nd edn. Stoughton & Hodder, London

Gugerty L J 1997 Situation awareness during driving: explicit and implicit knowledge in dynamic spatial memory. Journal of Experimental Psychology: Applied 3(1): 42–66

Halligan P W 1995 Drawing attention to neglect. The contribution of line bisection. Psychologist 8(6): 257–263

Hayes N 1994 Foundations of psychology. Routledge, London

Henry J, Pickering J, Stevens R et al 1997 Towards a psychology of experience. The Psychologist 10(3): 117–120

Hiskins J 1995 Health education: what anthropology can teach us. Professional Care of Mother and Child 5(1): 25–27

Holaday B, Swan J H, Turner-Henson A 1997 Images of the neighbourhood and activity patterns of chronically ill school age children. Environment and Behaviour 29(3): 348–373

Jandt F E 1998 Intercultural communication, 2nd edn. Sage, Thousand Oaks

Johnson F C, Smith L D 1994 Cognition. In: Thompson T, Mathias P (eds) Lyttle's mental health and disorder, 2nd edn. Baillière Tindall, London, p 185

Lowe G 1998 Crime and violence. Psychologist 11(3): 137

Lusher J, Martin N 1998 Disgust and the neuropsychology of face perception. The Psychologist 11(1): 33

McConnell J V, Philipchalk R P 1992 Understanding human behaviour, 7th edn. Harcourt Brace Jovanovich, Fort Worth

Milisen K, Foreman M D, Godderis J et al 1998 Delirium in the hospitalized elderly. Nursing Clinics of North America 33(3): 417–434

Mitchell G 1996 A qualitative study of older women's perceptions of control, health and ageing. Health Education Journal 55(3): 267–274

Murphy N 1998 Perceiving social signals. Psychologist 11(2): 64

Nasar J L, Jones K M 1997 Landscapes of fear and stress. Environment and Behaviour 29(3): 291–324

O'Kane B L, Cooper E E, Biederman I, Nystrom B 1997 An account of object identifications confusion. Journal of Experimental Psychology: Applied 3(1): 21–41

Pembroke L 1998 Echoes of me. Nursing Times 94(9): 30–31

Perret D 1995 Seeing and pulling faces. Psychologist 8(2): 77

Rakover S S, Teucher B 1997 Facial inversion effects: parts and whole relationship. Perception and Psychophysics 59(5): 752–761

Romme M 1998 The invisible intruders. Nursing Times 94(9): 30–31

Roth-Roemer S, Fann J, Syrjala K 1997 The importance of recognizing and measuring delirium. Journal of Pain And Symptom Management 13(3): 125–127

Smith L B, Quittner A L, Osberger M J, Miyamoto R 1998 Audition and visual attention: the developmental trajectory in deaf and hearing populations. Developmental Psychology 34(5): 840–850

Staniszewska S, Ahmed L 1998 Patient expectations and satisfaction with health care. Nursing Standard 12(18): 34–38

Stead M, Wimbush E, Eadie D, Teer P 1997 A qualitative study of older people's perceptions of ageing and exercise: the implications for health promotion. Health Education Journal 56(1): 3–16

Stevenage S 1997 Face facts: theories and findings. Psychologist 19(4): 163–167

Stockman R 1994 Mental health care in Central Africa and China. British Journal of Psychiatry 165(2): 145–148

Wenger A F 1993 Cultural meanings of symptoms. Holistic Nursing Practice 7(2): 22–35

Westacott M 1995 Strategies for managing auditory hallucinations. Nursing Times 91(3): 35–37

Whitehead M 1997 Do stereotypes get in the way of effective health promotion? Health Education Journal 56(1): 1–2

Wilkinson J A 1996a Psychology 2: message received and understood? British Journal of Nursing 5(14): 852–855

Wilkinson J A 1996b Psychology 3: 'Don't give me that attitude!' British Journal of Nursing 5(15): 933–936

Williams S A 1997 Caring in patient-focused care: the relationship of patients' perceptions of holistic nurse caring to their levels of anxiety. Holistic Nursing Practice 11(3): 61–68

Young A 1997 Finding the mind's construction in the face. Psychologist 10(10): 447–452

Young A, Bruce V 1998 Pictures at an exhibition: The science of the face. Psychologist 11(3): 120–125

FURTHER READING

Charters P J 1999 The religious and spiritual needs of mental health clients. Nursing Standard 13(26): 34–36

Hoffman R E, Rapaport J, Mazure C M et al 1999 Selective speech perception alterations in schizophrenic patients reporting hallucinated 'voices'. American Journal of Psychiatry 156(3): 393–398

Meyer J, Taieb M, Flascher I 1997 Correlation estimates as perceptual judgments. Journal of Experimental Psychology: Applied 3(1): 3–20

Schofield I 1997 A small exploratory study of the reactions of older people to an episode of delirium. Journal of Advanced Nursing 25(5): 942–952

Wichowski H C, Kubsch S M 1997 The relationship of self-perception of illness and compliance with healthcare regimens. Journal of Advanced Nursing 25(3): 548–553

Wunderlich R J, Perry A, Lavin M A 1999 Patients' perceptions of uncertainty and stress during weaning from mechanical ventilation. Dimensions in Critical Care Nursing 18(1): 2–8

Memory is one of the important concepts in psychology. It is a multi-faceted set of structures. Several theories have been put forward to explain its nature. In this chapter the aims are to:

- **describe such structures**
- **explain the perspectives associated with its features**
- **introduce some disorders that can affect memory integrity**
- **discuss the role of care providers in supporting clients with memory loss.**

WHAT IS MEMORY?

It is quite common for people to take their memory for granted. Prior to reading the first line of this chapter, were you pondering over the meaning of memory and its usefulness? The answer is most likely to be non-affirmative. Yet without memory our whole being disintegrates; the word personality itself would be void of meaning. It is a person's memory that makes their personality: it guides behaviour; it is motivating; it enhances learning and perception; it helps to develop knowledge and intelligence, and other mental functioning associated with being human. In fact, memory is the hub of cognitive processes.

Memory, Dye (1989) emphasized, is probably of greater importance to humans than any other mental functions. A person's memory makes

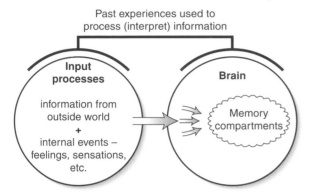

Fig. 14.1 How memory acquires information.

individuals what they are (Cohen 1990). The study of memory has preoccupied psychologists for decades; they intepret memory as a complex phenomenon of human cognitive processes. Memory refers to one's ability to use information stored (retained) in the brain and concerns the mechanisms one uses to retrieve the information and input processes (the acquisition of information from outside world) (Fig. 14.1).

Both the external and our internal (physiological, psychological) environments feed the brain with information, which is subsequently analysed from past experience (stored in long-term memory) before being transferred into the memory compartment. Cohen (1990) explained that people's daily lives consist of coping with the vast amount of information bombarding their memory. It is not surprising, therefore, that a filtering mechanism is in position to assess and prioritize the information before storage takes place. Nevertheless, it is known for one's memory to store vast amounts of unimportant information. The 1990s television programme, 'You Bet', is testimony to this: in this programme some contestants proved their memory skills in recalling, for example, the numerous designs of cars' rear lights, or who said what in a movie in the 1960s.

MEMORY MECHANICS
Biology and memory

In the search for a better understanding of the memory process, psychologists have investi-

gated the role of biology in the scheme of things.

Memory performance relies on both anatomical and physiological integrity. As the brain is the organ where memory resides, neuroscientists have concentrated their efforts on researching the brain neurochemistry and its role in memory formation. Rosenzweig (1996), in his exploration of the connection between memory and neural mechanisms, has highlighted some important neurochemical issues that affect memory. He began with the premise that the plasticity of the nervous system must be recognized; in particular, the relationship among learning, memory and nerve cells. Learning is dependent upon memory, and the latter relies on the proper functioning of neurochemical and neuroanatomical structures (the integration of cellular (structures) functioning with physiological functioning). The notion that training and experience are inter-related in these processes are central to this argument, as is the idea that long-term memory (LTM) is relevant to the changes occurring anatomically and neurochemically.

Rosenzweig explained that specific areas of the brain will undergo changes according to the types of learning, training and environmental conditions a person is exposed to. He pointed out that, as far back as the 1890s, research findings indicate support for the theory that changes at neural junctions (synaptic junctions) might account for memory. He argued that learning causes these changes. In fact, it is believed that intellectual exercise (learning, memorizing material and events from life) is likely to increase the size of neural networks.

In the 1960s (Rosenzweig 1996) experiments showed that formal training and varied environmental experiences can cause the rodent brain to undergo neurochemistry and neuro-anatomy changes. In addition, an association was established between 'brain chemistry and problem-solving ability'. The researchers discovered that an enzyme (acetylcholinesterase) level was higher in the cerebral cortex of rodents that had been trained and tested on more difficult problems. Moreover, an enriched environment (stimulating, secure, comforting, sophisticated) caused specific changes in specific regions (the cortex) of the brain. These changes have been consequent to learning and formation of memory. Memory development is contingent on sound physiological and anatomical structures (a biological perspective) and the quality of the environment (a social perspective) – i.e. is it deprived or enriched – which determines the quality/standards of learning and problem-solving skills (psychological perspective).

Rosenzweig pointed out that the quality of training and/or differential exposure to learning situations will have an effect upon the 'number of synapses, their sizes' etc., thus giving an indication of memory capacity. It appears, hence that memory, unless stimulated by exposure to learning, can remain underdeveloped.

In attempting to explain this argument, experimenters have discovered that when animals are deprived of light in one eye, cortical cells in that eye remain underdeveloped and unresponsive to subsequent stimulation. It appears that memory may be subjected to similar principles: lack of learning leads to poor memory skills. In fact, it is argued that LTM is reliant upon protein synthesis in the cortex, after training, to mature. Moreover, Rosenzweig explained that some drugs (opioid antagonists) can enhance memory formation.

These findings of Rosenzweig show that memory, although an abstract concept, does not exist in a vacuum, but hinges on brain functioning: neural activities in combination with chemical processes and healthy neuro-anatomical structures.

Activity 14.1

Recall events in your life – from childhood onwards – that could have helped your memory development.

??? Question 14.1

How could sickness or ill-health interfere with memory?

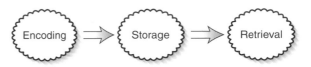

Fig. 14.2   Stages of memory.

Relationship between short-term memory and long-term memory

Memory is said to consist of three stages (Atkinson et al 1993) (Fig. 14.2):

1. The encoding stage: a process of interpreting incoming information/stimuli by creating some representations of the material, to deposit the new experience in memory.
2. The retention stage: storing and retaining the information.
3. The retrieval stage: accessing stored information at a later time.

The mechanisms that concern the above processes are, however, quite complex. People rely on their consciousness to hold information temporarily, while information that is permanently stored resides in the unconscious. The former refers to 'primary memory' and the latter 'secondary memory' (Healy & McNamara 1996). Primary memory is commonly known as short-term memory (STM); secondary memory is known as long-term memory (LTM).

Eysenck (1996) and Healy and McNamara (1996) explain that research theories indicate the presence of three distinct memory stores or a multi-store model of memory:

1. Sensory registers memory, with the specific functions of storing individual sensory experiences, e.g. visual, auditory, touch, taste etc. separately (Fig. 14.3).
2. Short-term store (STS).
3. Long-term store (LTS).

Using computer terminology as analogy, STS and LTS represent the 'hard drive'; they are the permanent features of the system (Healy & McNamara 1996). The control processes (strategies to remember and the cognitive mechanisms) are seen as the software.

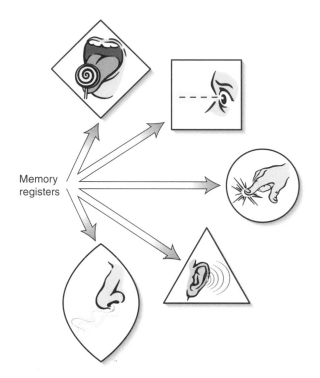

Fig. 14.3   A memory compartment for each sensory experience.

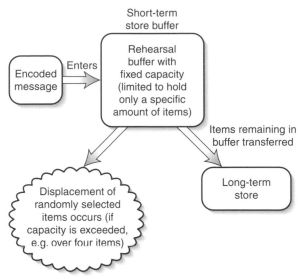

Fig. 14.4   Fixed capacity rehearsal buffer.

Encoded messages (information from outside world and/or internal subjective states) enter a fixed capacity rehearsal buffer (Fig 14.4). If the capacity buffer is overloaded items are displaced, making way for new input. Information remaining in buffer are 'rehearsed' and transferred to LTS. It is, however, assumed that items may be retained in the STS buffer as well as LTS. Retrieving any item relies on information in both LTS and STS. For example, you hear on the radio that two school girls who were abducted three days ago have been found by the police. You have been following developments on this topic since their initial disappearance. As you listen to the latest news, you quickly search your short-term and long-term stores, to give meaning to the new messages. Your long-term store may contain news items from three days ago; your short-term store may relate to what was read in the morning papers. A full picture emerges as you retrieve memories from both short-term and long-term stores.

Recall can be affected by distraction, a fast presentation rate, and the number of items, because messages remain in the buffer zone for a shorter time, which means that less is transferred to long-term memory (Healy & McNamara 1996).

Research shows that attempts to learn two sets of material interfere with the retention of such material (Mann & Brenner 1996). The authors point out, for example, that retroactive interference (new set of material learned interferes with previously learned information), caused decreased recall. Retroactive interference can be further explained by the 'response-set suppression theory', which postulates that a subject learns to suppress items from an original list when learning a second list. The second list (or new material) assumes greater importance and demands focused attention, displacing the old information.

Distinction is established in the two types of processing: a shallow level of processing occurs when an item is temporarily encoded (short-term memory (STM)) and a deeper level of encoding (Healy & McNamara 1996) takes place with the transfer to LTM, which is pivotal to the time spent in the rehearsal buffer. STM and LTM should not be interpreted as antagonistic cognitive processes, but as associates in the complex phenomenon of learning, remembering and forgetting.

In a review of current thinking on issues connected with the links between STM and LTM, Healy and McNamara explained that LTS is accessed via retrieval cues (Box 14.1), which are broad categories of concepts. Success in retrieval is reliant upon rehearsal and coding mechanisms conducted in STM. A retrieval attempt, they argue, consists of sampling one memory image (visual representations) based on its strength (i.e. degree of impact, importance, relevance etc.), relative to that of all other images stored in LTM. Additionally, STM activation is considered to be a subset (a secondary element) within LTM. Activation of STM causes activation of LTM.

Box 14.1 Some categories of retrieval cues

Animals, diseases, lung conditions, cardiovascular problems, trees, housing, architecture, antiques, computers, medicine, nursing.

STM is considered to be efficient at storing *recent* input. This is called the recency effect (Eysenck 1996), i.e. one is able to recall the last few words in a list, but not the first. LTM, on the other hand, is to do with the storage of earlier information and, according to Eysenck, has a vast capacity. Moreover, LTM has differing functional systems in that LTM stores *declarative* knowledge (e.g. 'knowing how' to drive a car), and also becomes the 'owner' of knowledge after feedback from STM.

Atkinson et al (1993) pointed out that the role of STM in the equation of memory mechanics should be recognized: STM is seen as a 'way-station' to LTM. Information remains in STM, is encoded and transferred to LTM, a process described as a 'dual-memory model', i.e. a two-memory systems model. Healy and McNamara (1996) felt that there are additional memory systems operating concurrently with conventional STM and LTM (Box 14.2).

Box 14.2 Additional memory systems

Working memory: this theory accepts STM as an active worker rather than a passive one, i.e. information-processing in STM is active. The features of a working memory in short-term store are:

- a limited attention capacity
- a central executive (a coordinating system)
- an auditory (acoustic) buffer
- a visual buffer.

These buffers will temporarily store auditory, visual and phonological (speech-based) stimuli in STM, co-ordinated by the central executive (Fig. 14.5).

Conceptual short-term memory (CSTM): this system plays a role in everyday reading, scene perception and sentence processing. It is a transient memory (subject to rapid decay). Visual stimulus (e.g. a sentence/a picture) reaches CSTM. Although CSTM holds considerable material, the latter is rapidly lost unless it is relevant to a conceptual structure (past images/representations) consolidated in LTM. Experiments show that words spoken at a fast rate enter CSTM but not conventional STM. CSTM is considered to be the basis for encoding information in LTM, or is viewed as an activated part (a subset) of LTM.

Long-term working memory (LTWM): LTWM is activated when future memory demands are anticipated. It becomes useful for skilled activity and storage of information relevant to the task to be performed. Comprehension of reading material is stored in LTWM. Experimenters suggest that superior text comprehension is due to increased ability to encode information in LTWM, making it accessible via cues in short-term working memory. Moreover, previous input is kept accessible in LTWM. This allows new knowledge to be encoded and integrated with previous one.

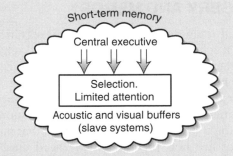

Fig. 14.5 The central executive is an attentional control system: it selects and integrates information from various sources.

ASSOCIATIVE MEMORY

The process of learning is associated with our ability to make associations with knowledge stored in LTM and STM. Associative memory is a fundamental cognitive process (Salthouse 1995). In addition, associative learning, which is memory-dependent, relies on the ability to be vigilant and alert to environmental stimuli. Sustained attention has a major role in daily activities (Tomporowski & Tinsley 1996).

When presented with a task, individuals quickly search their memory stores for the best approach to tackle the problem. In other words, people rely on past experience and knowledge. This searching is similar to opening a file cabinet to access specific file(s) (e.g. procedures, policies, memos, messages) *associated* with the task to be performed. However, distraction can disrupt one's attention, while one is making associations. For instance, as the file cabinet is opened, someone enters the office and says that our attention is needed urgently. Cognitive processes are temporarily disturbed. When the person returns to the task of making associations by using memory skills – they will probably use the familiar words 'Now where was I?'.

Higher mental functions, according to Gross (1992), such as cognition (thinking, reasoning, learning, memory and perception), are closely linked to the 'association cortex' in the brain. It can be argued hence that ageing and pathology of the brain can cause memory impairment.

IMAGERY AND MEMORY

Mental imagery is of psychological significance since it relates to learning, retention and retrieval of material from memory. Complex images consist of conceptual structures (a framework with many attributes, ideas and their representations) with memory as their foundation (Saariluoma & Kalakoski 1997). It is also pointed out that mental images are not 'pictures in the head' and that perception has a role in the creation of mental images, although research is lacking to prove the extent of this role.

Without memory, a human's conceptual system will not produce imaging. People formulate images from the vast store of concepts accumulated from life experience, residing in memory. Dopkins (1996) claimed that a number of

research findings have shown the role of imagery in memory for propositional knowledge. The latter applies to language understanding: the meaning that people associate with particular sentences, statements/assertions. Moreover, Saariluoma and Kalakoski (1997) wrote that experiments show a relationship between memory and conceptual aspects of mental images such as in skill acquisition. The more skilled a person is, the better developed will be this conceptual framework, and the more elaborated and integrated will be the images. 'Skilled imagery' (mental images of skills learned stored in long-term working memory) – as it is called – relies on the activation of LTWM.

In an experiment in which chess players were blindfolded, mental imagery and visual memory were depended upon to play the game (Saariluoma & Kalakoski 1997). The researcher showed that experienced players are speedier at retrieving knowledge from LTM (because expert players use their vast stores of pre-learned chunks). They construct complex images, keeping them in memory, while updating knowledge as needed (Saariluoma & Kalakoski 1997), highlighting the fact that LTWM and skilled imagery are associated structures.

Activity 14.2

Think of a skill you have; how complex is it? Write down how your past knowledge and experience help you to carry out a task efficiently.

??? Question 14.2

How would you describe imagery and memory using a diagram?

AUTOBIOGRAPHICAL MEMORIES

Autobiographical memory may be defined as the recall of personal experience (Atkinson et al 1993). It is a particular memory style with diverse features, such as childhood memories, emotional memories, painful experiences, smells and dreams (Sehulster 1995). Because autobiographical memory is a subjective experience, divergent recollections of events are expected (Ross et al 1998). Such memories, which are internally generated experiences, are more thought-oriented or constructively imagined, i.e. fantasy construction (McGinnis & Roberts 1996).

Autobiographic memory accounts for the experience history of a person. Some people claim to have superior autobiographic memory, i.e. that they can remember events long forgotten by others. It is also argued that these people have frequent dreams with a strong emotional content. From a phenomenology perspective (according to the person's lived experience), their memory experiences are rated more intensely. This memory style is also associated with a personality affined to intense emotional relationships. Sehulster (1995) believed that such individuals have a propensity to report intense private experiences. Other additional features, according to Sehulster, are:

1. people with autobiographic memory believe they are aesthetically sensitive (they like music, dancing, painting, films and other arts)
2. as music is emotionally arousing, they may point out that it is an important aspect of their lives
3. from a cognitive perspective, such individuals may possess a 'unique cognitive "space"' for processing and remembering their 'emotional and experiential material'.

Research findings indicate, however, that memories attributed to imagined childhood talked about, with uncertain reality characteristics, are less clear and less intense than memories linked to a previous *external* (objective) event (McGinnis & Roberts 1996). The memory of an experience is considered plausible when its content has distinct 'sensory and contextual attributes' corresponding to the reality of an event.

Autobiographic memory accounts may not be accurate, and are considered to be questionable when the details are unclear and the descriptions are mainly cognitive-based, i.e. lacking in sensory details and emotional intensity. Some experiments have been conducted (Ross et al 1998) to assess the accuracy of autobiographical memories. The findings are relevant to the criminal justice system. Additionally, professionals in health care practice need accurate information from their clients to make clear clinical decisions.

It is a challenging task for investigators and diagnosticians to detect the plausibility of event recollections when conflicting accounts exist. Recollections of events one has personally experienced are prone to diverge from earlier perceptions, Ross et al (1998) postulated. The reason could be due to information decay as time lapses, or to changes in beliefs that accompany changes in recall or decreased importance.

In view of conventional beliefs that autobiographic accounts can change over time and are prone to conflicting recollections, researchers have attempted to assess their validity and reliability by using varied strategies:

1. assessing the coherence and intuitive consistency of the events, and how convincing the descriptions are
2. external consistency: seeking other people's accounts of similar events
3. evaluating the content according to one's own knowledge and experience, by looking for normative behaviour (i.e. do people normally behave like this in such situations?)
4. assessing behavioural consistency: is the story teller's action/account plausible (i.e. consistent with their personality traits, intentions, motives)?

Ross et al discovered from experiments that autobiographic recollection tellers are liable to perceive their own account as accurate, in spite of divergent versions. Further, people may be inclined to convince others of the truth of their memories, to receive public acceptance. It is also human nature to avoid being seen as a liar. The understanding is hence, the more one adheres to one's own initial account of events, the less likely one is going to be judged as being deceptive.

Activity 14.3

Attempt to recall your childhood experiences at school. Can you list any varied recollection of sensory images?

???   ### Question 14.3

How useful is it to professionals to have an awareness of autobiographical memory theories?

FALSE MEMORIES SYNDROME

False memories may be defined as the recollection of events from the past which never occurred; they are considered false because the accounts have been imagined or uncertain. It is a controversial subject matter, particularly in cases of child sexual abuse (CSA). Some writers have provided alternative arguments on the topic. Hodgson (1995) posed the question whether memories of CSA are false or repressed; Trevelyan (1995) believed there was evidence of widespread CSA. Reports from clients undergoing counselling (Case example 14.1) point to the possibility that memories could be dictated

Case example 14.1 Dictated memories

'Helen is a professional, middle-aged woman. In 1992 she was advised to seek counselling to help her husband cope with post-traumatic stress disorder. She was referred to a community psychiatric nurse.

Helen expected a few brief sessions. She had no idea that she was about to embark on something at least as traumatic as her husband's experience.

The psychiatric nurse started to probe into Helen's childhood during the sessions. Using a mixture of direct questions and insinuations, he took her back into memories of her early childhood until he eventually made her 'recall' being abused by a friend of her brother at the age of seven.

Helen says she was never hypnotized. But she believes she was put into a heightened state, which allowed the CPN virtually to dictate her memories to her' (Hodgson 1995).

(Hodgson 1995) or implanted. Alternative argument alludes to the belief that recovered memories are possible representations of past traumatic experiences (Farrants 1998), or that poor psychotherapeutic technique could influence suggestible clients to believe that they did experience trauma in the past. Toon (1995) argued that CSA is widespread and a huge body of evidence supports the notion that false memories syndrome is unrelated.

However, in the USA, one extreme position is adopted by a movement named the False Memory Syndrome Foundation (FMSF), to treat any assertions of past childhood trauma as 'false memories' unless 'they meet legal criteria for rules of evidence' (Hall & Kondora 1997). The same group has attempted to exert pressures on health care organizations to view 'false memories' as a psychiatric diagnosis.

Negative views on false memories syndrome could undermine sensitive recognition of genuine memories of past trauma. From a professional viewpoint, the expertise of practitioners may be questioned, causing doubt as to their credibility. In addition, the traumatized person may delay seeking counselling or fail to comply with therapeutic regimen, due to disbelief in the authority of the caregiver. It is clear, from a psychoanalytic perspective, that genuine past traumatic experiences can be repressed. Hall and Kondora (1997) make allusion to the 'amputation of terrorizing experiences from awareness'. However, such feelings may resurface in adulthood when the individual confronts events reminiscent of childhood encounters.

Proponents of false memories syndrome, Farrants (1998) pointed out, explain that abusive situations can be constructed or fictionalized by adults from exposure to media coverage of child abuse. They have a 'pre-existing script' for common events; however, young children may not possess such a script. Should their account of traumatic events be given more credibility?

The issue nevertheless is how to prevent the implantation of false memories. Other real issues concern an attitude change towards victims accused of fabricating memories. To those who have memories diagnosed as false, they face the problem of how to cope with feelings that their memories could be true. They therefore have a need for emotional support; professional counselling is recommended. They should be encouraged to talk freely about their subjective experiences. As insight is gained into their cognitive processes, other pertinent personal issues may be revealed, allowing professionals to seek specialist help if needed. The act of remembering should not be discouraged; on the contrary, active reminiscing, concurrent with clients' wishes, should be allowed. Hall and Kondora (1997) emphasized the healing powers of remembering; they saw it as an empowering phenomenon. McCourt (1994), on the other hand, explains that the process of reviewing life and perhaps of coming to terms with the past has a positive psychological value.

Professionals use their clinical expertise and judgement, as each client's needs differ. Some people may decide to continue repressing aspects of memories they find too personal and traumatic to reveal; forgetting, in this context, becomes a therapeutic tool. In other cases, repression can be damaging to health. Hall and Kondora explained how unresolved mental conflict can cause bodily changes; a process described as somatization; the displacement of past trauma from conscious awareness, and channeled into a specific body area. Trevelyan (1995) made reference to the theory that emotional problems stored in memory can cause physical ills, manifested in body tension.

AGEING AND MEMORY

It is widely accepted that ageing causes not only physical changes but intellectual alterations as well. Forgetfulness is common in old age. In particular, evidence shows that as one ages, STM capacity reduces accordingly, while LTM remains relatively unchanged. The older adult's readiness to engage in recalling events from many years ago is familiar. Conversely, there are occasions when an older person's memory for recent events, such as remembering what they had for breakfast, shows their fallibility.

Some writers on ageing (Goor et al 1995) have established a link between cobalamin deficiency

and mental impairment in old age. The deficiency is caused by malabsorption of the protein due to intrinsic factor deficiency, thus showing low serum level on examination. It is argued that the resulting altered mental status circumscribes memory impairment, reduced attention span and learning skills. Cobalamin replacement therapy may help reduce cognitive decline if initiated within 6 months of onset (Goor et al 1995).

It is important to be aware that memory impairment can sometimes be caused by drug therapy. As the older person is prone to having multiple pathology (polypharmacy is therefore common), some of their medications could affect their memory. For example in the early 1990s, the drug triazolam (to treat insomnia) was found to cause impaired memory (Community File 1991).

Vascular changes due to arteriosclerosis are common in old age; reduced blood supply to the brain can affect cognition. Intellectual changes may be accompanied by behavioural problems: confusion, agitation, aggression. It is difficult to assess whether forgetfulness is due to reduced cognitive skills – a consequence of healthy ageing – or the insidious onset of cerebral pathology.

Older adults count on wisdom and experience when undertaking tasks. As their life experiences are extensive, it is anticipated that their LTM store will contain a vast amount of knowledge. Retrieval can, however, be slow for this reason. Others theorize that the effects of ageing affect cognitive function, which can impede retrieval from skill memory, due to fewer recollective experiences and a failure to encode material (Perfect & Dasgupta 1997). This may explain why older people take longer when carrying out a task.

Learning in old age, which is memory-dependent, is not impeded unless some organic dysfunction is present. There is evidence of people doing degree courses and learning foreign languages successfully in their 80s. Although they make take longer than a younger person to achieve their ambition, their success proves that memory remains active in old age. Motivational factors may explain this technical ability.

Problem-solving skills and intellectual attainment in early years may facilitate memory performance in later years. In fact, some researchers have argued that the degree of cognitive decline in old age might be dependent upon the amount of education in the early critical periods (Lyketsos et al 1999a). A good formal education of at least 8 years, they argued, could bestow some protection against decline. Stuart-Hamilton (1994) suggests that socio-economic and educational background are possible determinants of intellectual performance. On the other hand, memory fallibility may be attributed to central nervous system failure in information processing.

AMNESIA

Amnesia can be caused by drugs. Anterograde amnesia (STM impairment present in blackouts) has been linked to triazolam (Community File 1991, Lehne & Scott 1996). If patients complain of forgetfulness, an evaluation of drug therapy should be done. Other causes of amnesia are:

1. **Alcohol-induced**: prolonged heavy drinking causes brain damage, a pathology described as Korsakoff's syndrome, which worsens when alcohol consumption is coupled with malnutrition and thiamine deficiency (Austin 1995).
2. **Brain lesions**.
3. **Viral encephalitis**.
4. **Acute traumatic episode** causing hysterical amnesia (Wakeham & Barre 1988) (Case example 14.2). There are different types of amnesia (Stafford 1996) (Box 14.3).

Stafford (1996) pointed out that in alcoholic abuse some severe features are found. The person affected may 'confabulate responses' to questions, in order to camouflage memory gaps.

Patients who have amnesia need a safe and supportive environment. This encompasses physical and psychological safety. Therapeutic interpersonal relationships must be developed gradually. It can be frustrating for both client and therapist to establish a rapport in the early stages. The reduction of anxiety is necessary, as the client will be better able to cooperate with care providers. Signs of depression must be identified and antidepressant medications may be administered if required. While drug therapy is useful,

Case example 14.2 Hysterical amnesia

Peter's case is a modern example of someone whose accumulated problems became apparently too traumatic to cope with on a conscious level.

Peter came to the ward from the accident and emergency department, accompanied by his GP and a neighbour; he was exhibiting confusional state and gross memory loss. Although middle-aged, Peter insisted he was 7 years old, talked as if World War II was still in progress (he could hear the sound of 'doodlebugs' above) and displayed no awareness of where he was or how he got there. Although he seemed to be profoundly disoriented in time, place and person, he was alert, able to communicate and his level of consciousness seemed unimpaired.

Despite being surprised when he was told the present year and date, Peter did not seem overtly distressed or upset, rather demonstrating a childlike wonder at the news.

He showed no recognition of his neighbour and gave an address which was that of his childhood home (Wakeham & Barre 1988).

Box 14.3 Classifications of amnesia

- **Localized**: a common type of amnesia. The person is unable to remember events for a short time – a few hours to a few days.
- **Global**: a rare type. When it occurs there is complete memory loss of a whole lifetime and experience.
- **Selective**: inability to recall some events for a short time. The person may remember coming to hospital, but not what happened during his stay.
- **Anterograde**: short-term memory impairment – occurs in alcohol abuse.
- **Retrograde**: a failure to recall past events that occurred before the onset of the amnesia-producing events.

the causes of depression must be sought. Spending time to listen to the client's version of events may provide insight into the source of amnesia. As the causes are varied, individual differences in responses to therapy are to be expected. Therapy should be tailored according to each client's special needs.

MEMORY DISORDERS

Memory disorders constitute some of the cognitive impairment processes allied with brain

Activity 14.4

Make a list of the possible complications the amnesic person may experience in relation to social and psychological factors.

??? Question 14.4

1. How should the care professional assess the needs of the amnesic client?
2. Should relatives be included in the assessment procedure?

physiology alterations and pathology. Disordered memory is equally connected with personality change and learning reduction. Intellectual weakening therefore incapacitates the person: participation in activities of daily living becomes a major challenge. In this section, a common condition known as dementia is described.

Dementia

Dementia is characterized by a progressive intellectual deterioration. There are different types of dementia (Box 14.4). During the early stages of the disease, the person begins to experience forgetfulness and the realization that something is wrong (Robinson et al 1997). The sufferer subsequently attempts to seek meaning for the changes, while making efforts to conceal the

---

Box 14.4 Types of dementia

- **Alzheimer's disease (AD):** the Alzheimer's Disease Society sees AD as the commonest form of dementia, responsible for about half to two-thirds of all cases
- **Multi-infarct dementia (vascular dementia):** a type of dementia caused by reduced vascularity to tiny areas of the brain, leading to death of nervous tissues
- **Creutzfeldt-Jacob disease (CJD):** a rapidly progressing form of dementia caused by viruses. Inoculation with infected tissue is linked to the disease.
- **Alcoholic dementia:** chronic heavy drinking can cause damage to the brain
- **Lewy body dementia:** impairment of the brain parietal lobe caused by neural cell changes.

---

deterioration from significant others. Azuma and Bayles (1997) point out that a striking feature of dementia is the insidious memory impairment. This deficit, they explain, reduces the client's ability to communicate and understand language.

While the features outlined in Box 14.4 are common presentations, the presence of mood disturbance is also consistent with mild dementia (Valentine et al 1998). Feelings of depression can heighten cognitive sluggishness and affect memory integrity. In addition, researchers have discovered that depression is very often present with physically aggressive behaviour (Lyketsos et al 1999b). Caregivers are at the forefront of the sufferer's anger, and are prone to mental distress. The progressive deterioration in memory, intellectual function and adaptive ability (O'Brien 1994) becomes a challenge to the client's families' and professionals' caring skills. From the patient's perspective, in the early stage of dementia, feelings of insecurity and uncertainty are prominent (Phinney 1998). They have a need to maintain normal social activities and to control the disease process. They have an awareness of their failings initially: their inability to remember ordinary events, their disorientation and communication problems (Phinney 1998).

The chronic nature of dementia means that the sufferers and their families will be regular service users. Services in the community should be deployed to ensure that carers receive adequate support to undertake the task of caring, including respite care to allow carers time to recuperate. Community mental health workers need to liaise with other agencies to ensure that care programmes and evaluation reports are disseminated widely to prevent fragmentation of services.

The impairment in STM and LTM (Arnold 1996a), a common feature in dementia, disables the person. There is evidence that personal hygiene suffers, and clients often need constant reminders to wash and dress. Global decline in cortical functioning, it is believed (Arnold 1996a), affects not only cognitive control, but bodily functions too. Although the level of consciousness is not affected in dementia (Breitner & Welsh 1995), informal and professional carers have difficulties in developing the client's responsibility for basic self-care. Significant personality changes distress families as they watch their loved ones deteriorate.

The combination of communication problems, loss of judgement, agitation and aggressive behaviours frustrate carers and increase their feelings of helplessness. Global memory loss (Arnold 1996a) and global changes in cognition and other capacities (Breitner & Welsh 1995) accentuate the client's vulnerability towards self-harm.

There are several principles professionals utilize in dementia care (Box 14.5).

MEMORY FACILITATION

To the individual on the verge of memory loss, intense feelings of anxiety and depression are debilitating. Attempts to self-restore memory capacity become futile as cognitive deficits worsen; a professional input to memory facilitation is then required.

Latest research findings from the Alzheimer's Disease Society show the beneficial effects of art therapy in people with dementia (Open Mind 1999). Art therapy lowers depression and makes the client more alert, an important feature in memory facilitation. Control of depression increases a client's cooperation in working with professionals and carers who aim to reduce memory deficits.

Pharmacological treatment is also recommended in memory facilitation. In the past, reliance on drug treatment, at the expense of a person-centred approach to care, was criticized. The new culture of dementia care has somehow displaced the value of medication in alleviating symptoms (Norman 1998). Advances in pharmacological treatment (e.g. memory-enhancing medications) for dementia are often not acknowledged by nurses (Norman 1998). The culture has shifted from overmedication to reduced drug therapy; the ideal position is to balance the two extremes, with drug therapy as an ally of person-

---

Box 14.5 Principles of care

Personhood: Although personality changes cause behavioural problems, the client should be treated with dignity and respect. Privacy is paramount, and the preservation of identity and individuality must be maintained. This is a clear departure from a biomedical focus of the past. As the effects of the disease differ from one person to another, so the care is adapted accordingly (Phair 1996a). Some clients may show occasional insight into their conditions, particularly in the initial phase, arousing fears about the future; others may be oblivious. A person-centred approach is a requisite to preserve dignity (Norman 1998). Using the client's name during interactions, for example, is an acknowledgement of their individuality.

Phair (1996b) wrote that the new culture of dementia care has contributed to protecting the client from impersonal intervention. As clients have personal beliefs, interests and existing abilities, full recognition has to be given. Their subjective experience needs attention; people with memory disorders have a need to discuss their fears and feelings to professional carers (Willis 1996). In the early phase of dementia, the client's need for non-informal support must be anticipated (Bennett et al 1997).

Informed care: Clients and their carers must be kept informed. Failure to communicate with them regarding their right to access pertinent community services will lead to disempowerment. As home care is at the heart of community care, a variety of services should be mobilized

to achieve this goal. Support groups are resources to be utilized. Educational programmes for both carers and carees can develop insight of the disease process, and facilitate problem-solving skills.

Needs assessment: The identification and treatment of depression in dementia patients is recommended. Armstrong (1997) points out that depression is prevalent among people with dementia. Inability to carry out activities of daily living is associated with being depressed, and may lead to aggression (Lyketsos et al 1999b). The researchers point out that aggression occurs during caregiving situations, and suggest that an evaluation of the technique used by carers should be done to identify shortcomings. Further, other pathology may be present instigating violent behaviour (e.g. urinary tract infections), or the excessive use of medications.

Blood pressure (BP) assessment is indicated. Some research findings have begun to establish a complex relationship between BP and cognition (Glynn et al 1999). It is posited that as BP elevates, decline in cognition is possible. This mechanism may, however, be due to other variables requiring further investigations.

The assessment of cognition demands a thorough knowledge of age-related changes (Dellasega 1998). Moreover, empathetic communication is essential. Observing their non-verbal messages is a requirement as clients can quickly become tired during the procedure. Short periods of interactions are hence necessary.

centred therapy. Norman (1998) asserts the use of medication as 'consistent with a person-centred approach to dementia care'.

Medications to improve memory and cognition are available (Norman 1998). Improving memory skills reduces primary symptoms, such as language, attention, orientation and knowledge problems. The aim is to enhance functional abilities, so that the sufferer can exercise better control over activities of daily living. The drug Aricept (Box 14.6), introduced in 1997 to treat mild to moderate symptoms of Alzheimer's disease (Packer 1998), reduces cognitive decline. Noticeable improvement in the level of alertness and verbal fluency has been observed, Packer pointed out.

Box 14.6 Aricept

In about 40% of patients, Aricept may slow the rate of cognitive and non-cognitive deterioration. It is used for the symptomatic treatment of mild to moderate dementia in Alzheimer's disease.

Dose 5 mg once daily at bedtime. Can be increased after 1 month to 10 mg daily; maximum 10 mg daily. Side-effects: nausea, vomiting, insomnia, fatigue, muscle cramps, diarrhoea (British National Formulary 36 1998).

By slowing the rate of decline, medications provide clients and carers with opportunities to discuss present and future needs; for example, the direction the treatment will take, planning for future personal needs: finance, insurance, making a will, pensions, personal preferences regarding care provision and so on. Sensitive communication is essential, as is an empathetic attitude. Fitzgerald and Parkes (1998) explained that patients with progressive cognitive loss are sensitive, and are often aware of their mental ability deficiency. Staff who are tactless, by reminding clients of their memory deficits, can trigger explosive reactions.

MEMORY CLINICS

Memory clinics are becoming popular settings to enhance the care of people with Alzheimer's disease (Payne 1998). The philosophy of memory clinics is to promote the skills of nurses and other care professionals in delivering care to empower clients and their carers.

A knowledge of psychology is relevant. An awareness of cognitive functioning supported with psychological theories is necessary, as clinic nurses have the complex task of carrying out 'cognitive assessment'. In fact, Wilkinson (1997) felt that an understanding of the conceptual framework of memory will aid nursing practice. He posited that memory can be aided by effective communication skills. Clients have a need to access information unambiguously. Clear and concise language to address sensory difficulties and cognition problems can facilitate the input of messages.

The need for clear information applies to carers as well, who rely on professional guidelines to participate in memory-enhancing activities; one such activity is reality orientation, known to alleviate memory difficulties (Allen & Brown 1996). This approach may consist of using memory aids: clocks, calenders, notice boards, posters etc., known as external memory aids.

Memory aid groups are useful for participants. Coping skills are discussed and stress-related factors associated with memory difficulties are identified. The sharing of experiences widens the knowledge base of participants, as alternative strategies are learned to be applied in home settings.

Memory clinic staff are responsible in encouraging the use of different memory aid strategies; e.g. 'internal memory' methods: mnemonics (using visual imagery and method of loci). Psychologists, such as Atkinson et al (1993), describe mnemonics as the skill to memorize items (e.g. bread, egg etc.) by linking and visualizing them to be in specific locations, e.g. a slice of bread nailed to the door, an egg dangling from the ceiling.

While the utilization of varied methods to ease memory difficulties is encouraged, some clients may not be able to control their cognition to achieve the required results. Patience and perseverance must be exercised, as progress may be laboured. The client must be made to feel valued, and positive reinforcement for small successes given. As memory deficits arouse clients' concerns (Cromwell 1998), learning can become impaired. It is hence necessary to prevent unnecessary anxiety by providing continuing support and encouragement.

REMINISCENCE GROUPS

Reminiscing is the act of recollecting past memories. Reminiscing has an affective component that distinguishes it from the recalling of historical facts (McCourt 1994). It is a therapeutic activity: the person who is reminiscing may choose to select from memory events with a pleasurable impact on the senses. However, it is known for many people to recall negative events too: war, famine and destruction. For example, in the late 1990s regular television programmes focus on natural disasters across the world: tornadoes, earthquakes, floods and hurricanes; on these programmes people reminisce their bad experiences.

Although such events are negative in nature, positive benefits can be reaped for the person reminiscing. It allows the uncovering of repressed emotions, which when shared and compared with similar experiences from group members, permits the individual to come to terms with past adversity and to be perceived as a survivor. The revisiting of past trauma through life review permits the person to reframe the experience in a positive way (Arnold 1996b). The older person, Arnold surmised, prefers groups that focus on past events rather than current ones.

Armstrong (1999) described the positive outcomes of a reminiscence project to help enhance communication among people with dementia. Group members were invited to bring mementos as retrieval cues (e.g. photographs, slides, audio tapes). Some clients may respond to these triggers with expressions of sadness, anxiety, depression or happiness. When distress becomes overpowering, McCourt (1994) suggests seeking the expertise of a counsellor, following informed consent. Equally important, the client should be made to feel valued, and any contribution acknowledged.

To the facilitator of reminiscence groups, individual reactions indicate that reminiscing can be a worrying and disturbing process (Coleman 1993). Once disturbing materials have been recovered, reminiscing should be redirected to focus on positive memories. It is important for the person concerned to terminate on a positive note.

The advantage of group reminiscing lies in fostering social interactions; knowledge and experience are shared. Moreover, older people and their carers learn to view each other as individuals with unique life experiences (McCourt 1994), reducing social isolation and anxiety, and elevating self-esteem (Armstrong 1999). McDougall and Balyer (1998) recommended that, when assessing clients, issues related to depression and self-confidence in their ability should be examined before initiating memory enhancement treatment programmes.

Activity 14.5

1. List the advantages of reminiscence therapy.
2. In small groups of 4–6 talk about some past events that were meaningful to you. Write down your thoughts and feelings after the group work.
3. Read Armstrong's (1999) article: identify the methods used in the project and describe the benefits gained by the participants.

??? **Question 14.5**

1. How important is it to recall past memories?
2. What steps would you take in organizing a reminiscence group?

SUMMARY

Memory is a complex concept in psychology. An analysis of its nature reveals that memory formation is dependent on the integrity of neural structures and healthy physiology. Scientists have discovered that training, knowledge and experience impact on specific areas of the brain, increasing cell sizes.

Memory is conventionally divided into short-term memory (STM) and long-term memory (LTM). It is believed that these two systems operate concurrently. LTM has a vast store of information; STM holds material temporarily: some is discarded, while other items are transferred to LTM after a rehearsal mechanism.

There are, however, additional memory systems:

- a **working memory** (STM as an active rather than a passive system)
- a **conceptual short-term memory** (CSTM), which is concerned with everyday reading, scene perception and sentence processing. This system is prone to rapid decay

- a **long-term working memory** (LTWM), which is useful for skilled activity and is activated when future memory demands are anticipated.

Memory disorders affect communication and learning. Individuals who suffer from dementia show signs of cognitive decline, which they find distressing. Depression is often present in dementia. People with memory problems and other cognitive impairment due to dementia can be supported with medications and a person-centred care approach.

GLOSSARY

Acetylcholinesterase   an enzyme found in the grey matter of nervous tissue, in red blood cells and in skeletal muscle

Arteriosclerosis   degenerative changes in arteries causing thickening and hardening, with loss of elasticity

Dissociative disorders   the fragmentation of consciousness, when memory and other cognitive functions become impaired

Experiential material   knowledge gained from personal experience and practice

Intrinsic factor   a chemical substance (enzyme) secreted within an organ necessary to stimulate a result or change (e.g. for the satisfactory absorption of vitamin B$_{12}$)

Method of loci   a method in psychology used to aid memory by focusing images of concepts to be remembered on specific objects and situations

Opioid antagonists   an agent that opposes the action of narcotics on the nervous system

Polypharmacy   a person who is on many medications

Pre-learned chunks   a group of items (categorized and classified) that has been learned previously

Synaptic junctions (neural junctions)   the site between neurons at which an impulse is transmitted from one neuron to another by either electrical or chemical means

Viral encephalitis   inflammation of the brain by a virus

REFERENCES

Allen C, Brown N 1996 G-P based memory aid group benefits clients and carers. Nursing Times 92(40): 42–44

Armstrong M 1997 Dementia: supporting the patient and the carer. Nursing Times 93(32): 44–45

Armstrong M 1999 Remembering yesterday, caring today. Elderly Care 11(1): 18–20

Arnold E N 1996a The journey clouded by cognitive disorders. In: Carson V B, Arnold E N (eds) Mental health nursing. W B Saunders, Philadelphia, p 977

Arnold E N 1996b Group psychotherapy. In: Carson V B, Arnold E N (eds) Mental health nursing. W B Saunders, Philadelphia, p 385–420

Atkinson R L, Atkinson R C, Smith E et al 1993 Introduction to psychology, 11th edn. Harcourt Brace Jovanovich, Fort Worth

Austin N 1995 Memory information and meaning. In: Messer D, Meldrum C (eds:) Psychology for nurses and healthcare professionals. Prentice Hall, London, p 157

Azuma T, Bayles K A 1997 Memory impairments underlying language difficulties in dementia. Topics in Language Disorders 18(1): 58–71

Bennett A, Jones B, Murphy M, Riordan J 1997 Informed care. Nursing Times 93(24): 30–31

Breitner J C, Welsh K A 1995 Diagnosis and management of memory loss and cognitive disorders among elderly persons. Psychiatric Services 46(1): 29–35

British National Fomulary 36 1998 Aricept 4.11. Royal Pharmaceutical Society and British Medical Association, London, p 232

Cohen G 1990 Memory. In: Roth I (ed) Introduction to psychology. Open University Press, Milton Keynes, vol 2, p 571–620

Coleman P 1993 Adjustment in later life. In: Bond J, Coleman P, Peace S (eds) Ageing in society. Sage, London, p 106

Community File 1991 Memory impairment associated with triazolam. Professional Nurse 6(9): 542

Cromwell S L 1998 Development and testing the elder concerns about memory scale. Archives of Psychiatric Nursing 12(3): 148–153

Dellasega C 1998 Assessment of cognition in the elderly. Nursing Clinics of North America 33(3): 395–405

Dopkins S 1996 The role of imagery in the mental representation of negative sentences. American Journal of Psychology 109(4): 551–565

Dye C A 1989 Memory and aging: a nursing responsibility. Recent Advances in Nursing 23: 53–65

Eysenck M 1996 Simply psychology. Psychology Press, Hove

Farrants J 1998 The 'false memory' debate: a critical review of the research on recovered memories of child sexual abuse. Counselling Psychology Quarterly 11(3): 229–238

Fitzgerald R G, Parkes C M 1998 Blindness and loss of other sensory and cognitive functions. British Medical Journal 316(7138): 1160–1163

Glynn R G, Beckett L A, Hebert L E et al 1999 Current and remote blood pressure and cognitive decline. JAMA 281(5): 438–444

Goor L P, Woiski M D, Lagaay A M et al 1995 Review: cobalamin deficiency and mental impairment in elderly people. Age and Ageing 24(6): 536–542

Gross R D 1992 Psychology: the science of mind and behaviour, 2nd edn. Hodder & Stoughton, London, p 89

Hall J M, Kondora L L 1997 Beyond 'true' and 'false' memories: remembering and recovery in the survival of childhood sexual abuse. Advance Nursing Science 19(4): 37–54

Healy A F, McNamara D S 1996 Verbal learning and memory: does the modal model still work? Annual Review of Psychology 47: 143–172

Hodgson J 1995 The making of memories? Nursing Standard 9(43): 22–24

Lehne R A, Scott D 1996 Psychopharmacology. In: Carson V B, Arnold E N (eds) Mental health nursing. W B Saunders, Philadelphia, p 551

Lyketsos C G, Chen L, Anthony J C 1999a Cognitive decline in adulthood: an 11.5 year follow-up of the Baltimore epidemiologic catchment area study. American Journal of Psychiatry 156(1): 58–64

Lyketsos C G, Steel C, Galik G, Rosenblatt A et al 1999b Physical aggression in dementia patients and its relationship to depression. American Journal of Psychiatry 156(1): 66–70

McCourt V 1994 Cherish the memory. Nursing Times 90(29): 63–64

McDougall G, Balyer J 1998 Decreasing mental frailty in at-risk elders. Geriatric Nursing American Journal of Care for the Aging 19(4): 220–224

McGinnis D, Roberts P 1996 Qualitative characteristics of vivid memories attributed to real and imagined experiences. American Journal of Psychology 109(1): 59–77

Mann T, Brenner L A 1996 Improving text memory by organising text at retrieval. American Journal of Psychology 109(4): 539–549

Norman I 1998 Treating dementia. Elderly Care 10(1): 13–16

O'Brien M E 1994 The dementia syndromes: distinguishing their clinical differences. Postgraduate Medicine 95(5): 91–93

Open Mind 1999 News digest: art therapy benefits dementia sufferers. Open Mind 95: 5

Packer T 1998 Rationing. Elderly Care 10(1): 16–17

Payne D 1998 Memories are made of this. Nursing Times 94(24): 17

Perfect T J, Dasgupta C K 1997 What underlies the deficit in reported recollective experience in old age? Memory and Cognition 25(6): 849–858

Phair L 1996a Dementia: knowledge for practice. Nursing Times 92(24): 1–4

Phair L 1996b Dementia: the role of the nurse. Nursing Times 92(25): 5–7

Phinney H 1998 Living with dementia: from the patient's perspective. Journal of Gerontological Nursing 24(6): 8–15

Robinson P, Ekman S, Meleis A I et al 1997 Suffering in silence: the experience of early memory loss. Health Care in Later Life 2(2): 107–120

Rosenzweig M R 1996 Aspects of the search for neural mechanisms of memory. Annual Review of Psychology 47: 1–32

Ross M, Buehler R, Karr J W 1998 Assessing the accuracy of conflicting autobiographical memories. Memory and Cognition 26(6): 1233–1244

Saariluoma P, Kalakoski V 1997 Skilled imagery and long-term memory. American Journal of Psychology 110(2): 177–201

Salthouse T A 1995 Selective influences of age and speed on associative memory. American Journal of Psychology 108(3): 381–396

Sehulster J R 1995 Memory styles and related abilities in presentation of self. American Journal of Psychology 108(1): 67–88

Stafford L 1996 The journey compartmentalized by dissociative disorders. In: Carson V B, Arnold E N (eds) Mental health nursing. W B Saunders, Philadelphia, p 866

Stuart-Hamilton I 1994 The psychology of ageing, 2nd edn. Jessica Kingsley, London

Tomporowski P D, Tinsley V F 1996 Effects of memory demand and motivation on sustained attention in young and older adults. American Journal of Psychology 109(2): 187–204

Toon K 1995 False ideas about syndrome. Nursing Times 91(18): 23

Trevelyan J 1995 The uncharted mind. Nursing Times 91(14): 44–45

Valentine A D, Meyers C A, Kling M A et al 1998 Mood and cognitive side-effects of interferon-alpha therapy. Seminars in Oncology 25(Suppl 1): 39–47

Wakeham A, Barre T 1988 Escaping from the past. Nursing Times 84(46): 52–54

Wilkinson J 1997 Understanding memory to enhance nursing practice. British Journal of Nursing 6(13): 741–744

Willis J 1996 New culture in dementia care. Nursing Times 92(34): 66–68

FURTHER READING

Gold A 1997 Cognitive functions and diabetes. Journal of Dementia Care 5(6): 25

Keady J 1999 Dementia. Elderly Care 11(1): 21–26

Allan K, Killick J 1999 The blind hunter of dementia. Elderly Care 11(1): 30

Adams T 1996 Kitwood's approach to dementia and dementia care: a critical but appreciative review. Journal of Advanced Nursing 23(5): 948–953

Zubenko G S, Winwood E, Jacobs B et al 1999 Prospective study of risk factors for Alzheimer's disease: results at 7.5 years. American Journal of Psychiatry 156(1): 50–55

Communication

We spend all our lives communicating. Communication has many dimensions of relevance to health care professionals. In this chapter we shall consider some of these dimensions. The aim is to:

- discuss issues of importance in a social, psychological and cultural context
- highlight underpinnings of the communication process
- pinpoint the role of professionals in the process of communication
- discuss the functions of effective communication in health care settings
- emphasize the importance of alliances and partnerships within the communication framework.

COMMUNICATION AS A MULTIDIMENSIONAL CONCEPT

A SOCIAL PERSPECTIVE

When people communicate they are performing a social activity; it is through social interactions that people learn social rules. People respond and react to others' verbal and non-verbal signals, and learn overt and covert messages from the language used and the choice of words of the speaker.

The social context of communication is a dimension well recognized by researchers and social scientists. Talking, writing and using signs are ways adopted by humans to transmit thoughts, feelings and moods. Hence, communication is said to possess a psychological component: the choice of words will convey specific messages abour one's affective states, cognitive processes, attitudes, educational background and personal beliefs. In addition, language reflects the socio-cultural context of communication.

When one hears a spoken language – English or French, for example – images are created of the speaker's social origin; a person's accent will also confirm an estimate of such origin. The diversity of languages and accents in one society should be acknowledged. An individual may resort to a definite dialect to communicate in some circumstances; others may attempt to conceal their accents if they feel that the listener may act differently when their native voice is heard. Sociologists have long accepted that there is a difference in the way working-class and middle-class people communicate: the former use a 'restricted code' while the latter speak with an 'elaborated code'. Such use of language has implications for clinical practice (Béphage 1997). It is pointed out, for instance, that nurses must exercise sensitivity when communicating with clients from diverse social class systems. Whether the communication style is restricted or elaborated, important needs are being communicated, and when necessary, an interpreter to decode the information should be sought.

Language and culture

To the communicator, language is not only a vehicle for self-expressions, but also represents social identity. Talking in one's language is comforting. People who are bilingual have recourse to their native language, or mother tongue, when addressing their countrymen. Additionally, Roberts (1994) points out that at times of stress, bilingual individuals prefer to impart information in their foreign language, a common strategy as it is felt that communication takes place more effectively.

Roberts (1994) posits that health professionals can enhance communication skills by being sensitive to clients' style of verbalizing needs.

The quality of the nurse–patient relationship is contingent on language choice and 'language switching'; the latter applies to the utilization of alternative language during interactions, as it is easier to express certain thoughts in one's own native speech.

When bilingual nurses interact with bilingual patients from a similar social background, language switching (Case example 15.1) is common.

Case example 15.1 Language switching (Roberts 1994)

Patient: Sorry
Nurse: Iawn bach (All right dear)
Patient: Oh! its sore
Nurse: Be careful now, byddwch yn ofalus (be careful now, be careful)
Patient: Thanks bach
Nurse: Wedi gorffen bach? (Finished dear?)
Patient: Ydw, wedi gorffen (Yes, finished).

Such an approach reaffirms values and cultural attitudes. Moreover, clients and caregivers 'promote interpersonal and ethnic harmony'. The advantage of this strategy resides in fostering a spirit of mutual understanding. It ensures better cooperation: the clients feel more secure and at ease to talk about their fears.

The language of ethnic minority Asians is an issue medical and nursing literature makes reference to in communication debates (Johnson 1999). It is explained that Asians are not homogeneous groups; they have a diversified culture, religion and there is a multiplicity of linguistic styles and educational experiences. Johnson argued that 'cultural variations' and 'religion' mean that clients' understanding of health and ill-health matters will also be communicated in a variety of ways. While it is recommended that ethnic health workers are recruited to help combat communication problems, their bilingual or multilingual skills may be limited, due to clients' language and cultural diversity.

The task of ascertaining that communication is clear and easily understood becomes even more challenging when the ethnic clients have severe learning disabilities. Chatterton (1998) believed that the communication environment should be evaluated to ensure that interactions with clients who have learning difficulties are productive and empathetic. In a small-scale study of seven *non-ethnic* residents with severe learning difficulties, Chatterton discovered that:

1. a communication workshop for staff:
   a. raised their awareness of non-effective communication
   b. encouraged the development of strategies to be applied in practice
   c. increased the duration of interactions with their clients
2. speech and language therapy empower clients to initiate communication with their care providers
3. after training, care providers responded to clients' needs with more immediacy.

An application of the principles outlined above to ethnic groups with learning disabilities should be considered. As speech and language patterns could be different – even among second-generation ethnic Asian groups – staff should be equipped to deal with language issues. Interpreters, families and health workers with multilingual skills should be involved in the process. Johnson (1999) pointed out, however, that the recruitment of ethnic workers, although pertinent, is not a 'complete solution to issues of communication'.

Occupational culture and language

In a consumer-driven society, it is becoming imperative for organizations to communicate with their clients clearly. Banks, law firms, insurance companies and health care organizations are known for their complex use of words, both written and spoken. It is not surprising that clients become mystified and preoccupied with searching for meanings. In a health care setting, complex communication heightens anxiety.

Some writers (Crawford et al 1995) have commented on the importance professionals attach to the acquisition of technical language. They assert, however, that professional discourse can have inadvertent social functions. Nurses'

language style in practice is influenced by three different cultural sources:

1. a professional language obtained from health training and reading academic textbooks
2. clinical practice socialization: the acquisition of technical jargon from other professionals at work
3. basic language concepts assimilated during primary socialization and the wider Western culture (Crawford et al 1995).

Technical language in clinical practice is either consciously or unconsciously used to demonstrate authoritative knowledge. It is perceived as affirming the position of power, in particular the power of professionals over their patients (Crawford et al 1995). It is interesting to note, for example, in the late 1990s, a plethora of new technical terminologies appearing in the nursing literature (Box 15.1).

Box 15.1 Nursing terminologies

- Clinical effectiveness
- Clinical governance
- Clinical supervision
- Concordance
- Critical care pathways
- Evidence-based practice.

While clients are encouraged to verbalize their needs and problems through language as a therapeutic strategy, the effects of professional language on clients' care have not been investigated (Crawford et al 1995). In fact, Crawford et al (1999) asserted that when language is used 'artlessly', nurses in practice may not be aware of the impact of words on care. A lack of sensitivity in the choice of words can exert a detrimental effect on clients' psychological well-being. Further, the imposition of professional wording on care recipients' description of experiences may not always be a true reflection of the person's bio-psycho-social health status. In some cultures, the spirit world has more significance than religion; consequently, reference to a metaphysical being who communicates personal messages to the believer may be mis-diagnosed as hallucinatory states – one of the features of schizophrenia. Some researchers (Koffman et al 1997) have observed discrepancies in medical notes, which they argued are often incomplete and may be inaccurate in regard to clinical diagnosis. Other observers have noted health clinic physicians' lack of skills to diagnose and treat common mental disorders (anxiety states and depression) (Patel et al 1998).

Imposition of medical labels in these cases took priority over the clients' socio-economic deprivation status, which predisposed to distress and despair. The identification of 'psychopathology' appears to assume greater importance than an identification of social ills, which could be the source of the problem. Crawford et al (1995) suggest health workers show awareness of 'linguistic interaction': the merging of lay knowledge (language style, experiences, narratives) with professional knowledge. An acknowledgement of this process, they assert, will help prevent the pathologization and/or the psychologization of problems that might be founded within a socio-political framework.

There is evidence too that clients' thinking regarding their health status – their subjective states – to be incongruent with their doctors' explanations (Salmon et al 1999). Salmon et al explain that there are two parallel dimensions:

- the lay person's style of communicating information on health status, founded on health beliefs and cultural values
- the medical model of viewing health/illness.

Reconciling the two sets of beliefs can prove difficult for care professionals. Subsequently, Salmon et al found that information-giving from doctors was parsimonious, and any explanations given to clients were interpreted as medical reluctance to encourage self-care management.

When the causes of the clients' complaints could not be proven by investigations, doctors were unable to reassure their clients and were inclined to psychologize the sufferers' problems.

The nomenclature and knowledge of medical conditions may not be infallible, which explains medical professionals' occasional inability to pinpoint accurately the cause of a patient's distress.

To communicate a sense of powerlessness and failure is not professionally desirable. This may explain some of the behavioural characteristics of professionals confronted with somatization disorders (Box 15.2).

Box 15.2 Types of explanations for patients' symptoms given by doctors (Salmon et al 1999)

- **Rejection**: denies reality of symptoms; implies imaginary disorder or stigmatizing psychological problem.
- **Implications**: unresolved explanatory conflict: doctor distrusted with future symptoms.
- **Collusion**: acquiescence by doctor to explanation offered by patient.
- **Implications**: questioning of doctors' openness and competence.

Lack of information can be a reason for a patient's recalcitrant behaviour. Hence, non-compliance may be a safety mechanism for the client who feels that commital to treatment may jeopardize their future health status when communication concerning options available is lacking. Inconsistencies in communication between professionals can compound the problems (Jarman 1995) (Case example 15.2).

Case example 15.2 Communication problems

'When my husband was admitted to hospital he noted inconsistencies between the registrar and the consultant. The registrar would advise one course of action but a day or two later this would be reversed by the consultant …

'The registrar suggested that my husband be transferred to a specialist unit in a teaching hospital in London, which is outside our region … However, when the consultant came back he told my husband that if he did not wish to move he could stay in our local hospital. He did not ask us any questions nor did he ask if we had any' (Jarman 1995).

As well as inconsistencies, communication breakdown occurs when professionals are unable or unwilling (Singleton 1995) to discuss sensitive and emotive care issues with clients' significant others (Case example 15.3).

Case example 15.3 Consultation

'My mother was admitted to hospital for what every-body expected to be a routine cholcystectomy but after two days post-op, the consultant informed us that he was not happy with his findings and had sent the gallbladder for histology.

'The nurses at the hospital were unwilling (or unable) to discuss the findings with me, and I was left to make my own diagnosis when my mother was given MST for her pain' (Singleton 1995).

Communication, Jarman (1995) asserted, is concerned with empathetic listening: the recognition of individual differences in perception of health–ill-health founded in personal knowledge. Language differences and socio-cultural origins are equally important issues to consider. Interpersonal communication among diverse health care professionals is an issue receiving increased attention. A diverse occupational culture predisposes to fragmentation of communication (Milligan et al 1999). Several factors have been identified as barriers to effective communication.

1. The prevention of direct communication through distinct language style.
2. The perennial sociological and occupational issues concerned with power–subservience relationships, between the medical and nursing profession – rooted in past and present professional role conflict.
3. Communication problems perpetuate as professional collaboration widens to include other agencies that utilize their own specific and technical language systems; e.g. biologists, psychologists, sociologists and others communicate contrastingly on similar subjects due to their divergent scientific background.
4. A high-tech competence emphasis at the expense of basic 'hands-on' efficiency.
5. A conflictual arena where social causes of ill-health clash with a bio-medical focus on ill-health issues.

It is evident that the educational programmes of specialist personnel do not prepare them to communicate adaptively in changing clinical situations. While a technical language is necessary to convey information on specialized topics (e.g. sociological concepts, biological concepts etc.), the receivers of messages need support to encode meanings.

As far back as the late 1980s, studies have established both the differences in language use among medical and nursing personnel (Bourhis et al 1989), and the implications for patient care. Health professionals, Bourhis et al wrote, adopt 'different registers' to patients' method of communication: the latter use everyday language, the former use medical language. Doctors and nurses are 'bilingual': they can use both everyday language and medical language. Their clients, on the other hand, are unilingual, as they do not possess medical knowledge. Nurses may, nevertheless, be initially disadvantaged in some specialized clinical situations (e.g. operating theatres, intensive care units etc.) where they lack expertise knowledge of the technical language applied to these settings.

Since there are contrasting language uses in clinical practice, evidence shows that clients and some professionals may become disadvantaged during the communication process. In addition, expert language causes confusion and incomprehension in patients. Hence, it is anticipated that lack of clarity by not using everyday language will undermine effective care provision.

Bourhis et al's (1989) study highlighted some issues with implications for clinical practice:

1. Clients' subservient status may prevent them from communicating effectively with medical staff. Their everyday language may not empower them to express needs and problems adequately. It is therefore essential for nurses to utilize their communication skills to mediate interactions between clients and their physicians.
2. As doctors have a tendency to use medical language, nurses can intervene to translate complex terminologies for their patients. Additionally, it is widely accepted that anxiety and apprehension prevent patients from assimilating information. Information-giving should always be accompanied with constant reassurance.

3. The diversity of speech registers in clinical settings should be recognized: personnel training that focuses on developing sensitivity to language usage is a requisite.

The reconciling or integration of differing training programmes can prove challenging. As Grundstein-Amado (1992) pointed out, medical personnel's approach to information-giving tends to be 'impersonal' and 'universal' following a medical practice tradition. Nursing knowledge, in contrast, is rooted in 'personal touch' and daily involvement in bedside practice. It is to be anticipated that interpretations of clinical events will therefore be at variance.

Milligan et al (1999) assert that an effective communication framework can be cultivated, despite diversity among disciplines. To achieve this objective, Milligan et al suggest the pooling of expertise – the integration of knowledge when assessing and diagnosing – to present a 'consistent message'. Consensus regarding the clinical picture is, in any case, necessary. Clear and sensitive communication, with mutual exploration of divergent opinions is recommended to alleviate interprofessional conflict.

Equally important is to be conscious of patients' endeavour to *appear* that they are grasping the meanings of medical language, by adopting the speech patterns of the communicator. It is a strategy observed by Bourhis et al (1989), and could create a false impression, i.e. that comprehension is being achieved. Professionals have a role in not making assumptions that their clients fully understand the communication. Regular tactful evaluation is hence needed to ensure that meaningful and understandable communication is taking place.

As health care systems develop, it is envisaged that, while new communications systems (e.g. internet, e-mail, computerized care plans, hospital intranet systems etc.) achieve prominence and become enhanced, complex language cultures will simultaneously expand. New wording in the everyday professional language is becoming the norm. Although nursing and medicine have to keep pace, there is fear that new terminologies can exacerbate communication breakdowns

(Alexander 1998, Clarke 1998), undermining patient care. Clarke (1998) made reference to a plethora of terms (Box 15.3) applied to varied clinical situations – from descriptions of clients' behaviour to management terminologies – which obscure real meanings and may mask the real problems.

Box 15.3 Euphemisms, which obscure real meanings

- Challenging behaviour: tendency to be aggressive.
- Downsizes: redundancies.
- Rationalization: cutbacks or shortages.
- Temporary and involuntary immobility contingent upon environmental assault (these terms were used to refer to a 'patient immobilized in traction because of a broken leg caused by an accident with a lorry').

Jennings and Staggers (1998), in a critical review, evaluated the meanings attached to the word 'outcomes'. They explained that clarity of meaning is necessary to achieve effective communication, and refer to the haziness of outcomes linguistics. For example, managers may apply such terms as 'performance outcomes' and 'management outcomes', which in reality are outcomes studies. Jennings and Staggers emphasize the need to enlighten consumers of outcomes literature (i.e. nurses, doctors, managers etc.) concerning the specific meanings attached to the variety of outcomes models used. If outcomes are related to performance measures, a lexicon of terminologies should be adopted to specify the criteria associated with what constitutes 'good outcomes'. A failure to do so would confuse health professionals in their implementation of effective care, which should be founded on communication clarity.

Intercultural communication

Communication is a shared process (Report of the 4th Annual Conference 1998). Talking with others from diverse cultures on an agreed foundation of mutual trust, value and respect, forms the essence of intercultural communication.

Although language barriers can block commu-

Activity 15.1

1. Read the nursing and medical literature of the past 3 years. Identify the use of new terminologies. Can you define them?
2. Observe the interactions between nurses and patients, and medical staff and patients while on placement. Record the frequency of medical language used. Does the patient use any medical terminology?
3. Arrange with the ward manager for you to attend a doctor's round. At the end of the round, spend some time talking with your patients. Invite them to talk about their understanding of what the doctors had told them. How accurate is the patients' version of events? Did the medical staff use any technical language?
4. Read the doctor's case notes. Now read the nursing notes. How different are they? Can you highlight any issues that may have implications for practice?

??? Question 15.1

1. What makes the communication process complex?
2. Should nurses and doctors adopt an everyday language style with all their clients? Can you think of situations when a medical/nursing language should only be used in communicating with a client?
3. How would you facilitate a better understanding of information by the clients in your care? List the strategies you would use.
4. It is becoming the norm in clinical practice for patients and their relatives to access medical case notes. What are the implications in terms of effective communication?
5. What is sensitive communication?
6. How can the use of effective language help to reassure clients?

nication, professionals can still communicate empathetically and non-verbally. Smiling, nodding, opening doors respectfully and drawing curtains at the bedside for privacy are some measures demonstrating that effective communication takes place in the absence of bilingual or multi-lingual skills. To communicate interculturally – in its broadest sense – entails recognizing heterogeneous health beliefs, as the style of communication will be accordingly determined. Understanding lay health beliefs, for instance, will direct professionals to communicate in ways that can be interpreted most effectively.

The aim of good communication, according to Wilkinson (1999), is to ascertain clear understanding of meanings to the language used. In addition, verbal communication should be congruent with non-verbal behaviour as clients from all walks of life are sensitive to professionals' non-verbal signals.

When values and beliefs are conflictual between care providers and their clients, communications assume a contradictory nature. Problems are accentuated when misunderstanding of clients' feelings exist. Richards and Constable (1998) found some Bangladeshi women reluctant to use children or other relatives as interpreters; they concluded several things: first, children are not ideal interpreters: it is difficult for them to translate physical signs and symptoms accurately for someone else; secondly, it is embarrassing for the client to divulge personal health matters to children; thirdly, relatives may experience similar difficulties being privy to others' personal problems. Medical interpreters can help to reduce communication problems.

As intercultural communication emphasizes culture (Dodd 1995), lack of cultural awareness predisposes to misunderstanding, negative stereotypes and labels. These factors erect barriers in the communication process. Dodd (1995) proposes a model (Fig. 15.1) of intercultural communication, consisting of the following concepts:

1. the role and influence of culture
2. personality
3. perceived group
4. perceived difference
5. uncertainty–anxiety
6. drive or motivation and adaptive culture.

The influence of culture applies to the presence of group identities: ethnicity, practices, habits, values, beliefs that influence group behaviour. Personality as a psychological component refers to individual differences, which can affect communication style. Perceived difference is an automatic response, when we notice cultural differences and begin to 'assess others internally'; in other words, we begin to evaluate similarity and dissimilarity based on 'internal'/personal experiences. Dodd said this process induces

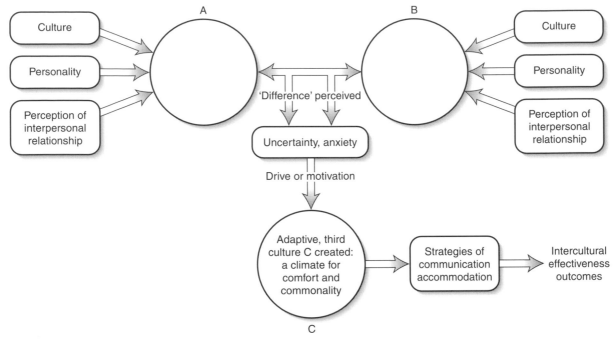

Fig. 15.1 Perceived dissimilarity model of intercultural communication. (Redrawn with kind permission of the McGraw-Hill Companies from Dodd C H 1995, Dynamics of Intercultural Communication. Brown & Benchmark, Madison, WI.)

social categorizing, whereby assumptions are made concerning the other person's motives, personality and social practices. Negative social categorization can precipitate racism, prejudice and ethnocentric attitudes. Uncertainty and anxiety are possible psychological reactions (Dodd 1995). The uncertainty motivates the observer of cultural difference to seek 'information to fill the gaps': a drive to know another person, to find out more, while drawing on our own cultural knowledge and identities during the evaluating. Dodd sees the adaptive culture of the model as crucial. In many social settings, attempts are made to achieve stability, integration and harmony between diverse interacting cultures. Some adaptive cultural behaviours (Dodd 1995) are positively motivated, leading to positive social outcomes; others, however, can cause cultural conflict and communication failure.

To work and communicate with people from other cultures (Brislin 1994) is a skill, which can be refined to prevent intercultural conflict and communication breakdown. Brislin pointed out several approaches to be considered:

1. Attempt to learn some basic cultural practices of the group (e.g. local language, modes of greeting etc.). Effort to communicate in someone's native language is reassuring to the listener, and will enhance 'ice-breaking' more effectively.

2. Develop knowledge of local non-verbal modes of communication, an important aspect, because Western non-verbal behaviour is markedly different from some cultural contexts. Brislin (1994) points out, for instance, the Asians' 'inscrutable' external behaviour.

3. An understanding of local culture is recommended, i.e. a community's mode of thinking, their perception of social and work practices; their world views of social organizations; perceptions of health, illness, disease.

4. Tolerance and openness: cultural sensitivity is a requirement, and the avoidance of ethnocentric attitudes is recommended.

5. Cooperation and collaboration: working and communicating with other cultural groups facilitates better understanding and acceptance of other cultures, their values and beliefs, and their understanding of one's own culture.

These are some of the principles adopted by anthropologists, who spend years immersing themselves into the cultures of ethnic societies (Béphage 1997).

For intercultural communication to be effective, other strategies must be utilized, in addition to the ones outlined above. For example, ongoing research into the behaviour of ethnic minorities will develop better insight of their societies. Positive ethnic monitoring is an accepted health care practice.

Recent research in ethnic monitoring (Box 15.4), focusing on community family planning clinics (Christopher 1999), provides invaluable insight into the sexual behaviour of diverse ethnic groups and their needs for professional support.

Box 15.4 Ethnic monitoring in Haringey Health Care Trust

Sixty-two per cent of female respondents (1673) were between 20 and 34 years old. Fewer than 20% of Caribbean, West African and Turkish Cypriot women, and only 6% of Turkish/Kurdish women born in Turkey, had not had children. Thirty-three per cent of women admitted to having one or more terminations; 49% West African, 43% Kurdish and 40% Kurdish/Cypriot women had one or more abortions. The lowest percentage (12%) of women admitting to a termination were Irish.

The majority of women did choose a method(s) of contraception. The oral contraceptive pill and condom were popular methods, often used together (Christopher 1999).

Community clinics, Christopher (1999) concluded, are found to be beneficial for ethnic women. In such clinics, linkworkers and female doctors are present, to communicate sensitively with their clients and meet their needs accordingly; uptake of services is hence expected to increase. The researcher did not point out, however, whether the linkworkers and female doctors were of ethnic origins, which could have facilitated the communication and increased attendance.

Cortis (1998), in a small-scale, qualitative study of ten elderly Pakistani men and seven women, pinpointed the major role of intercultural communication in clinical practice. To the clients

studied, the essence of nursing was located in the skill of communication between nurses and their patients. The male respondents felt their needs were unmet: communication was inadequate and poor (Box 15.5). Although an interpreting service was available, there was evidence of insensitive preparation due to the interpreters not being pre-booked (Cortis 1998). To the clients, interpreters were invaluable resources in an unfamiliar environment, since they could give reassurance. The nurses' ethnocentrism prevented them from communicating effectively and learning from their patients. Cortis also observed that nurses' behaviour was influenced by stereotypic beliefs such as 'they (Pakistani (Urdu) community) look after their own' and the view that ethnic communities are 'static' and not subjected to dynamic cultural change.

Box 15.5 Clients' feelings caused by poor communication (Cortis 1998)

Male respondents: 'This was really bad'; 'I felt uptight inside'; 'Nobody wanted to bother with me'; 'They try to fob me off'. Female respondents: 'Inability to communicate in English meant failing to express one's feelings to a stranger'.

Patients, according to this study, showed great sensitivity to nurses' non-verbal communication. Patients felt, for instance, that nurses' interventions did not always appear to be congruent with their non-verbal expressions of feelings, i.e. that nurses were caring in a mechanistic way, lacking in warmth.

Bynom (1997) extends the application of intercultural communication to the perioperative setting within the operating department. Qualified interpreters with surgical knowledge were found to be useful, as well as the implementation of a suitable skill mix in languages and the participation of linkworkers to bridge the gap between the health care workers and the clients.

Dawkins and Ingram (1998) discussed how important it is to maintain culturally sensitive care in the theatre suite, by communicating empathetically and avoiding judgemental attitudes. Other writers (Brown & Duxbury 1997) have emphasized a person-centred approach in communicating and interviewing patients in day surgery areas. It is recognized that day surgery patients have a need to talk about their anxieties and apprehension.

In a health care climate where clinical effectiveness is paramount to patient care (McClarey 1998), findings obtained from intercultural communication research provide evidence for practice improvement. As McClarey pointed out, once evidence is used in practice, the impact of the use of the evidence must be evaluated 'in terms of improved patient outcome'.

The literature on intercultural communication provides a wealth of knowledge and strategies to facilitate communication in health and social contexts. Cushner (1994), for example, examined ways to prepare teachers to meet the needs of a multicultural group of students. He suggested that assessing the perspective (subjective view: emic) of the person is *critical* to any functional relationship. In addition, he postulated that social isolation can be prevented by creating an environment conducive for 'newcomers' to establish new 'ingroups' membership. Similar principles can be applied in a health care context: ethnic groups can be helped to feel part of the health care team by seeking *their* advice on what and how *they feel* they could be helped. Quereshi (1998) recommends that care providers avoid 'over-assertiveness', because it is 'counter-productive', particularly in the context of 'cross-religious' interactions. For many ethnic groups, religion is integral to their socio-cultural beliefs. It is a sensitive aspect of care, and painstaking consideration should be given to this dimension during the process of communication.

While influencing positive attitude change to promote health is a health care priority, it is important for nurses, health educationalists and health promoters to seek alternative methods of communicating important information. In a study undertaken in Bangladesh, Hussain et al (1997) found that some simple communicative approaches can be used in health education programmes (Box 15.6).

The strategies outlined in Box 15.6 are culture-oriented, non-ethnocentric and take place within

---

Box 15.6 Communication channels to promote health

- **Folk singers**: singers use modified texts containing health promotion information, while preserving the original 'rhymes and tunes' of traditional music and songs.
- **Local leaders**: community leaders recruited, as they have a role in group integration.
- **'Mother groups'**: women's health matters (pregnancy, lactation, infants' and mothers' nutrition) discussed by women.
- **Neighbourhood groups**: local people meeting with each other, to discuss health issues, with health promoters acting as facilitators.
- **Women volunteers**: local women, after some training, will convey required information to their communities.

---

a context the targeted groups can identify with. In such forums, ethnic community workers can exercise considerable influence. Their knowledge of health issues is communicated in the language with which their audience is familiar.

Activity 15.2

1. List as many dialects in your region as you can.
2. Prepare a teaching programme you would use in clinical practice to help colleagues communicate interculturally.
3. Using a reflective diary, comment on how your thoughts and attitude have changed since reading on intercultural communication.

 Question 15.2

1. Should professionals learn other languages to help them communicate better with ethnic groups?
2. If communication is the essence of nursing, what do you consider to be good qualities in a nurse?

A PSYCHOLOGICAL PERSPECTIVE

Personality

The process of communication is inextricably linked with psychology. For example, personality traits such as introversion and extroversion will determine a person's communication style. Some believe that introverts make better listeners (Hargie et al 1987) because their attention level is better, and that extroverts are prone to distraction and are more communicative, i.e. they are more vocal in their interactions. This does not mean that they are not good listeners, but their listening ability may not be as intense.

Extroverts are overtly communicative and express their thoughts and feelings readily. They tend to be reactive to what is being said. Introverts, on the other hand, use many pauses during conversations, pondering over the content before venturing into some discussions. They may question more often to check their understanding of the message.

It is during interactions that people make casual inferences about others' personality, based upon 'how they look' (Hargie 1997). Impressions that we obtain can therefore impinge upon how we interact and communicate with them.

Emotion

Humans express emotions through language (verbal communication) as well as in non-verbal ways. The English vocabulary has many words denoting emotions, e.g. 'depressed', 'sad', 'angry', 'uptight', 'resentment', 'jovial', 'happy' etc. Arnold (1995) believed, however, that people communicate more often and more truly non-verbally, e.g. through facial expressions: smiling, laughing, crying or by making gestures such as rubbing the forehead, clenching the fists, biting the lips. Arnold explained that emotions are important 'message carriers'. However, some messages can be communicated in ways that go unnoticed. Some clients in care settings, Arnold pointed out, may refuse to comply with treatment regimen because of 'emotional barriers', i.e. anger, fear and anxiety.

Although people use language to communicate emotions, it should be remembered that language can also be used to arouse emotions in people (Box 15.7).

In health care practice, it is essential to avoid negative emotion-arousing communication, which can exacerbate a client's feelings of uncertainty

Box 15.7 Emotion-arousing communication

The three infants were found in the woods after their attackers had left them for dead. The infants came from a broken home. They were very often beaten by their parents. Their small bodies were covered in bruises. They were too frail to escape their torturers.

and anxiety. Careful choice of words is hence necessary.

Some writers (Mallett & A'Hern 1996, Bain 1997) have examined the place of humour in communication. Bain suggested that humour is a therapeutic intervention if used sensitively. When humour is introduced in the process of communication, concerned with sensitive health matters, it helps to reduce the effects of stress in these situations (Bain 1997).

Mallett and A'Hern, in their research studies on the 'distribution and use of humour within nurse–patient communication', concluded that a humorous framework may be utilized to avoid conflict. Humour, they remarked, has a facilitative function in clinical practice, during nurse–patient interactions.

Humour in selected contexts can counteract strong negative emotions and defuse conflictual situations. Spontaneous unplanned humour intervention is most effective. Nurses who have developed a good rapport with their clients are able to use humour confidently; in addition, some clients may use humour as a channel to communicate some deep emotional need or problem, a dimension of which professionals must be conscious.

Cognition

Cognitive processes (thinking, memorizing, reflecting, perceiving) are relevant to communication. During social interactions one is constantly processing the information one receives (Hargie 1997). Additionally, new information is compared with that stored in memory stores, before one decides how to impart one's ideas. People are constantly thinking as they communicate. This is important, as inadequate thinking could interfere with the logic, sequence, structure and meanings of the conversation.

In an interview situation candidates cognitively appraise the content of the interviewers' communication before answering. In an informal encounter, two friends will communicate light-heartedly, without having recourse to intense cognitive processing. When mistakes are made (e.g. wrong choice of words used) they may comment jokingly on the distorted message.

Encoding and decoding are key concepts in communication. Messages must be understood in their context and interpreted accordingly. Kreps and Kunimoto (1994) interpret these two concepts of cognition as translation processes. They explain that we have a need to search for meanings in the messages we receive. They assert that encoding and decoding are the building blocks of human communication.

Encoding is defined as the integration of one's personal knowledge and meaning into the message, how one interprets the message from one's vast store of ideas and knowledge. Decoding is the 'translating of the messages' (Kreps & Kunimoto 1994) to make sense of the content according to one's personal experience.

Motivation

In a commentary article, Bishop (1999) pointed out that effective communication is the 'key to staff motivation' and to improving patient care in clinical setting. Health care environments are stressful arenas. As professionals aim to achieve a high standard of performance within a constrained resource environment the motivation to communicate effectively, to prevent substandard care and litigation, assumes considerable significance.

It is becoming increasingly important for the client in an evolving and dynamic NHS setting to be a participator in care. The media constantly reinforces this notion. Caregivers are hence motivated to ensure that individuals under their care are given information according to needs. A client-centred approach to care signifies the recognition that the person as an individual has a need to communicate. Ill-health and disease are spectres to the sick person. Being nursed in an alien setting compels the client to seek information to alleviate feelings of anxiety.

Hargie (1997) posits that clients in need of care in varied settings – a dental surgery, an outpatient clinic, a surgical ward, for example – are in high states of arousal and should be encouraged to voice their fears. A demanding care climate impacts on the personnel too. There are needs to seek peer support and communicate feelings regarding meeting deadlines in stressful clinical circumstances. Provision for counselling is a management responsibility. Failing to identify low morale and communication needs could precipitate burnout.

Attention and listening

In the chapter on psychology (p. 241), it was noted that attention is an important concept. This feature is highly significant in communication. When people listen, they are paying attention. The concept of listening will therefore be discussed since it cannot be demarcated from the process of communication.

Bostrom (1997) views listening as one of the many cognitive mechanism frameworks. The listener acquires information, retains it temporarily in memory, assesses its importance, compares it with stored information in long-term memory and decides whether to give a response or not.

To listen, however, does not necessarily mean that the person has a good retention capacity. Bostrom explains that listening is a demonstration of an attitude. People listen for many reasons:

- to show politeness
- it is an unwritten social rule
- to be manipulative: it encourages the speaker to be more vocal and cooperative.

Some organizations may use 'listening' as their motto, because consumers prefer 'good listeners'.

The literature on listening appears to focus primarily on attention to the spoken words. The art of listening also entails listening to a person's silence and understanding it. Lomax (1998) comments that 5–10 seconds of silence during interactions can be uncomfortable to people, spurring them to restart the conversation. Lomax asserts that important messages will be lost if the silence is disrupted.

Personality characteristics and cultural styles will determine how some individuals will use silence. Some ethnic groups will make more use of silences, e.g. Asians, Inuit, Chinese and Japanese (Lomax 1998). Socially isolated individuals (who live in remote places far from civilization) are prone to be reticent and use long pauses during communication. Burnard (1998) argued that listening is not only a skill, but is a personal quality. To Burnard, a good listener:

1. uses non-verbal cues moderately during interactions
2. concentrates on the speaker using the right degree of attention 'without losing sight' of the main message
3. is able to avoid listening to their own thoughts ('forgetting ourselves')
4. recognizes their own shortcomings in listening to people of varied temperament, as they may be less inclined to listen to some people.

Ford (1997) advised professionals to listen to the hidden message behind the spoken words. Patients with chronic and life-threatening illnesses communicate their needs in subtle ways (Case example 15.4), according to Ford. Listening to the tone and expression, and noticing body language signals is essential.

In Case example 15.4, the professional suddenly gained insight into the patient's meaning of 'going home' from the 'force of her words, blazing through' … Attending to the verbal, non-verbal and paralinguistic aspects of the message (Kacperek 1997) will enhance understanding of the subtleties of communication.

Social reinforcement

When two persons are communicating, they become aware of each other's verbal and non-verbal cues. Not listening, for example, shows that the other person is distracted, not interested, or may be bored. In many cultures, smiling, nodding and responding positively by making vocal noises (i.e. mms, yeh, yeh, uh, oh yes etc.) urges the speaker to continue talking.

Cairns (1997) describes the use of non-verbal

Case example 15.4 Tillie is going home

'Tillie was a frequent flyer in our intensive care unit. Her heart had been ravaged by high blood pressure, coronary heart disease and infarctions. During her two previous admissions – for heart failure and pulmonary oedema – Tillie had required ventilatory assistance. … Before Tillie allowed her family to call emergency medical services to transport her from home to the hospital, she made them swear that she would not be placed on the 'breathing machine again'.

'For 4 days we worked to remove fluid from Tillie's heart and lungs … Several times a day she implored, "I want to go home" … On her fifth day in hospital … Tillie grabbed my arm and pleaded, "I want to go home" … I finally understood. I spoke with her to confirm that I had received the message she had been trying to convey. It occurred to me that we hadn't listened well enough to what Tillie had been saying all along. The home of which she spoke was a place of peace and comfort, but it was not the one with her street address. Her message now understood, Tillie was transferred to a private room … It was from this room that Tillie finally went home'. (Adapted from Ford F S 1997 Tillie is going home. American Journal of Nursing 97(12): 55, with kind permission of Lippincott, Williams & Wilkins, Philadelphia, PA.)

cues as social reinforcement: they confirm to the speaker that the conversation is meaningful and one is interested. Negative reinforcement will, evidently, terminate a conversation much earlier. Some people, when in a hurry for example, are quite adept at using negative reinforcement. They may listen but from time to time will glance at their watches. Or they may speed the communicator along by suggesting they 'come to the point'; 'can you put it in a nutshell'; or 'maybe we should talk about this later'.

There are many instances of negative social reinforcement in care settings due to work pressures. In addition, the choice of environment can act as a negative reinforcement: a busy ward corridor is unsuitable for effective communication and clients may therefore be unable to express fully their feelings. A quiet room is more conducive to better communication as the client is most likely to feel relaxed and to be listened to.

At the time of writing, some practitioners (Kennedy 1999) are examining approaches to improve handover communication at the bed-side. This may prove invaluable for both nurse–patient and nurse–nurse relationships. Since handover reports concern clients' progress, it is another opportunity to impart information to the clients. The use of positive verbal and non-verbal reinforcement should be used to encourage the verbalization of feelings as required.

TEAMWORK AND COMMUNICATION

A traditional view of teamwork has been concerned with professionals working together to attain certain aims, while the targeted groups (clients/patients) assume a non-participatory role. Yet clients should be included as team members; without their cooperation health outcomes would be undermined.

Communication studies in health care settings have pinpointed clients' dissatisfaction with the amount of information they receive. Good communication skills are beneficial to patients, especially when staff members (porters, ward clerks, nurses, doctors, domestic staff) pool their expertise to maximize patients' satisfaction (Woods et al 1998).

Recognizing the barriers to communication can help staff develop methods to erase communication problems. Any strategies used should consider the central role of the client in the model of communication being designed. The literature on communication studies identifies several major concerns with implications for the implementation of effective teamwork in the field of communication. The issues are linked to the following:

- role conflict between physician and nurse (Larson 1999)
- complex communication patterns in hospital setting (Coiera & Tombs 1998), which impair the efficiency of information-giving with consequences for patient care
- problems with inter-organizational communication associated with discharge planning (Anderson & Helms 1998)
- fragmentation of communication in primary health care settings (Ford et al 1997; McDonald et al 1997; McCann 1998; Baptiste & Drennan 1999)
- the inadequacy of nurse-designed information leaflets for patients (Mumford 1997).

Role conflict

Communication impairment occurs when inter-professional collaboration is poor (West 1999), an issue affecting the relationships between the nurse and the physician. Situations arise in clinical settings (e.g. not including nursing staff in decision-making concerning patients with fatal illnesses), which create tensions and conflicting communication.

Larson (1999) identified some possible factors causing interprofessional conflict:

1. historical perceptions of the doctor as decision-maker and expert, and the nurse as subservient
2. diverging professional viewpoints:
   a. nurses' perception of clinical events differs to the doctors'
   b. medical and nurse training differ
   c. evidence of a hierarchy of values in health care with pathology and curing assuming greater significance
   d. gender differences.

Although professional training does consider communication skills, the application of theory into practice has always been difficult. In reality, interpersonal skills are acquired in clinical settings, through trial and error.

Collaborative working entails respecting each others' differences in approaches to care delivery. It applies to the integration of knowledge via effective communication channels (e.g. workshops, seminars, conferences, discussion groups etc.) to erase conflicting ideals. Larson used the term 'collegiality', implying the development of a 'meaningful sense of community'.

Unless professionals are prepared to look critically at their own practices – with reflective evaluation – and acknowledge their collective responsibilities, effective team communication will not be achieved.

Activity 15.3

Organize a workshop with your course manager, with the aim to explore ways to implement effective communication in a health care setting of your choice.

??? Question 15.3

What do you consider to be the major barriers to communication?

Complex communication patterns

Health workers in hospital and community settings rely upon the telephone system to communicate with other departments and colleagues in their daily tasks. Moreover they utilize opportunities to establish face to face communication as much as possible during the course of their work. These two methods of communication have been described as '**synchronous**' (because they demand immediate responses between the speakers) and are considered to be interruptive (Coiera & Tombs 1998). Coiera and Tombs argued that time spent conversing disturbs care continuity, and causes distraction and diversion. Their research in an Australian hospital setting showed that doctors and nurses relied too much on the telephone system on many occasions, when written communication, e-mail or voicemail could have been used. They refer to the latter forms of communication as '**asynchronous**'. This approach to communication, they wrote, is less interruptive as the receiver of the message chooses when to reply.

Coiera and Tombs's (1998) study showed that many telephone calls had to be made to book a clinical investigation; on some occasions several administrative staff had to be contacted before a booking was made. When messages were verbally conveyed to intermediaries, distortion (caused by Chinese whisper effect) of information had occurred. Telephone communication skills are, nevertheless, essential since patients and relatives are dependent upon this channel of communication (Farrell 1996).

Communication in primary care settings

Both US and UK health care systems have problems with communication in primary care settings. Anderson and Helms (1998), in an American study, reported poor written information received by community care organizations from hospital departments. Discharge documentation showed a lack of detail on clients' psychosocial needs, which constrained effective care delivery by community staff. In the UK, McCann's (1998) study reported inadequate information on cancer patients' needs when discharged in the community. Poor discharge information can mean that continuing care is disrupted.

In other cases, general practitioners have been criticized for the poor quality of referral letters (Allan 1997). It is suggested that 'information transfer skills' should be taught to prevent communication failures. Other issues refer to the nature of communication between general practitioners and other primary care workers. Baptiste and Drennan (1999) discovered that school nurses are not included in the primary care team framework by general practice. This issue has implications for joint working and collaborative partnerships advocated by government and policy makers.

In the mental health field, similar communication problems have been identified. Ford et al (1997) found mental health workers unable to work collaboratively with other professionals and agencies. It is anticipated that, as more agencies

Activity 15.4

Arrange a visit with the local school nurse. Discuss issues related to their role within the primary care teams in the area.

??? Question 15.4

Is the new climate of joint working and collaboration working in your community health trust?

adopt a care providing role, complex organizational structures will develop, increasing the density of communication channels. As McDonald et al (1997) pointed out, a diversity of care providers – from community, acute and social services – heightens anxiety over communication issues.

Information leaflets for patients

The preparation of informative leaflets in patient care is important. Research shows, however, that the readability of the leaflets is inadequate (Mumford 1997), i.e. patients are unable to understand the content of leaflet information due to the complexity of language used.

Short hospitalization demands that complex messages and advice are written clearly to allow the clients and relatives to manage care at home. It is also relevant to ensure that leaflets are available for inpatients. Some clients may find reading instructions material more useful than seeking advice directly from care professionals; others may find leaflets a supplement to verbally given information. The aims of written information must nevertheless be kept in focus:

- to aid better understanding
- to reassure and inform
- to encourage adherence to treatment in a friendly non-imposing way.

The preparation of leaflets and brochures should be carried out after consultation with team members, and by listening to users and their relatives.

NETWORKING, ALLIANCES AND PARTNERSHIPS

Networking may be defined as the avoidance of insularity by establishing links with other people – locally, nationally and internationally. At its most fundamental level, networking occurs when colleagues communicate with other professionals. It is a dynamic process (Hughes 1999) with the aim to share knowledge and expertise; it is also a powerful tool for disseminating good practice (Hughes 1999).

Networking has no boundaries because professionals have the freedom to set up global links with any agencies they feel are pertinent to needs. Networking is, however, not a new phenomenon. For example, the International Council of Nurses (ICN) was created in 1899 (Murphy 1998) with the goal to share information worldwide. Links with the World Health Organization (WHO) demonstrate how collaboration is promoted between governmental and non-governmental agencies and the ICN (Murphy 1998). In Europe, an international group of health care professionals is networking with the aspiration to demystify cultural taboos that affect health care practice (Humm 1998).

Intercultural networking is a productive forum to develop better cultural awareness of diverse health care cultures. Networkers have several methods they can use in addition to face to face communication. Accessing the internet, web pages, e-mail and fax systems, the dissemination of newsletters and research papers are instrumental. Salvage (1999) comments that good practice information can be distributed worldwide to networkers according to needs by making topical issues accessible in the form of books and monographs. Health promoters use networking to make their research results known.

Health promotion

Some researchers (King et al 1998) have put forward the argument that there is deficiency in the system of disseminating new research findings about health-promoting programmes. An approach that builds upon mutual involvement (cooperation between researcher and practitioner) by linkage systems is recommended.

With this outlook, health promotion specialists will adopt a two-way process in disseminating crucial research findings. They propose to implement this strategy by the following measures:

1. critically evaluating the researchers' characteristics: their role and methods in health promotion programmes
2. creating a climate compatible for researchers and practitioners (those involved in putting into practice findings) to work in partnerships

3. establishing links with the ultimate aim to foster trust and identify common interests. Collaboration can dispel negative views, with the development of shared understanding about the value of and limitations of applying research into practice
4. the prevention of premature dissemination of findings, before evidence of effectiveness has been founded. This can be done by liaising with targeted organizations to discuss issues connected with the research process
5. discussing with practitioners the practicality of changing work practices to adopt research programmes.

At the time of writing, contemporary health issues in society – such as BSE (bovine spongiform encephalopathy or 'mad cow disease') virus in beef and the debates over GM (genetically modified) food, provide evidence of the distrust, confusion and contradictory arguments generated by politicians, research scientists, consumers and medical organizations. While the Government explains that their agreement with scientists is based on compelling scientific evidence that GM food is safe, uncertainty and anxiety are widespread among food providers and consumers. These cases highlight examples of the imposition of scientific research findings on targeted groups – the consumers – without consultation and involvement in the decision-making process.

For health-promotion programmes to be effective, better partnerships – with involvement of users – will reduce strong resentment when new environmental health and food production initiatives are introduced. Furthermore, as Professor Patrick Bateson of King's College asserted in a Radio 4 interview (23 February 1999), the publishing of scientific findings (e.g. on GM food) should be properly evaluated before reaching public domain. However, failure to consult users arouses resentment and non-cooperation amongst food associations and pressure groups.

Alliances and partnerships in health promotion (Gillies 1998) do work when lay people are involved, and when public, private and non-government agencies are consulted in research policy initiatives. Gillies emphasizes that making

use of social capital (a community-driven approach) will ensure a sharing of power and knowledge, with a degree of shared control as well. By networking across boundaries to involve businesses, corporations, the public and employers the promotion of good health practices is more likely to be uniform.

 Activity 15.5

1. Do a literature search on 'promoting health through partnerships'. Identify the differing perspectives and discuss your findings in a seminar group.
2. Talk to the managers of your health education and health promotion departments. Describe their views concerning their role as 'health promoters'.

??? Question 15.5

What are your views on how researchers should disseminate information to health care professionals?. Can you identify any constraints in clinical practice that can prevent the application of (evidence-based) research into practice?

SUMMARY

Communication is a social and psychological need. How people express themselves is influenced by social background as well as sociocultural beliefs. It has been observed that, in the workplace, professionals use technical language during interactions, explained by the fact that a training culture encourages the use of professional language. Nevertheless, it is acknowledged that patient care can be affected by over-use of technical terminologies, without clear explanations. There is evidence that professional language between professionals from different training cultures and social backgrounds will affect understanding.

Some authors have emphasized the importance of intercultural communication. The notion that differing cultural influences impinge on communication styles is central to the concept of intercultural communication. Proponents of intercultural approaches to communication urge professionals in various care settings to exercise sensitivity and understanding when interacting with multicultural groups.

Psychology forms part of the communication process. For example, psychological concepts such as personality, emotions, cognition, motivation, attention and social reinforcement are attributes in the conceptual framework of communication.

Good teamwork is dependent upon effective communication. It is, however, shown that role conflict and complex communication patterns (e.g. in a hospital setting) can interfere with the effective transmission of information. Communication in primary care settings is considered to be inadequate, due to professionals being unable to implement joint-working and collaborative partnerships. Establishing alliances and partnerships are accepted as the way forward in the new health care climate. Effective health promotion programmes are more likely to be possible when researchers and practitioners work together in research to ensure that findings can be implemented realistically.

GLOSSARY

BSE   bovine spongiform encephalopathy – degenerative brain changes caused by a virus that normally affects cattle
Cholecystectomy   removal of gall bladder
Clinical effectiveness   care interventions founded on evidence, sound clinical guidelines, education and cost-effectiveness
Clinical governance   standards of performance in clinical practice linked with evidence-based interventions, continuing education, and risk management to improve quality of care
Clinical supervision   supportive behaviours from an appointed experienced professional with the role and responsibility to ensure ongoing support to individual practitioners, with the aim to enhance patient care
Concordance   a non-paternalistic approach, which aims to develop partnerships with clients during treatment and

care interventions. It is a clear departure from 'compliance', which is practitioner-led. Concordance is patient-centred.
Critical care pathway   strategic stages of a person's illness which demand specific assessment followed by required care interventions
Elaborated code   explicit style of speech, characterized by elaboration of sentences and in the amount of information imparted
Histology   the study of microscopic tissues structure
Paralinguistic (paralingual)   the vocal rather than the verbal aspects of speech (e.g. intonation, rate, volume, fluency)
Restricted code   a pattern of speech understood by people with shared assumptions and an implicit understanding of the content of the message in a conversation
Somatization disorders   bodily symptoms believed to originate from mental states

REFERENCES

Alexander J 1998 Confusing debriefing and defusing postnatally: the need for clarity of terms, purpose and value. Midwifery 14(2): 122–124
Allan A N 1997 Effective communication from general practice: the referral letter. Health Informatics 3(1): 37–45
Anderson M A, Helms L 1998 Comparison of continuing care communication. Image 30(3): 255–260
Arnold E 1995 Self-concept in the nurse-client relationship. In: Arnold E, Boggs K (eds) Interpersonal relationships, 2nd edn. W B Saunders, Philadelphia, p 59
Bain L 1997 The place of humour in chronic or terminal illness. Professional Nurse 12(10): 713–715
Baptiste L, Drennan V 1999 Communication between school nurses and primary care teams. British Journal of Community Nursing 4(1): 13–18
Béphage G 1997 Social science and healthcare: nursing applications in clinical practice. Mosby, London, p 95
Bishop V 1999 Commentary. Communication: the key to staff motivation and improved healthcare. NT Research 4(1): 43
Bostrom R N 1997 The process of listening. In: Hargie O D (ed) The handbook of communication skills, 2nd edn.

Routledge, London, p 236
Bourhis R Y, Roth S, MacQueen G 1989 Communication in the hospital setting: a survey of medical and everyday language use among patients, nurses and doctors. Social Science and Medicine 28(4): 339–346
Brislin R W 1994 Working cooperatively with people from different cultures. In: Brislin R W, Yoshida T (eds) Improving Intercultural Interactions. Sage, Thousand Oaks, p 23
Brown A, Duxbury J 1997 Day surgery-communication and interviewing skills. British Journal of Theatre Nursing 7(4): 10–15
Burnard P 1998 Listening as a personal quality. Journal of Community Nursing 12(2): 32–34
Bynom S 1997 Perioperative communication in a multicultural society. British Journal of Theatre Nursing 7(5): 14–16
Cairns L 1997 Reinforcement. In: Hargie O D (ed) The handbook of communication skills, 2nd edn. Routledge, London, p 135
Chatterton S 1998 An investigation of speech and language therapy to improve the communication environment of

people with severe learning disabilities who have communication difficulties and behaviours that challenge services. Journal of Learning Disabilities for Nursing and Social Care 2(4): 203–211

Christopher E 1999 The relevance of ethnic monitoring in the experience of Haringey healthcare NHS Trust community family planning clinics. British Journal of Family Clinics 24(4): 123–127

Clarke L 1998 What's in a name? Nursing Times 94(22): 38–39

Coeira E, Tombs V 1998 Communication behaviours in a hospital setting: an observational study. British Medical Journal 316(7132): 673–676

Cortis J D 1998 The experiences of nursing care received by Pakistani (Urdu speaking) patients in later life in Dewsbury, UK. Clinical Effectiveness In Nursing 2(3): 131–138

Crawford P, Nolan P, Brown B 1995 Linguistic entrapment: medico-nursing biographies as fictions. Journal of Advanced Nursing 22(6): 1141–1148

Crawford P, Brown B, Nolan P 1999 Nursing language: uses and abuses. Nursing Times 95(6): 48–49

Cushner K 1994 Preparing teachers for an intercultural context. In: Brislin R W, Yoshida T (eds) Improving Intercultural Interactions. Sage, Thousand Oaks, p 109–128

Dawkins M, Ingram D 1998 Ethnic and cultural awareness. British Journal of Theatre Nursing 8(6): 16–17

Dodd C H 1995 Dynamics of Intercultural Communication, 4th edn. Brown & Benchmark, Madison, WI

Farrell G 1996 Telephoning a nursing department: callers' experiences. Nursing Standard 10(33): 34–36

Ford F S 1997 Tillie is going home. American Journal of Nursing 97(12): 55

Ford K, Middleton J, Palmer B, Farrington A 1997 Primary healthcare workers: training needs in mental health. British Journal of Nursing 6(21): 1244–1249

Gillies P 1998 Effectiveness of alliances and partnerships for health promotion. Health Promotion International 13(2): 99–117

Grundstein-Amado R 1992 Differences in ethical decision-making processes among nurses and doctors. Journal of Advanced Nursing 17(2): 129–137

Hargie O D 1997 Interpersonal communication: a theoretical framework. In: Hargie O D (ed) The Handbook of Communication Skills, 2nd edn. Routledge, London, p 50

Hargie O D, Saunders C, Dickson D 1987 Social skills in interpersonal communication, 2nd edn. Croom Helm, Cambridge, p 172

Hughes M 1999 The missing link. Nursing Times 95(5): 28–29

Humm C 1998 Talking taboos. Nursing Standard 12(45): 27

Hussain A, Aaro L E, Kvale G 1997 Impact of a health education program to promote consumption of vitamin A-rich foods in Bangladesh. Health Promotion International 12(2): 103–109

Jarman F 1995 Communication problems: a patient's view. Nursing Times 91(18): 30–31

Jennings B M, Staggers N 1998 The language of outcomes. Advances in Nursing Science 20(4): 72–80

Johnson M 1999 Communication in healthcare: a review of some key issues. NT Research 4(1): 18–30

Kacperek K L 1997 Non-verbal communication: the importance of listening. British Journal of Nursing 6(5): 275–278

Kennedy J 1999 An evaluation of non-verbal handover. Professional Nurse 14(6): 391–394

King L, Hawe P, Wise M 1998 Making dissemination a two-way process. Health Promotion International 13(3): 237–243

Koffman J, Fulop N J, Pashley D, Coleman K 1997 Ethnicity and use of acute psychiatric beds: one-day survey in North and South Thames regions. British Journal of Psychiatry 171: 238–241

Kreps G L, Kunimoto E N 1994 Effective communication in multicultural care settings. Sage, Thousand Oaks, p 14

Larson E 1999 The impact of physician–nurse interaction on patient care. Holistic Nursing Practice 13(2): 38–46

Lomax B 1998 Learning to understand a patient's silence. Nursing Times 93(17): 48–49

McCann C 1998 Communication in cancer care: introducing patient-held records. International Journal of Palliative Nursing 4(5): 222–229

McClarey M 1998 Implementing clinical effectiveness. Nursing Management 5(3): 16–19

McDonald A, Langford I H, Boldero N 1997 The future of community nursing in the UK: district nursing, health visiting and school nursing. Journal of Advanced Nursing 26(2): 257–265

Mallett J, A'Hern R 1996 Comparative distribution and use of humour within nurse–patient communication. International Journal of Nursing Studies 33(5): 530–550

Milligan R A, Gilroy J, Katz et al 1999 Developing a shared language: interdisciplinary communication among diverse health care professionals. Holistic Nursing Practice 13(2): 47–53

Mumford M E 1997 A descriptive study of the readability of patient information leaflets designed by nurses. Journal of Advanced Nursing 26(5): 985–991

Murphy S 1998 Global links. Nursing Management 5(5): 25–27

Patel V, Pereira J, Coutinho L et al 1998 Poverty, psychological disorder and disability in primary care attenders in Goa, India. British Journal of Psychiatry 172: 533–536

Quereshi B 1998 Religion and family planning. Family Medicine 2(2): 24–25

Report of the 4th Annual Conference 1998 Adolescents and chronic illness. Paediatrics Today 6(4): 90–91

Richards C, Constable M 1998 Primary healthcare in a Bangladeshi community. Primary Health Care 8(4): 10–15

Roberts J W 1994 Nurse/patient communication within a bilingual health care setting. British Journal of Nursing 3(2): 60–67

Salmon P, Peters S, Stanley I 1999 Patients' perceptions of medical explanations for somatisation disorders: qualitative analysis. British Medical Journal 318 (7180): 372–376

Salvage J 1999 Joined-up thinking. Nursing Times 95(5): 26–27

Singleton C 1995 Communication breakdown. Nursing Standard 9(48): 45

West M 1999 Communication and team working in healthcare. NT Research 4(1): 8–17

Wilkinson J A 1999 Understanding patients' health beliefs. Professional Nurse 14(5): 320–322

Woods M, Brown H, Filler M 1998 Using teamwork to improve communication. Nursing Times 94(40): 48–49

FURTHER READING

Crane J A 1997 Patient comprehension of doctor–patient communication on discharge from the emergency department. Journal of Emergency Medicine 15(1): 1–7

Delaney F, Adams L 1997 Preventing skin cancer through mass media: process evaluation of a collaboration of health promotion agencies. Health Education Journal 56(3): 274–286

Hatim B 1997 Communication across cultures. University of Exeter, Exeter

Jandt F E 1998 Intercultural communication. Sage, Thousand Oaks

Tanno D V, Gonzàlez A 1998 Communication and identity across cultures. Sage, Thousand Oaks

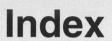

Index